Persister Cells and Infectious Disease

Kim Lewis

Editor

Persister Cells and Infectious Disease

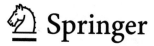 Springer

Editor
Kim Lewis
Antimicrobial Discovery Center
Northeastern University
Boston, Massachusetts, USA

ISBN 978-3-030-25243-4   ISBN 978-3-030-25241-0   (eBook)
https://doi.org/10.1007/978-3-030-25241-0

This Springer imprint is published by the registered company Springer Nature Switzerland AG.
The registered company address is: Gewerbestrasse 11, 6330 Cham, Switzerland

Introduction

This volume brings together leaders of the emerging field of persistence and antibiotic tolerance to present the state of the art and provide a roadmap for future studies. Drug-tolerant persisters form stochastically in bacterial populations, and were first described by Joseph Bigger in 1944. However, it took a long time for the importance of persisters to be recognized. This recognition is still a work in progress—for one, the attention of the scientific community and the public has been focused on the antimicrobial resistance (AMR) crisis we are currently experiencing. Antibiotic discovery lags behind the rapid acquisition and spread of resistance, and we now have pan-resistant pathogens such as *Acinetobacter baumannii*. Very considerable resources have been dedicated to fight AMR by governments and private Foundations. This is a subject that is commonly discussed at the UN and the WHO. After a long dry spell, we are finally seeing promising new lead compounds to treat AMR pathogens, such as teixobactin and arylomycin. At the same time, most infections are caused by drug-susceptible pathogens. Most patients in the hospital have challenging infections, which require lengthy treatment regimens, often with multiple antibiotics. The inability to rapidly eradicate a drug-susceptible pathogen is the main problem in the clinic. This problem stems from bacterial tolerance, the ability to survive a lethal dose of antibiotic, and is often associated with biofilms forming on indwelling devices and soft tissues. Persister cells confer tolerance to a population of bacteria in chronic infection.

The significant burden of chronic infections in the developed world is dwarfed by the global epidemic of tuberculosis. The disease requires an unusually lengthy treatment, and the consensus is that dormant cells are responsible for this. So far, the study of persisters, with a focus on conventional pathogens such as *Escherichia coli*, *Pseudomonas aeruginosa*, and *Staphylococcus aureus*, happened very much in isolation from the work on drug-tolerant *Mycobacterium tuberculosis*. This volume for the first time brings these two fields together—we have two chapters on *M. tuberculosis* drug tolerance. This should really be a single field, and we hope that this volume will serve as a link for researchers working on the same problem with different pathogens.

While we have a good understanding of the mechanisms of antibiotic resistance, this is not the case with antibiotic tolerance. Similarly, and perhaps not surprisingly, approaches to eradicate persisters are lagging. Once the AMR crisis is behind us, we will still be facing the daunting task of combatting persister cells.

The relatively slow pace in the study of persisters has been not only due to the late realization of their important role in chronic infections but also due to objective difficulties in studying a small subpopulation of cells with a fleeting phenotype. Advanced tools for the study of single cells have become available, and several chapters in this book describe experiments with persisters using cell sorting, microfluidics, and microscopy, in addition to traditional molecular and biochemical approaches. Studies of persister formation point to two types of mechanisms—specialized and general. Toxin/antitoxin modules represent the specialized mechanisms operating under particular conditions, while relative dormancy, with metabolic inactivity and low ATP, is emerging as a possible general mechanism of persister formation.

This volume also covers early advances in the discovery of anti-persister compounds. The mechanisms of action of the first anti-persister compounds provide a blueprint for additional discoveries, and are a cause for optimism in achieving the ultimate goal of developing sterilizing antibiotics.

This is an exciting time to be joining the field of persister studies—the tools have been developed, the knowledge base has been established, but the big discoveries are still waiting in the wings.

Boston, MA   Kim Lewis

Contents

Contributors

Robert B. Abramovitch Department of Microbiology and Molecular Genetics, Michigan State University, East Lansing, MI, USA

Nathalie Q. Balaban Racah Institute of Physics, The Hebrew University, Jerusalem, Israel

Bork A. Berghoff Institute for Microbiology and Molecular Biology, Justus Liebig University Giessen, Giessen, Germany

Maikel Boot Department of Microbial Pathogenesis, Yale University, New Haven, CT, USA

Mark P. Brynildsen Department of Chemical and Biological Engineering, Princeton University, Princeton, NJ, USA

Iliana Escobar Division of Infectious Diseases, Rhode Island Hospital, Department of Medicine, Warren Alpert Medical School of Brown University, Providence, RI, USA

Nathan Fraikin Cellular and Molecular Microbiology, Faculté des Sciences, Université Libre de Bruxelles (ULB), Gosselies, Belgium

Beth Burgwyn Fuchs Division of Infectious Diseases, Rhode Island Hospital, Department of Medicine, Warren Alpert Medical School of Brown University, Providence, RI, USA

Frédéric Goormaghtigh Cellular and Molecular Microbiology, Faculté des Sciences, Université Libre de Bruxelles (ULB), Gosselies, Belgium

Alexander Harms Biozentrum, University of Basel, Basel, Switzerland

Sophie Helaine Department of Medicine, MRC CMBI Imperial College London, London, UK

Pauline Herpels VIB, Center for Microbiology, Leuven, Belgium
KU Leuven, Centre of Microbial and Plant Genetics, Leuven, Belgium

Peter W. S. Hill Department of Medicine, MRC CMBI Imperial College London, London, UK

Arvi Jõers Insitute of Technology, University of Tartu, Tartu, Estonia

Niilo Kaldalu Insitute of Technology, University of Tartu, Tartu, Estonia

Wooseong Kim Division of Infectious Diseases, Rhode Island Hospital, Department of Medicine, Warren Alpert Medical School of Brown University, Providence, RI, USA

Kim Lewis Antimicrobial Discovery Center, Department of Biology, Northeastern University, Boston, MA, USA

Jiafeng Liu Racah Institute of Physics, The Hebrew University, Jerusalem, Israel

Hannes Luidalepp Quretec OÜ, Tartu, Estonia

Sylvie Manuse Antimicrobial Discovery Center, Department of Biology, Northeastern University, Boston, MA, USA

Jan Michiels VIB, Center for Microbiology, Leuven, Belgium
KU Leuven, Centre of Microbial and Plant Genetics, Leuven, Belgium

Wendy W. K. Mok Department of Chemical and Biological Engineering, Princeton University, Princeton, NJ, USA
Department of Molecular Biology and Biophysics, UConn Health, Farmington, CT, USA

Eleftherios Mylonakis Division of Infectious Diseases, Rhode Island Hospital, Department of Medicine, Warren Alpert Medical School of Brown University, Providence, RI, USA

Marta Putrinš Insitute of Technology, University of Tartu, Tartu, Estonia

Hesper Rego Department of Microbial Pathogenesis, Yale University, New Haven, CT, USA

Tanel Tenson Insitute of Technology, University of Tartu, Tartu, Estonia

Laurence Van Melderen Cellular and Molecular Microbiology, Faculté des Sciences, Université Libre de Bruxelles (ULB), Gosselies, Belgium

Natalie Verstraeten VIB, Center for Microbiology, Leuven, Belgium
KU Leuven, Centre of Microbial and Plant Genetics, Leuven, Belgium

E. Gerhart H. Wagner Department of Cell and Molecular Biology, Biomedical Center, Uppsala University, Uppsala, Sweden

Dorien Wilmaerts VIB, Center for Microbiology, Leuven, Belgium
KU Leuven, Centre of Microbial and Plant Genetics, Leuven, Belgium

Huiqing Zheng Department of Microbiology and Molecular Genetics, Michigan State University, East Lansing, MI, USA

Chapter 1
Evolution Under Antibiotic Treatments: Interplay Between Antibiotic Persistence, Tolerance, and Resistance

Nathalie Q. Balaban and Jiafeng Liu

Abstract In this chapter, we describe the experimental evolution of antibiotic tolerance and persistence under antibiotic treatments and how these phenomena can speed up the subsequent evolution of resistance. The first two parts are dedicated to defining the difference between antibiotic resistance, tolerance, and persistence with qualitative definitions and quantitative metrics. The third part describes experimental observations of the evolution of tolerance and persistence under antibiotic treatments. The fourth part shows that tolerance and persistence speed up the evolution of antibiotic resistance. In each part, mathematical subsections can be skipped by the reader without losing the qualitative understanding of the effects.

1.1 Distinguishing Between Resistance, Tolerance, and Antibiotic Persistence

Following our recent works (Balaban et al. 2019; Brauner et al. 2016), we briefly characterize below antibiotic resistance, tolerance, and persistence. Within the antibiotic persistence phenotype, three main archetypes have been observed in vitro. We outline these archetypes in Sect. 1.1.4 and describe in Sect. 1.2 the differences in the experimental protocols required to measure the persistence levels for each type. We note that these definitions do not preclude the existence of other types of antibiotic persistence, but we chose to focus on those characterized already in several labs. Finally, we briefly describe a phenomenological mathematical model that allows identifying parameters that vary among different modes of survival.

N. Q. Balaban (✉) · J. Liu
Racah Institute of Physics, The Hebrew University, Jerusalem, Israel
e-mail: nathalie.balaban@mail.huji.ac.il

© Springer Nature Switzerland AG 2019
K. Lewis (ed.), *Persister Cells and Infectious Disease*,
https://doi.org/10.1007/978-3-030-25241-0_1

1

1.1.1 Antibiotic Resistance

"Antibiotic resistance" is the *inherited* ability of bacteria to reproduce consecutively in the presence of a drug that would otherwise prevent the growth. The most widespread measure of the level of resistance is the Minimum Inhibitory Concentration (MIC) of the antibiotic, which prevents the replication of the bacteria. Higher resistance points to a higher MIC (Fig. 1.1a). Resistance is largely acquired by horizontal transfer of resistance gene cassettes (e.g., antibiotic inactivating enzymes (Jacoby 2009) or efflux pumps (Du et al. 2018)) or de novo mutations (e.g., altering the antibiotic target or reducing the uptake of antibiotics through the membrane (Blair et al. 2015)). Importantly, all these mechanisms result in a lower effective antibiotic concentration.

1.1.2 Antibiotic Tolerance

"Tolerance" is a transient ability of an *entire* population of bacteria to survive a bactericidal antibiotic treatment, without a change in the MIC, by slowing down a process that is required for antibiotic activity. Often, this slowing down also results in significantly slower growth and even growth arrest. The survival advantage of tolerant bacteria is often seen in treatments by drugs belonging to different classes,

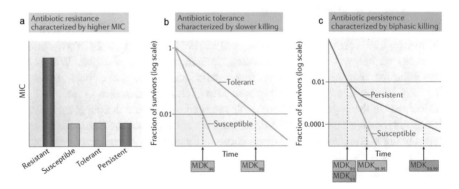

Fig. 1.1 Antibiotic resistance, tolerance, and persistence are distinct responses to antibiotic treatment that lead to increased survival compared with susceptible cells. (**a**) Resistant bacteria are characterized by a higher minimum inhibitory concentration (MIC). Antibiotic persistence and tolerance do not lead to an increase in the MIC compared with susceptible bacteria. (**b**) Tolerance is characterized by an increase in the minimum duration for killing [MDK; e.g., for 99% of bacterial cells in the population (MDK$_{99}$)] compared with susceptible bacteria. (**c**) Persistence is a heterogeneous response of the bacterial population with a population of susceptible bacteria and a subpopulation of tolerant bacteria. Therefore, the MIC is the same as for susceptible bacteria and the MDK is different, depending on the subpopulation size. Here, a subpopulation of ~1% of tolerant bacteria leaves the MDK$_{99}$ unchanged but affects the MDK$_{99.99}$. Adapted with permission from Balaban et al. (2019). Springer Nature Limited (this material is excluded from the CC-BY-4.0 license)

for example, β-lactams and fluoroquinolones (Wolfson et al. 1990), and even phages (Pearl et al. 2008). However, strains highly tolerant to these antibiotics may still be killed efficiently by other drugs. Although their survival under the antibiotic treatment to which they are tolerant is much higher than in non-tolerant strains, their MIC is unchanged (Fig. 1.1a), and another measure is introduced to characterize their slower killing: the Minimum Duration of Killing 99% of the bacterial population (MDK$_{99}$) (Fridman et al. 2014) (Fig. 1.1b).

1.1.3 Antibiotic Persistence

"Antibiotic persistence" (henceforth termed simply "persistence") enables a *subpopulation* of tolerant bacteria to survive in the presence of a bactericidal antibiotic. Persistent cells re-cultured on the fresh medium will demonstrate the same susceptibility to the same antibiotic as the initial culture, that is, only a subpopulation of the new culture will exhibit the persistent phenotype.

Unlike resistant cells, persisters cannot replicate in the presence of the drug any better than other cells but are killed at a lower rate than the susceptible population from which they are derived. This feature distinguishes persistence from heteroresistance, a phenomenon in which a small subpopulation transiently displays a substantially (>8-fold) higher MIC (El-Halfawy and Valvano 2015).

The hallmark of antibiotic persistence is the biphasic killing curve during the time-kill assays (Fig. 1.1c). On this curve, persisters correspond to the significantly slower killing phase after the bulk of the bacterial population is eliminated during the first phase of rapid killing.

Antibiotic tolerance and persistence are similar epigenetic traits that enable bacterial survival in the presence of bactericidal drugs. In some qualitative studies, the two terms may be interchangeable (Meylan et al. 2018). Nonetheless, differences do exist between persistence and tolerance. Persisters basically represent a *subpopulation* (typically <1%) of tolerant bacteria (thus, the phenomenon could have been called "heterotolerance") that can survive drug concentrations much higher than the MIC. Not surprisingly, mechanisms responsible for tolerance, such as dormancy, reduced metabolism, and ATP levels, have also been identified for persistence (Lewis 2007). What differentiates tolerance from persistence is the heterogeneous killing seen in the latter, that is, not all bacteria in a clonal culture are killed at the same rate. A subpopulation of persister cells is able to survive much better the antibiotic treatment than the majority of the population, as attested by the biphasic killing curve. Antibiotic persistence is not restricted to just two subpopulations. In the general case, more than one persister subpopulation may coexist and, thus, a multimodal killing curve is observed (Balaban et al. 2004). When studying persistence, two aspects are particularly interesting, the first one being pertaining to tolerance, and the second is specific to persistence: (1) the molecular mechanism(s) that enables tolerant bacteria to survive, and (2) the mathematical principle that generates heterogeneity in the population (Ackermann 2015), for example, nonlinear mechanisms leading to bimodality by amplifying stochasticity (Tsimring 2014; Huang et al. 2018).

1.1.4   Different Types of Persistent Bacteria

It is still a subject of hot debates whether a single general or multiple specific molecular mechanisms underlie the persistence phenotype (Levin et al. 2014; Michiels et al. 2016; Radzikowski et al. 2017), and the reader is referred to other chapters of this book. However, major mechanistically distinct ways for generating persisters in a culture have been identified. Distinguishing between the types of persistence is crucial, for each type requires a different procedure to measure the persistence level.

1.1.4.1   Triggered Persistence [Previously Called Type I (Balaban et al. 2004)]

In most observed cases, antibiotic persistence in bacteria is induced by external conditions, the commonest one being starvation. Even when the pressure is removed, for example, by diluting a starved overnight culture in fresh medium, some cells may still remain in the dormant state for extensive periods of time and may be found in the survival fraction. Even when the culture is regrown for a few hours and reaches what seems to be "exponential growth," a fraction of the persisters triggered by starvation may still be in a lag phase. Therefore, the lag time distribution of individual cells after exposure to a stress is an important factor that may determine the persistence level (Jõers et al. 2010; Levin-Reisman et al. 2010).

Numerous stress conditions have been identified to induce triggered persistence, among them starvation for various nutrients (Gutierrez et al. 2017), cell number (Vega et al. 2012), oxidative and acid stress, subinhibitory concentrations of drugs, immune factors, and exposure to immune cells (Helaine et al. 2014).

A further complication of the phenomenon is associated with high concentrations (Eagle and Musselman 1948) of antibiotics that trigger growth arrest, and cause a paradoxical lower killing rate and *drug-induced persistence* (Dörr et al. 2010). In this scenario, a bactericidal antibiotic becomes bacteriostatic for a subpopulation of cells that respond to the antibiotic signal itself, for example, by activating a stress response that enables them to survive (Dörr et al. 2010; Audrain et al. 2013). This type of response does not depend on the history of the culture prior to exposure to the drug (Johnson et al. 2013), and, therefore, may be attributed to spontaneous persistence. However, it may be more specific to the applied antibiotic and its concentration compared to other forms of persistence.

1.1.4.2   Spontaneous Persistence [Previously Called Type II (Balaban et al. 2004)]

Persistence may occur spontaneously in a steady exponentially growing culture. This form of persistence seems to be significantly less common than Type I persistence, and at present, no direct observations of spontaneous persistence have been clearly reported at the single-cell level in wild-type strains.

1.2   Quantification of Antibiotic Tolerance and Persistence

Tolerance is poorly characterized due to the lack of a quantitative and easily measured indicator similar to the MIC. The MDK_{99}—the minimum duration for killing 99% of the bacteria—can be defined when the killing rate reaches saturation at high concentration, for example, in Eq. (1.2) (Fridman et al. 2014; Brauner et al. 2017) (Fig. 1.1b). The MDK_{99} can be deduced from kill curves measured under antibiotic concentrations above the saturation regime (Brauner et al. 2017).

For characterizing the persistence of a bacterial population, a similar indicator such as $MDK_{99.99}$, can be used (Fig. 1.1c). However, if the persistence level itself is needed, the fraction of the tolerant subpopulation (α in Eq. 1.3) should be measured by extrapolating to slower killing curve to the initial measurement.

Predictive models of the survival of microorganisms under bactericidal drugs show that the MIC metric is insufficient to characterize the behavior, although it is widely used (EUCAST 2019; Barry et al. 1999). Common phenomenological models for the dependence of the survival, S, versus the concentration, c, or duration of treatment, t, are the Zhi function (Zhi et al. 1986), or E_{max} or Hill models (Levin and Udekwu 2010). Within the framework of these models, the killing rate, ψ, is described by three main parameters, which represent distinct underlying physico-chemical mechanisms: (1) the MIC, (2) MDK_{99}, and (3) the Hill coefficient for the steepness of the concentration dependence, k.

$$S(c,t) = e^{\psi t} \tag{1.1}$$

$$\psi(c) = \frac{\ln(0.01)}{MDK_{99}} \cdot \frac{1 - \left(\frac{c}{MIC}\right)^k}{\frac{\ln(0.01)}{\psi_{max} \times MDK_{99}} - \left(\frac{c}{MIC}\right)^k} \tag{1.2}$$

This general function predicts how the concentration of the antibiotic and its duration will affect the growth or death of a strain with growth rate without antibiotic, ψ_{max}. Note that the common notation of the model uses $\psi_{min} = \frac{\ln(0.01)}{MDK_{99}}$.

In this model, resistance is defined as an increase in the MIC, whereas tolerance is defined as an increase in the MDK_{99}. So far, the parameters describe a uniform population. When the population is heterogeneous, at least one of the parameters is heterogeneous.

Heteroresistance means that a subpopulation(s) of cells have a higher MIC than most bacteria in the population. In typical reports of heteroresistance, it is also assumed that the heritability of the increased MIC is long enough to create detectable colonies (Nicoloff et al. 2019).

Antibiotic persistence (which in this context could have been called heterotolerance) means that a subpopulation(s) of cells have a higher MDK_{99} than the major portion of the population. If we assume that the fraction of persisters is α, then the survival can be presented as the sum of the survival of two subpopulations with different killing rates:

$$S(c,t) = (1 - \alpha)e^{\psi t} + \alpha e^{\psi^* t} \tag{1.3}$$

where ψ is the killing rate of the normal population as in (1.1), and ψ^* is the killing rate of the persisters with a longer MDK_{99}.

1.3 Evolution of Antibiotic Tolerance Under Intermittent Antibiotic Treatments

Most evolutionary assays in antibiotic treatments usually consist of a constant exposure of the bacterial population to the drug starting with an initial dose below the MIC and a gradual daily dose increase until high MIC, that is, high resistance, is reached (Sun et al. 2009; Toprak et al. 2012). However, tolerance would mainly be selected if the antibiotic treatment is transient because tolerant bacteria do not grow under antibiotic treatments above the MIC (Fig. 1.1a) and have an advantage only under transient treatments. In effect, the pharmacokinetics of many antibiotics show intermittent, rather than constant concentrations in patients. Even when the goal of the treatment procedure is to reach a concentration above the MIC for at least 50% of the time, for example, for treatment with β-lactams, this is not always achieved in practice (Roberts et al. 2014). Therefore, the evolution under intermittent antibiotic exposures is of general interest (Moreillon et al. 1988). The examples below demonstrate that mutations leading to high tolerance or persistence are very rapidly selected in various protocols under intermittent treatments.

1.3.1 Tolerance and Persistence-by-Lag Evolve to Match the Duration of the Antibiotic Treatment

Intermittent exposure to antibiotics in vitro, coupled with high mutagenesis, led to isolation of mutants of *Escherichia coli* with elevated persistence (Moyed and Bertrand 1983) or tolerance (Tomasz 1979). To test how common would be the appearance of tolerant mutants without mutagenesis, we subjected parallel cultures to daily intermittent treatments with ampicillin. The way the antibiotic was administered had a profound impact on the evolutionary outcome. The bacteria were exposed to the drug when they were taken from an overnight culture and diluted into fresh medium with the antibiotic. Within ~7 daily intermittent exposures to the antibiotic, the bacterial population evolved a very high level of antibiotic tolerance (Fridman et al. 2014). The tolerance could be explained by the extension of the lag time, an often overlooked phenotype (Baranyi et al. 2009) that may evolve also under other stress factors (Zhou et al. 2012) and is linked to many cases of tolerance (Jõers et al. 2010) and persistence (Scherrer and Moyed 1988). As long as bacteria remained in the lag phase under the antibiotic treatment, despite the supply of

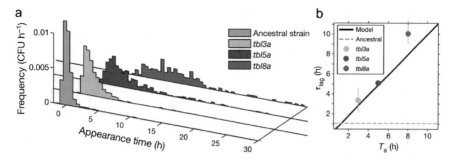

Fig. 1.2 Optimization of lag time in evolved *E. coli* populations under different durations of ampicillin exposure. (**a**) Lag time distribution measured by monitoring the appearance time of colonies continuously by ScanLag, an automated scanner system (Levin-Reisman et al. 2010), of the tolerant clones evolved under 3 h (green), 5 h (red), or 8 h (blue) of daily antibiotic exposures. (**b**) The measured mean lag-time (circles) of the distributions shown in (**a**) versus T_a, the antibiotic exposure duration. Solid line: model predictions for lag-time optimization reflecting the trade-off between a long lag that confers tolerance but delays the regrowth. The dashed line is the mean lag time of the ancestral strain. Figures are adapted with permission from Fridman et al. (2014)

nutrients, they could survive. Strikingly, the lag time duration evolved to match the duration of the antibiotic treatment (Fig. 1.2). This evolved tolerance-by-lag was shown to solve an evolutionary trade-off between staying dormant to survive the antibiotic treatment, and being able to grow fast once the concentration of antibiotics falls below the MIC.

Whole genome sequencing of the evolved clones and reconstruction of the ancestral alleles in the mutants allowed identifying mutation leading to increased tolerance. The "tolerome," that is, the assemblage of genes in which mutations responsible for the tolerance level are found, is very broad. These genes are found to be related to various cellular functions, including major metabolic pathways (Table 1.1). Thus, the large target size for mutations leading to increased tolerance is the main reason for the rapid evolution of tolerance.

In some mutants found in the parallel evolution cultures, the tolerance mutation had partial penetrance, that is, affected only a subpopulation, which resulted in antibiotic persistence with an increased lag time. Since antibiotic persistence is a particular case of tolerance, which concerns only part of the population, it is not surprising that the mutations evolved under this protocol in the high-persistent lines were similar to those found in tolerant strains (Table 1.1).

Interestingly, the tolerance mutations evolved under ampicillin treatment conferred high tolerance to other antibiotics such as norfloxacin (Fridman et al. 2014), cefazolin, ertapenem, and imipenem (Gefen et al. 2017). However, kanamycin was found to be as potent against the high-tolerant strains as against their wild-type ancestral strains (Gefen et al. 2017). Thus, high-tolerant strains evolved under certain classes of antibiotics may still be fully susceptible to other drug categories.

Table 1.1 High tolerance/persistence mutations identified in evolution experiments in vitro under intermittent high concentration antibiotic treatment

Organism	Antibiotic	Type of high tolerance/ persistence	Trigger	Mutated genes	References
E. coli K12	Ampicillin	Triggered, tolerance by lag	Stationary phase	*vapBC, prs*	Fridman et al. (2014)
E. coli K12	Ampicillin	Triggered, persistence by lag	Stationary phase	*metG*	Levin-Reisman et al. (2017)
EPEC	Ampicillin	Triggered, persistence by lag	Stationary phase	*metG*	Levin-Reisman et al. (2017)
S. aureus	Daptomycin	Triggered, tolerance at stationary phase	Stationary phase	*pitA*	Mechler et al. (2015)
E. coli	Aminoglycosides	Triggered, tolerance at stationary phase	Stationary phase	*oppB, nuoN, gadC*	Van den Bergh et al. (2016)
S. gordonii	Penicillin	Antibiotic-induced tolerance	Penicillin	*EI*	Bizzini et al. (2010)

1.3.2 Evolution of Stationary Phase Triggered Antibiotic Persistence

Since the days of Jacques Monod (1949), who defined the exponential phase of bacterial growth and the way to measure it precisely, microbiological studies have been primarily focusing on bacteria during this period. However, bacteria in natural circumstances are rarely present in the exponential growth phase (Bergkessel et al. 2016). In particular, bacteria colonizing the human body are growth arrested most of the time. Pathogenic bacteria are usually considered harmful when they multiply rapidly. Not surprisingly, most current detection techniques for pathogens in the clinical environment target the fastest growing bacteria, and antibiotics are selected for their ability to kill rapidly growing strains. Understanding the way bacteria evolve under drugs administered during their stationary phase is an important and overlooked question. In the experiments of van den Bergh et al., bacteria were exposed to antibiotic only after having reached stationary phase. After treating the stationary culture with antibiotic for several hours, the antibiotic was washed away and the culture regrown to stationary phase again (Van den Bergh et al. 2016). This work showed that mutations that elevate the level of tolerance and persistence rapidly occur also in this protocol. A similar exposure protocol led to a mutation resulting in high tolerance to daptomycin in *Staphylococcus aureus* (Mechler et al. 2015).

Interestingly, the mutations identified in the experiments of van den Bergh et al. had no overlap with those previously identified in the evolution experiments of Fridman et al. (2014). Whether this lack of overlap is due to the difference in the type of antibiotic classes used or to the different type of tolerance remains to be determined.

1.3.3 Evolution of Drug-Induced Tolerance

In the two studies described in Sects. 1.3.1 and 1.3.2, a stationary phase trigger was required for the tolerant or persistent phenotype. However, as mentioned in Sect. 1.1.4.1, certain antibiotics have been shown to be the trigger for tolerance (Dörr et al. 2010; Audrain et al. 2013; Moreillon et al. 1988). In cyclic exposure of *Streptococcus gordonii* to penicillin, Entenza et al. (1997) isolated high-tolerant mutants. Analysis of the way these mutants survive the antibiotics revealed that instead of causing lysis, as in the wild-type strain, the drug was inducing only growth arrest, which made the bacteria highly tolerant to penicillin. These lysis-defective mutants behaved under the bactericidal drug as if it were bacteriostatic (Table 1.1). Similar induction of tolerance or persistence by the antibiotic was observed for fluoroquinolone in *E. coli* (Dörr et al. 2010).

1.3.4 Antibiotic Tolerance in the Clinic

1.3.4.1 Evolution of Tolerance in the Clinic

During the 1970s, tolerant pathogenic bacteria were reported in clinical studies (Best et al. 1974; Sabath et al. 1977), especially in deep-rooted and chronic infections. These findings led to a burst of tolerance research during the next decade that identified tolerance in over 20 species, suggesting it to be a common feature in clinical bacterial pathogens (Handwerger and Tomasz 1985; Tomasz 1985). However, an important question that has been difficult to answer for a long time is whether the tolerant phenotype has clinical implications or not? Are the different tolerance levels measured in different species or strains the inevitable side effect of some intrinsic nature, or is it the result of evolution under antibiotic treatment as seen in in vitro strains evolved in the experiments described above? Some investigations were performed to check if patients infected by tolerant bacteria might have a worse treatment outcome (Denny et al. 1979; Rahal et al. 1986; Britt et al. 2017). Notwithstanding a potential correlation between tolerance and treatment failure, it seemed difficult to reach a conclusion yet.

Since the bacteriostatic drugs do not kill bacteria but merely inhibit their growth, all bacteria can be viewed as being tolerant to bacteriostatic drugs. Still, these drugs are effective at clearing bacterial infections in patients. If so, tolerant strains, that neither grow nor die under bactericidal antibiotics, should not be a threat. In 2014, a clinical work analyzed the cure rates of treatments with bacteriostatic and bactericidal drugs, and reported no statistically meaningful difference (Nemeth et al. 2015). However, these data did not focus on the infections where bactericidal effect was shown to be crucial, namely infections in immune-compromised hosts, or in niches where the immune system was ineffective (Nemeth et al. 2015). It is likely that in many infections, tolerance does not play a major role. However, identifying the subset of infections in which it does is a major goal.

With whole genome sequencing techniques, the evolution of pathogenic bacteria in the patients could be tracked. Through a series of pioneering research, evolution of tolerance was identified in patients with chronic infection (Mulcahy et al. 2010), compromised immune systems (Honsa et al. 2017), and biofilm-associated diseases (Dengler Haunreiter et al. 2019). These findings suggest that tolerance could evolve in the clinic, especially when the infection is difficult to eradicate. Thus, monitoring the evolution of tolerance might be important for these patients, and update the treatment accordingly with anti-tolerance antibiotics.

1.3.4.2 Techniques to Detect Tolerance in the Clinic

One major obstacle is how to detect tolerance quickly and accurately in clinical environments. For resistance, which can be identified by an increased MIC, disk diffusion assay can be easily and efficiently performed, as well as more precise technique such as the Etest (Joyce et al. 1992). For tolerance, though the killing assay was recognized as the gold standard for its detection, it was either too laborious to perform in a clinical laboratory or the results were so noisy that multiple replicates were required to reach a statistically meaningful conclusion. Therefore, an alternative method called MBC (minimum bactericidal concentration to reach killing of 99.9% of bacteria after 24 h of treatment) was applied in most studies dealing with tolerance in clinical research (Handwerger and Tomasz 1985). However, the MBC was shown to be a poor method to evaluate tolerance (Handwerger and Tomasz 1985). It is adequate to evaluate antibiotic-induced tolerance or persistence but fails to detect two major types of tolerance, namely tolerance-by-lag and tolerance-by-slow-growth.

Recently, a tolerance detection technique called TDtest was developed (Gefen et al. 2017). For high-throughput purpose, it might be an economic and easy method for monitoring tolerance in clinical settings. Briefly, the strategy behind the TDtest is to detect surviving bacteria without performing a killing assay. The TDtest consists of two steps. The first step is a disk diffusion assay, in which bacteria are exposed to antibiotics to form an initial inhibition ring. After a day, as the antibiotic concentration in the inhibition zone decreased, surviving bacteria should be able to grow. However, by then, most nutrients are used up by the peripheral bacteria. Therefore, the second step consists of adding nutrients to support the growth of the surviving tolerant bacteria to form a detectable colony (Fig. 1.3).

1.4 Antibiotic Tolerance and Persistence Promote the Evolution of Resistance

Most of the resistance evolution experiments were performed under gradually growing concentrations, where resistance mutations could gradually accumulate and reach a high resistance (Toprak et al. 2012; Baym et al. 2016). However, in

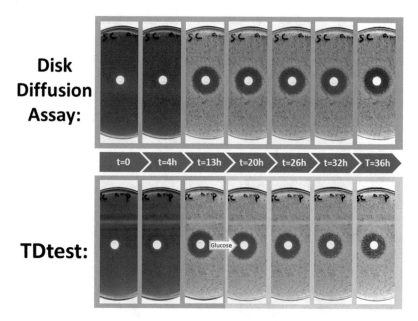

Fig. 1.3 Time-lapse imaging, using the Scanlag setup (Levin-Reisman et al. 2010) of the TDtest of a clinical isolate (*Enterobacter cloacae*) versus the regular disk diffusion assay. Top: Regular disk diffusion assay allows visualization of the inhibition zone. Even after 36 h of incubation, no growth is detected in the inhibition zone. Bottom: Same assay but with addition of glucose after 18 h, which allows surviving persister bacteria to form colonies in the inhibition zone. Adapted from Gefen et al. (2017)

the clinical setting, to avoid such gradual crawling of MIC, much higher concentrations are used, aiming to be above the MPC (mutant prevention concentration). This concentration is defined as being able to prevent growth, and even kill, single-step resistant mutants. The experiments described above show that tolerance evolves very rapidly under antibiotic concentration above the MPC when applied intermittently, for various protocols and different antibiotics. This suggests that the preferred evolutionary outcome under intermittent antibiotic treatment above the MPC is the establishment of a highly tolerant or persistent population. An important question is whether the now established tolerant strains impede or speed up the evolution of resistance factors. On one hand, the lower killing of tolerant strains implies that the number of generations that they undergo in each cycle is lower, suggesting that tolerant strains have a lower probability to evolve resistance. On the other hand, the increased survival of the tolerant strains may help reduce the drift.

In order to determine whether resistance establishes slower or faster on the background of tolerant strains, we subjected to the intermittent antibiotic treatment in parallel different *E. coli* ancestral strains (MGY, KLY, and EPEC) and their evolved respective tolerant mutant strains (Fridman et al. 2014; Levin-Reisman et al. 2017), and measured at each cycle the MIC of the populations. The results are shown in Fig. 1.4.

After enough cycles, resistant mutants were detected, with mutations in *ampC*, a beta-lactamase known to degrade ampicillin and which resulted in a $\times 4$ to $\times 20$

Fig. 1.4 Evolution
experiments with cultures
started from a tolerant strain
(dashed lines) evolved
resistance earlier than the
ancestral wt strain (solid
lines). Adapted from Levin-
Reisman et al. (2017)

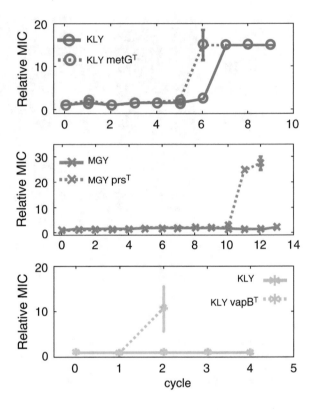

increase in the MIC. Resistance did not appear in all lines, but each time it did
appear, it was always earlier in the background of tolerant strains. Even when the
"ancestral" strains acquired resistance, we could actually detect that these lines had
acquired a tolerance mutation before acquiring resistance. Therefore, the predictive
path toward antibiotic resistance goes first through the evolution of tolerance and
only thereafter reaches resistance (Fig. 1.5).

This result demonstrated that tolerance could not only increase the survival under
antibiotic treatment, but also increase the probability of evolution of resistance.
Calculations (Fig. 1.6) show that tolerance increases the probability for the establishment of resistance by more than an order of magnitude. In order to understand the
main reason for such a high enhancement, one needs to realize that single-step
resistance mutations are not sufficient to allow the bacteria to grow at the high
concentration of antibiotics used in the experiment. In order words, although the
ampC mutations could increase the MIC by a factor of 10, the MIC of the resistant
mutants was still below the MPC antibiotic concentration. Therefore, resistant
mutants are constantly appearing in the ancestral strain background and being killed
by the high antibiotic concentration. However, when tolerance has established,
resistant mutations have now a much higher probability to survive the treatment
than when the same resistant mutation occurred on the ancestral background. This
intuitive thinking can be formulated mathematically to calculate the probability

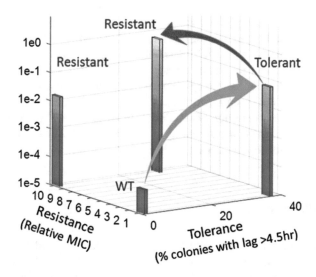

Fig. 1.5 Experimental evolutionary trajectory first passes through the high-tolerance peak (blue arrow) and then moves to resistance (red arrow). Height represents the survival under 4.5 h of ampicillin treatment at 50 μg/ml. Adapted from Levin-Reisman et al. (2017)

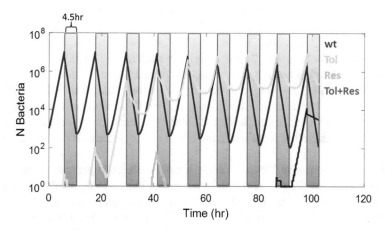

Fig. 1.6 An example of the dynamics in a simulation that includes all the details of the strains. The simulation shows the number of bacteria of each strain; *wt* (blue), tolerant (yellow), resistant (cyan), and tolerant + resistant (red) during intermittent antibiotic treatments of 4.5 h, and growth to stationary phase. Once the population reaches stationary phase, there is no change in the number of bacteria in each strain, therefore, in the simulation the killing starts immediately, while in the experiment a full cycle takes 24 h. During growth, the bacteria have a chance to gain mutations. During the antibiotic phase, each strain has a different killing rate. As predicted, when a resistance mutation occurs in the *wt* strain, it has less chances of establishment then on the background of tolerance. Note that the tolerant population coexists with the *wt* population for many cycles due to the long lag time that enables the *wt* recovery. Adapted from Irit Levin-Reisman—PhD thesis

of establishment of a resistance mutation, which is found to be more than an order of magnitude higher for resistance to establish on top of the tolerant strain (Levin-Reisman et al. 2017). A full simulation of the processes leading to the establishment of resistance faster on top of the tolerant strain can be seen in Fig. 1.6. The probability for the appearance of a resistance mutation is similar for *wt* and tolerant strains. When a resistant mutant appears (e.g., at 40 h in Fig. 1.6), it is killed by the high concentration of antibiotics. However, once the tolerant strain has established, a resistant mutant appearing at 85 h has a higher probability to survive and fix in the population in the next cycle.

1.5 Conclusion

In this chapter, we have shown that tolerance and resistance are orthogonal ways that bacteria can use to survive under bactericidal antibiotic treatments. Whereas resistance is achieved through mechanisms that decrease the effective concentration of the antibiotic, tolerance is due to a general slowing down of the killing. Antibiotic persistence is a special case of tolerance, in which only a subpopulation displays the tolerant phenotype. Both tolerance and persistence allow higher survival by a slowing down of essential processes in the bacterial cell.

Once bacteria acquire a resistant factor, their MIC increases and they may grow in concentrations that would otherwise be lethal. Increasing the concentration of antibiotic to above their MIC restores the killing. Therefore, the way to get rid of resistant strains is typically to increase the antibiotic concentration. However, bacteria that have become tolerant, either by a tolerance mutation or by external conditions, will often not respond to higher concentrations of antibiotics, but will eventually be killed by longer treatments. Therefore, understanding the reasons behind high survival is crucial in order to be able to decrease it. Furthermore, we have shown that tolerance and persistence lead to the rapid establishment of resistant mutants under intermittent antibiotic treatments, a major threat if proven to happen also in the clinic.

Whether tolerance facilitates the evolution of resistance in patients, or impedes it, is an open question with far-reaching implications. In pioneering works tracking the evolution of MRSA (methicillin-resistant *Staphylococcus aureus*) strains in a patient, tolerance was identified together with resistance (Sieradzki et al. 2003; Mwangi et al. 2007). However, dozens of mutations appeared in the resistant strains, making it difficult to assign specific mutations to the tolerance and relate them to this phenotype. To understand if tolerance can promote the subsequent evolution of resistance in patients, higher resolution of the evolution events needs to be captured.

Finally, the ability of bacteria to evolve tolerance strongly depends on a trigger provided either by environmental conditions or the antibiotic itself (Table 1.1). Therefore, measurements of the physiology of bacteria in the host, and its interplay with survival is a major gap that will need to be bridged if we aim to design better treatments, and to prevent the evolution of resistance.

References

Ackermann, M. (2015). A functional perspective on phenotypic heterogeneity in microorganisms. *Nature Reviews. Microbiology, 13*, 497–508.

Audrain, B., et al. (2013). Induction of the Cpx envelope stress pathway contributes to Escherichia coli tolerance to antimicrobial peptides. *Applied and Environmental Microbiology, 79*, 7770–7779.

Balaban, N. Q., Merrin, J., Chait, R., Kowalik, L., & Leibler, S. (2004). Bacterial persistenceas a phenotypic switch. *Science, 305*, 1622–1625.

Balaban, N. Q., et al. (2019). Definitions and guidelines for research on antibiotic persistence. *Nature Reviews. Microbiology, 1*, 441–448.

Baranyi, J., George, S. M., & Kutalik, Z. (2009). Parameter estimation for the distribution of single cell lag times. *Journal of Theoretical Biology, 259*, 24–30.

Barry, A. L., et al. (1999). *Methods for determining bactericidal activity of antimicrobial agents; approved guideline* (Vol. 19, pp. 1–3). Wayne, PA: Clinical and Laboratory Standard Institute.

Baym, M., et al. (2016). Spatiotemporal microbial evolution on antibiotic landscapes. *Science, 353*, 1147–1151.

Bergkessel, M., Basta, D. W., & Newman, D. K. (2016). The physiology of growth arrest: Uniting molecular and environmental microbiology. *Nature Reviews. Microbiology, 14*, 549–562.

Best, G. K., Best, N. H., & Koval, A. V. (1974). Evidence for participation of autolysins in bactericidal action of oxacillin on Staphylococcus aureus. *Antimicrobial Agents and Chemotherapy, 6*, 825–830.

Bizzini, A., et al. (2010). A single mutation in enzyme I of the sugar phosphotransferase system confers penicillin tolerance to Streptococcus gordonii. *Antimicrobial Agents and Chemotherapy, 54*, 259–266.

Blair, J. M. A., Webber, M. A., Baylay, A. J., Ogbolu, D. O., & Piddock, L. J. V. (2015). Molecular mechanisms of antibiotic resistance. *Nature Reviews. Microbiology, 13*, 42–51.

Brauner, A., Fridman, O., Gefen, O., & Balaban, N. Q. (2016). Distinguishing between resistance, tolerance and persistence to antibiotic treatment. *Nature Reviews. Microbiology, 14*, 320–330.

Brauner, A., Shoresh, N., Fridman, O., & Balaban, N. Q. (2017). An experimental framework for quantifying bacterial tolerance. *Biophysical Journal, 112*, 2664–2671.

Britt, N. S., et al. (2017). Relationship between vancomycin tolerance and clinical outcomes in *Staphylococcus aureus* bacteraemia. *The Journal of Antimicrobial Chemotherapy, 72*, 535–542.

Dengler Haunreiter, V., et al. (2019). In-host evolution of Staphylococcus epidermidis in a pacemaker-associated endocarditis resulting in increased antibiotic tolerance. *Nature Communications, 10*, 1149.

Denny, A. E., Peterson, L. R., Gerding, D. N., & Hall, W. H. (1979). Serious staphylococcal infections with strains tolerant to bactericidal antibiotics. *Archives of Internal Medicine, 139*, 1026–1031.

Dörr, T., Vulić, M., & Lewis, K. (2010). Ciprofloxacin causes persister formation by inducing the TisB toxin in Escherichia coli. *PLoS Biology, 8*, e1000317.

Du, D., et al. (2018). Multidrug efflux pumps: Structure, function and regulation. *Nature Reviews. Microbiology, 16*, 523–539.

Eagle, H., & Musselman, A. D. (1948). The rate of bactericidal action of penicillin in vitro as a function of its concentration, and its paradoxically reduced activity at high concentrations against certain organisms. *The Journal of Experimental Medicine, 88*, 99–131.

El-Halfawy, O. M., & Valvano, M. A. (2015). Antimicrobial heteroresistance: An emerging field in need of clarity. *Clinical Microbiology Reviews, 28*, 191–207.

Entenza, J. M., Caldelari, I., Glauser, M. P., Francioli, P., & Moreillon, P. (1997). Importance of genotypic and phenotypic tolerance in the treatment of experimental endocarditis due to Streptococcus gordonii. *The Journal of Infectious Diseases, 175*, 70–76.

EUCAST. (2019). *EUCAST reading guide*. The European Committee on Antimicrobial Susceptibility Testing.

Fridman, O., Goldberg, A., Ronin, I., Shoresh, N., & Balaban, N. Q. (2014). Optimization of lag time underlies antibiotic tolerance in evolved bacterial populations. *Nature, 513*, 418–421.

Gefen, O., Chekol, B., Strahilevitz, J., & Balaban, N. Q. (2017). TDtest: Easy detection of bacterial tolerance and persistence in clinical isolates by a modified disk-diffusion assay. *Scientific Reports, 7*, 41284.

Gutierrez, A., et al. (2017). Understanding and sensitizing density-dependent persistence to quinolone antibiotics. *Molecular Cell, 68*, 1147–1154.e3.

Handwerger, S., & Tomasz, A. (1985). Antibiotic tolerance among clinical isolates of bacteria. *Annual Review of Pharmacology and Toxicology, 25*, 349–380.

Helaine, S., et al. (2014). Internalization of salmonella by macrophages induces formation of nonreplicating persisters. *Science, 343*, 204–208.

Honsa, E. S., et al. (2017). Rela mutant Enterococcus faecium with multiantibiotic tolerance arising in an immunocompromised host. *MBio, 8*, 1–12.

Huang, G.-R., Saakian, D. B., & Hu, C.-K. (2018). Accurate analytic solution of chemical master equations for gene regulation networks in a single cell. *Physical Review E, 97*, 012412.

Jacoby, G. A. (2009). AmpC β-lactamases. *Clinical Microbiology Reviews, 22*, 161–182.

Jõers, A., Kaldalu, N., Tenson, T., & Jo, A. (2010). The frequency of persisters in Escherichia coli reflects the kinetics of awakening from dormancy. *Journal of Bacteriology, 192*, 3379–3384.

Johnson, P. J. T., Levin, B. R., Levin, B. R., Li, L., & Karger, B. (2013). Pharmacodynamics, population dynamics, and the evolution of persistence in Staphylococcus aureus. *PLoS Genetics, 9*, e1003123.

Joyce, L. F., Downes, J., Stockman, K., & Andrew, J. H. (1992). Comparison of five methods, including the PDM Epsilometer test (E test), for antimicrobial susceptibility testing of Pseudomonas aeruginosa. *Journal of Clinical Microbiology, 30*, 2709–2713.

Levin, B. R., Concepción-Acevedo, J., & Udekwu, K. I. (2014). Persistence: A copacetic and parsimonious hypothesis for the existence of non-inherited resistance to antibiotics. *Current Opinion in Microbiology, 21*, 18–21.

Levin, B. R., & Udekwu, K. I. (2010). Population dynamics of antibiotic treatment: A mathematical model and hypotheses for time-kill and continuous-culture experiments. *Antimicrobial Agents and Chemotherapy, 54*, 3414–3426.

Levin-Reisman, I., et al. (2010). Automated imaging with ScanLag reveals previously undetectable bacterial growth phenotypes. *Nature Methods, 7*, 737–739.

Levin-Reisman, I., et al. (2017). Antibiotic tolerance facilitates the evolution of resistance. *Science, 355*, 826–830.

Lewis, K. (2007). Persister cells, dormancy and infectious disease. *Nature Reviews. Microbiology, 5*, 48–56.

Mechler, L., et al. (2015). A novel point mutation promotes growth phase-dependent daptomycin tolerance in Staphylococcus aureus. *Antimicrobial Agents and Chemotherapy, 59*, 5366–5376.

Meylan, S., Andrews, I. W., & Collins, J. J. (2018). Targeting antibiotic tolerance, pathogen by pathogen. *Cell, 172*, 1228–1238.

Michiels, J. E., Van den Bergh, B., Verstraeten, N., & Michiels, J. (2016). Molecular mechanisms and clinical implications of bacterial persistence. *Drug Resistance Updates, 29*, 76–89.

Monod, J. (1949). The growth of bacterial cultures. *Annual Review of Microbiology, 3*, 371–394.

Moreillon, P., Tomasz, A., & Tomasz, A. (1988). Penicillin resistance and defective lysis in clinical isolates of pneumococci: Evidence for two kinds of antibiotic pressure operating in the clinical environment. *The Journal of Infectious Diseases, 157*, 1150–1157.

Moyed, H. S., & Bertrand, K. P. (1983). hipA, a newly recognized gene of Escherichia coli K-12 that affects frequency of persistence after inhibition of murein synthesis. *Journal of Bacteriology, 155*, 768–775.

Mulcahy, L. R., Burns, J. L., Lory, S., & Lewis, K. (2010). Emergence of Pseudomonas aeruginosa strains producing high levels of persister cells in patients with cystic fibrosis. *Journal of Bacteriology, 192*, 6191–6199.

Mwangi, M. M., et al. (2007). Tracking the in vivo evolution of multidrug resistance in Staphylococcus aureus by whole-genome sequencing. *Proceedings of the National Academy of Sciences, 104*, 9451–9456.

Nemeth, J., Oesch, G., & Kuster, S. P. (2015). Bacteriostatic versus bactericidal antibiotics for patients with serious bacterial infections: Systematic review and meta-analysis. *The Journal of Antimicrobial Chemotherapy, 70*, 382–395.

Nicoloff, H., Hjort, K., Levin, B. R., & Andersson, D. I. (2019). The high prevalence of antibiotic heteroresistance in pathogenic bacteria is mainly caused by gene amplification. *Nature Microbiology, 4*, 504.

Pearl, S., Gabay, C., Kishony, R., Oppenheim, A., & Balaban, N. Q. (2008). Nongenetic individuality in the host–phage interaction. *PLoS Biology, 6*, e120.

Radzikowski, J. L., Schramke, H., & Heinemann, M. (2017). Bacterial persistence from a system-level perspective. *Current Opinion in Biotechnology, 46*, 98–105.

Rahal, J. J., Chan, Y. K., & Johnson, G. (1986). Relationship of staphylococcal tolerance, teichoic acid antibody, and serum bactericidal activity to therapeutic outcome in Staphylococcus aureus bacteremia. *The American Journal of Medicine, 81*, 43–52.

Roberts, J. A., et al. (2014). DALI: Defining antibiotic levels in intensive care unit patients: Are current ß-lactam antibiotic doses sufficient for critically ill patients? *Clinical Infectious Diseases, 58*, 1072–1083.

Sabath, L. D., Laverdiere, M., Wheeler, N., Blazevic, D., & Wilkinson, B. J. (1977). A new type of penicillin resistance of Staphylococcus aureus. *Lancet, 309*, 443–447.

Scherrer, R., & Moyed, H. S. (1988). Conditional impairment of cell division and altered lethality in hipA mutants of Escherichia coli K-12. *Journal of Bacteriology, 170*, 3321–3326.

Sieradzki, K., Leski, T., Dick, J., Borio, L., & Tomasz, A. (2003). Evolution of a vancomycin-intermediate Staphylococcus aureus strain in vivo: Multiple changes in the antibiotic resistance phenotypes of a single lineage of methicillin-resistant S. aureus under the impact of antibiotics administered for chemotherapy. *Journal of Clinical Microbiology, 41*, 1687–1693.

Sun, S., Berg, O. G., Roth, J. R., & Andersson, D. I. (2009). Contribution of gene amplification to evolution of increased antibiotic resistance in Salmonella typhimurium. *Genetics, 182*, 1183–1195.

Tomasz, A. (1979). Escherichia coli mutants tolerant. *Journal of Bacteriology, 140*, 955–963.

Tomasz, A. (1985). Antibiotic tolerance among clinical isolates of bacteria. *Antimicrobial Agents and Chemotherapy, 7*, 368–386.

Toprak, E., et al. (2012). Evolutionary paths to antibiotic resistance under dynamically sustained drug selection. *Nature Genetics, 44*, 101–105.

Tsimring, L. S. (2014). Noise in biology. *Reports on Progress in Physics, 77*, 026601.

Van den Bergh, B., et al. (2016). Frequency of antibiotic application drives rapid evolutionary adaptation of Escherichia coli persistence. *Nature Microbiology, 1*, 16020.

Vega, N. M., Allison, K. R., Khalil, A. S., & Collins, J. J. (2012). Signaling-mediated bacterial persister formation. *Nature Chemical Biology, 8*, 431–433.

Wolfson, J. S., Hooper, D. C., McHugh, G. L., Bozza, M. A., & Swartz, M. N. (1990). Mutants of Escherichia coli K-12 exhibiting reduced killing by both quinolone and beta-lactam antimicrobial agents. *Antimicrobial Agents and Chemotherapy, 34*, 1938–1943.

Zhi, J., Nightingale, C. H., & Quintiliani, R. (1986). A pharmacodynamic model for the activity of antibiotics against microorganisms under nonsaturable conditions. *Journal of Pharmaceutical Sciences, 75*, 1063–1067.

Zhou, K., George, S. M., Li, P. L., & Baranyi, J. (2012). Effect of periodic fluctuation in the osmotic environment on the adaptation of Salmonella. *Food Microbiology, 30*, 298–302.

Chapter 2
Antibiotic Persisters and Relapsing *Salmonella enterica* Infections

Peter W. S. Hill and Sophie Helaine

Abstract Antibiotic persistence is defined as the ability of a subpopulation of bacteria within a clonal antibiotic-susceptible population to survive antibiotic treatment. Studies on antibiotic persistence have traditionally been carried out on bacteria cultured in laboratory media. However, over recent years, there has been a push to study antibiotic persisters in more physiologically relevant systems. Thus, the concept of antibiotic persistence during infection, which refers to the ability of a subpopulation of bacteria to survive combined host and antibiotic challenges, has emerged as a major new frontier of research. Here, we discuss the relevance and principles of this concept using relapsing *Salmonella enterica* infections as an example. We critically evaluate the clinical and experimental evidence for the existence and importance of antibiotic persisters in relapsing *Salmonella* infections; we outline our current understanding of the molecular mechanisms that enable successful antibiotic persistence during infection; and, finally, we discuss the challenges for this nascent field going forward.

2.1 Persistence of Infection, Antibiotic Persistence, and Antibiotic Persistence During Infection: What Is the Difference?

In this chapter, we discuss the relevance and principles of antibiotic persistence during infection in the relapse and recalcitrance of *Salmonella enterica* infections. In microbiology, persistence has acquired multiple definitions, each associated with a specific field. Thus, before discussing in detail the concept of antibiotic persistence during infection, for the sake of clarity, it is important to first understand what is meant by persistence in this context.

In the field of host–pathogen interactions, persistence refers to *persistence of an infection*. This is defined as the ability of bacteria to remain viable in the host for a

P. W. S. Hill · S. Helaine (✉)
Department of Medicine, MRC CMBI, Imperial College London, London, UK
e-mail: s.helaine@imperial.ac.uk

© Springer Nature Switzerland AG 2019
K. Lewis (ed.), *Persister Cells and Infectious Disease*,
https://doi.org/10.1007/978-3-030-25241-0_2

prolonged period of time (Monack 2013). Following infection by bacterial pathogens, the host usually responds by mounting first the innate and then the adaptive immune responses. These immune responses usually clear the invader. Some pathogenic bacteria, however, have evolved the ability to survive the initial robust immune response, resulting in persistence of the infection. This usually involves a complex interplay between host and pathogen, likely reflecting the coevolution and fine tuning of bacterial virulence mechanisms and host immune responses (Monack 2013).

On the other hand, in the field of fundamental bacteriology, persistence refers to *antibiotic persistence*. This is defined as the ability of a subpopulation of bacteria within a clonal antibiotic-susceptible population to survive antibiotic treatment (Fisher et al. 2017). The decreased susceptibility of cells of this subpopulation, known as antibiotic persisters, to killing by bactericidal antibiotics is achieved through phenotypic switching in which the antibiotic persisters enter into a slow-growing or growth-arrested state. This results in low target activity or low antibiotic uptake. Studies on antibiotic persistence have traditionally been carried out on bacteria cultured in laboratory media. However, over recent years, there has been a push to study antibiotic persisters in more physiologically relevant systems than defined laboratory media. Thus, a third field of persistence has emerged, one that in many ways bridges the fields of persistent infections and antibiotic persisters: *antibiotic persistence during infection* (Fig. 2.1). Antibiotic persistence during infection refers to the ability of bacteria to survive combined host and antibiotic challenges. It is this that we focus on here, using *Salmonella enterica* as an example.

2.2 A Brief Introduction to *Salmonella enterica* Infections

The bacterial pathogen *S. enterica* is a Gram-negative, facultative intracellular human and animal pathogen posing a major public health concern worldwide (Monack 2013). *S. enterica* Typhi, Typhimurium, and Enteritidis are three best characterized *Salmonella* serovars. Human-restricted *S.* Typhi causes a systemic infection, resulting in potentially life-threatening typhoid fever in humans (Monack 2013). In contrast, the non-typhoidal serovars (NTS) *S.* Typhimurium and *S.* Enteritidis infect a broad range of animals and are predominantly associated in humans with gastroenteritis, a disease normally self-limiting to the intestine (Monack 2013). However, bacteremia can occur even with these NTS serovars, a phenotype frequently associated in humans with malnutrition, coinfection with human immunodeficiency virus (HIV), or primary immune deficiencies (Feasey et al. 2012).

Infection of certain mouse strains with *S.* Typhimurium produces a systemic disease with some similarities to human typhoid fever (Carter and Collins 1974), and this has been used extensively over many years to study the pathogenesis of systemic *Salmonella* infections. *S.* Typhimurium first enters the murine host through the gastrointestinal tract and translocates by multiple mechanisms to deeper tissues (Monack 2013; Galán 2001) (Fig. 2.2). Like many Gram-negative bacterial

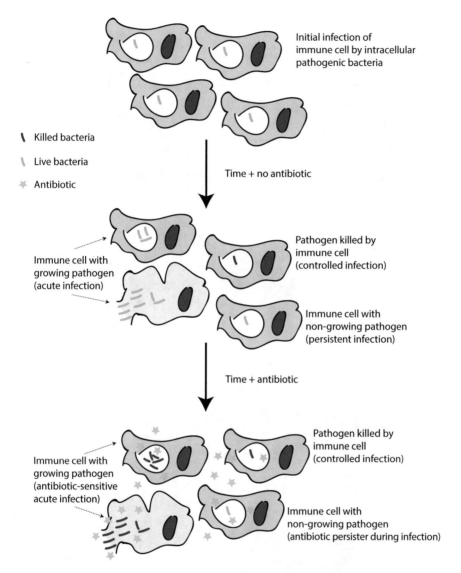

Fig. 2.1 Antibiotic persistence during infection. *Salmonella* Typhimurium is a facultative intracellular pathogen that preferentially resides in innate immune cells, such as macrophages or dendritic cells, during systemic infection. There, *Salmonella* is subjected to one of three fates: (1) immune-mediated death, in which the immune cells control the infection; (2) proliferation, which forms the basis of acute infection; or (3) entry into a non-growing persister state. During acute infection, the growing bacteria are susceptible to killing by antibiotics. In contrast, in the case of antibiotic persistence during infection, non-growing antibiotic-tolerant bacteria are able to survive challenge from both host immune response and antibiotic treatment

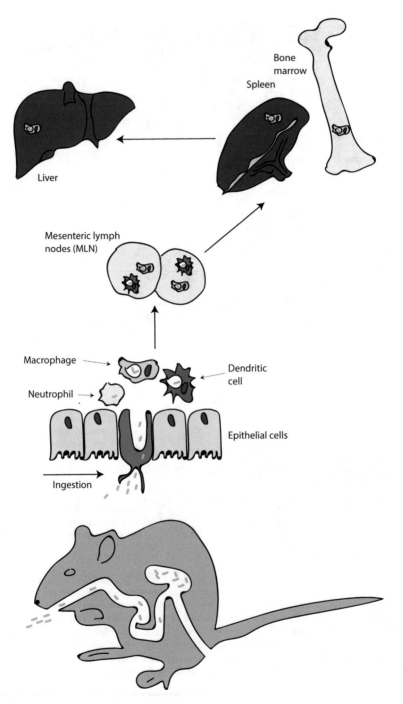

Fig. 2.2 Known sites of *Salmonella* infection and antibiotic persistence in the mouse: Bacteria are ingested in contaminated food or water and enter the gastrointestinal tract, where *Salmonella*

pathogens, *S. enterica* serovars, including Typhimurium, rely on Type III secretion system (T3SS) needle-mediated delivery of effector proteins from bacteria to host cells (Galán 2001). *S.* Typhimurium possess two T3SSs called *Salmonella* Pathogenicity Island 1 (SPI-1) and 2 (SPI-2) (Galán and Curtiss 1989; Shea et al. 1996). SPI1-dependent translocation of effector proteins into host epithelial cells enables the bacteria to traverse the small intestine epithelium barrier (Galán 2001). Although the *S.* Typhimurium SPI-1 T3SS has an important role in gastrointestinal disease (Galán 2001; Galán and Curtiss 1989), once the bacteria have crossed the gastrointestinal tract, it seems to be largely dispensable for the systemic phase of the infection in mice (Galán and Curtiss 1989; Jennings et al. 2017) (Fig. 2.2). In contrast, the SPI-2 T3SS functions both in intestinal and disseminated infection, and is required for growth within cells of different hosts (Figueira and Holden 2012; Jennings et al. 2017; Hensel et al. 1995). This includes cells of the monocyte/granulocyte lineage (Fields et al. 1986; Richter-Dahlfors et al. 1997; Salcedo et al. 2001), such as macrophages and dendritic cells, which represent a privileged niche that allows *Salmonella* to elude killing by the adaptive immune response (Figueira and Holden 2012; Monack 2013). When these *Salmonella*-infected phagocytes gain access to the lymphatics and bloodstream, the bacteria can spread to the liver, spleen, gall bladder, and bone marrow (Figueira and Holden 2012; Monack 2013) (Fig. 2.2).

Consistent with the SPI-1 T3SS role primarily in gastrointestinal disease, the corresponding genes are expressed in response to signals sensed by bacteria in the intestine of the infected host, and become active upon contact with epithelial cells (Figueira and Holden 2012; Galán 2001). Following this, the bacteria use SPI-1 to inject effector proteins across the host cell plasma membrane, several of which stimulate the assembly of actin filaments, resulting in localized membrane ruffling and bacterial invasion (Figueira and Holden 2012; Galán 2001). In *Salmonella* Typhimurium, SPI-1 T3SS effectors also trigger the activation of mitogen-activated protein kinase (MAPK) pathways; this results in the production of proinflammatory cytokines and stimulates the recruitment of polymorphonuclear leukocytes (PMNs), thus inducing acute intestinal inflammation (Figueira and Holden 2012; Galán 2001). While the SPI-1 T3SS is required for active invasion, expression of the SPI-2 T3SS promotes intracellular survival within a modified phagosomal compartment called the *Salmonella*-containing vacuole (SCV) (Figueira and Holden 2012; Jennings et al. 2017). After the early stages of infection, the SPI-1 system is generally downregulated, and the phagosomal environment (low pH, low Mg^{2+}, and Fe^{3+} content, low nutrient availability) triggers expression of the SPI-2 T3SS (Figueira and Holden 2012; Jennings et al. 2017; Monack 2013). Although the full

---

Fig. 2.2 (continued) invades epithelial cells. During systemic infection, *Salmonella* enters into the bloodstream, residing within dendritic cells and macrophages. The bacteria are disseminated through the lymphatics and bloodstream to the mesenteric lymph nodes (MLNs), which represents a major site of antibiotic persistence during infection. Subsequently, *Salmonella* are transported to the spleen, bone marrow, and liver, all of which represent further sites of antibiotic persistence during infection

repertoire of SPI-2 T3SS effectors is not present in all *S. enterica* serovars (Jennings et al. 2017), loss of function of the SPI-2 T3SS in different serovars invariably causes a strong virulence defect, usually associated with an intracellular growth defect regardless of host cell type (Figueira and Holden 2012; Jennings et al. 2017; Cirillo et al. 1998; Hensel et al. 1998; Khan et al. 2003). Effectors of the SPI-2 T3SS carry out a large number of functions (Jennings et al. 2017). These include maintaining the integrity of the SCV and its localization near the Golgi of host cells, modulating the host cytoskeleton, and interfering with immune signaling (Jennings et al. 2017).

2.3 Evidence for Role of Antibiotic Persistent *Salmonella* in Relapsing Infections

2.3.1 Clinical Evidence for Antibiotic Persistence During Infection in Humans

Broadly speaking, there are two possible clinical outcomes following initial *Salmonella* infection (Feasey et al. 2012): (1) failure to control the symptoms of infection, potentially resulting in death; or (2) resolution of the infection-associated symptoms, often aided by treatment with antibiotics. In the case of the latter, however, resolution of the symptoms associated with initial *Salmonella* infection does not necessarily equate with resolution of the infection itself (Monack 2013). For example, patients infected with *S.* Typhi can become asymptomatic carriers, shedding large amounts of bacteria from their gallbladder (Bhan et al. 2005; Levine et al. 1982; Shpargel et al. 1985; Sinnott and Teall 1987; Vogelsang and Boe 1948). This can result in typhoid fever being spread on to others. Alternatively, it is also well documented that acute relapse of infection can occur in patients previously infected with either *S.* Typhi or non-typhoidal *Salmonella* strains (such as Typhimurium or Enteritidis), including following antibiotic treatment (Marzel et al. 2016; Okoro et al. 2012; Wain et al. 1999). For example, in the case of *S.* Typhi, a 5% relapse rate was observed among 322 patients treated with broad-spectrum cephalosporins and a 1.5% relapse rate among 642 patients treated with fluoroquinolones at the Centre for Tropical Disease referral center in Ho Chi Minh City, Vietnam (Wain et al. 1999). Similarly, in a study of over 48,000 culture-confirmed non-typhoidal *Salmonella* infections that occurred in Israel between 1995 and 2012, 2.2% of all patients showed relapse of infection (with 65% of these being symptomatic with relapsing diarrhea) (Marzel et al. 2016).

Acute relapse may be due to *recrudescence* or *reinfection* (Fisher et al. 2017). In this context, recrudescence is defined by a failure to clear the initial infection (Fisher et al. 2017). Thus, although symptoms following initial infection may be temporarily abated, in the case of recrudescence, symptoms re-emerge due to reappearance of the same bacterial isolate that caused the initial infection. In contrast, reinfection refers to the reappearance of infection-associated symptoms due to a new infection with a different bacterial isolate following complete clearance of the initial infection (Fisher et al. 2017). A number of studies have suggested that recrudescence is a much greater source of relapse than reinfection, including following antibiotic treatment. For example, in a series of 10 patients in Vietnam with recurrent attacks of typhoid fever (and associated antibiotic treatment, as described in the above study), pulse-field gel electrophoresis (PFGE) and plasmid typing showed that nine of the ten patients suffered recrudescence of the original infection, while only one pair of acute- and relapse-phase stains were different from each other (Wain et al. 1999). In a study on relapsing invasive non-typhoidal *Salmonella* (iNTS), researchers used high-resolution single nucleotide polymorphism (SNP) typing and whole-genome phylogenetics to investigate 47 iNTS isolates from 14 HIV patients in Malawi with multiple recurrences of relevant symptoms following initial infection and antibiotic treatment (Okoro et al. 2012). They found that recrudescence with identical or highly phylogenetically related isolates accounted for 78% of recurrences, while reinfection with phylogenetically distinct isolates accounted for only 22% of relapses (Okoro et al. 2012). Similarly, whole genome phylogenetic analysis of *S.* Typhimurium isolates collected at two different time points (separated by a minimum of 33 days) from 11 non-immunocompromised patients with persistent relapsing infection in Israel revealed that, in all 11 cases, recrudescence was responsible for reappearance of the infection, with *Salmonella* isolates from the same person always clustering together in discrete nodes with high support values (Marzel et al. 2016). Finally, in an extreme example, analysis of the whole genome sequence of 11 *S.* Enteritidis isolates from a single patient, diagnosed with IL-12 β1 receptor deficiency, who had multiple recurrent systemic *S.* Enteritidis infections over a period of 9 years, revealed that each successive acute episode was due to relapse from the same infection rather than reinfection (Klemm et al. 2016).

In each of these cases, the conclusion that recrudescence is the primary factor driving relapsing *Salmonella* infections is based exclusively on observations from genotyping assays, which revealed highly similar genotypes between initial and relapsing isolates from the same patient. It remains formally possible, however, that, in some cases, a patient was infected more than once from the same sources (such as from a single typhoid carrier), resulting in apparent recrudescence, which may actually be reinfection. Nonetheless, the high incidence of recrudescence in patients with relapsing *Salmonella* infection is remarkable; the fact that recrudescence is frequently observed despite several courses of antibiotic treatment (Klemm et al. 2016; Okoro et al. 2012; Wain et al. 1999) is even more striking, and potentially implicates antibiotic persisters as a reservoir for relapsing *Salmonella* infection in humans. Another model remains possible, however, rather than needing to enter into a non-growing, non-dividing antibiotic persistent state prior to relapse, recrudescence following antibiotic treatment could be due to antibiotics failing to reach sufficient concentrations at specific sites within the infected host. In this case, bacteria at these sites could survive in a growing, antibiotic-sensitive state but never see antibiotic concentrations high enough to induce killing. This could result in relapse of the infection following antibiotic withdrawal. To distinguish between these two models—that is (1) antibiotic persistence or (2) insufficient antibiotic penetrance—in the role of relapsing *Salmonella* infections, researchers have turned to experimental models, which are discussed below.

2.3.2 Experimental Evidence for Antibiotic Persistence During Infection in Mice

The mouse is the preferred infection model for research into *Salmonella* pathogenesis, most commonly with the Typhimurium serovar (Monack 2013). As mentioned above, *S.* Typhimurium causes a typhoid-like disease in mice (Carter and Collins 1974). The severity of *S.* Typhimurium infection is highly contingent on the genetic background of the mouse, with so called resistant and sensitive mice expressing either a functional or non-functional allele of the Nramp1 (also known as Slc11a1) cation transporter, respectively (Cellier et al. 2007; Caron et al. 2002). In the case of resistant mice, such as those of the 129Sv genetic background, expression of the functional Nramp1 cation transporter in macrophages, dendritic cells, and neutrophils reduces cytoplasmic iron levels, thus, limiting the availability of iron for intracellular bacteria (Cellier et al. 2007). As a result, these mice readily control *Salmonella* proliferation, resulting in a persistent infection, with *Salmonella* residing in the gallbladder and within F4/80$^+$ MOMA-2$^+$ hemophagocytic macrophages in the mesenteric lymph nodes (Monack et al. 2004). Similar to what is frequently observed in humans infected with *S.* Typhi, these resistant mice can act as asymptomatic carriers of the disease (Monack et al. 2004; Caron et al. 2002). On the other hand, sensitive mice, such as those of the C57Bl6 genetic background, expressing a non-functional *Nramp1* allele due to two amino acid substitutions, are unable to limit iron availability to the same extent (Cellier et al. 2007). As a result, *S.* Typhimurium within these mice readily proliferate in innate immune cells, such as macrophages and dendritic cells, and sensitive mice rapidly succumb to overwhelming infection in the absence of prolonged antibiotic treatment (Caron et al. 2002; Griffin et al. 2011).

Over the last decade, scientists have used susceptible mice to develop robust animal models for the study of relapsing primary typhoid that initiates after apparently successful antibiotic treatment. Generally, in these models, susceptible mice are first infected either orally or intravenously, and the disease is allowed to progress for 24–72 h. This is then followed by days of antibiotic treatment with either fluoroquinolones (most commonly ciprofloxacin or enrofloxacin) or beta-lactamases (ampicillin), which are administered either intraperitoneally or in drinking water. A few days after cessation of the antibiotic treatment, relapse is typically observed (see below for details).

2.3.2.1 The Mesenteric Lymph Nodes and Spleen Are Preferred Niches for Antibiotic-Tolerant *S.* Typhimurium During Infection

In one of the first robust studies to explore relapsing *S.* Typhimurium infection in mice, McSorley and colleages attempted to determine the minimum period of antibiotic compliance for resolving murine typhoid (Griffin et al. 2011). They infected susceptible C57Bl6 mice orally and administered enrofloxacin in drinking water, beginning 2 days later (Griffin et al. 2011). In their experiments, all mice appeared to have resolved primary infection after only 4 days of antibiotic treatment: bacteria were no longer excreted in feces, and *Salmonella* was undetectable by conventional plating of intestinal [Peyer's patches and mesenteric lymph nodes (MLNs)] or systemic (spleen, liver, bone marrow, and gallbladder) tissues (Griffin et al. 2011). However, if antibiotic therapy was halted after a week, mice resumed shedding *Salmonella* in feces 3–8 days later, followed by development of obvious symptoms of systemic infection, and eventually death (Griffin et al. 2011). Relapsing infection was observed even following antibiotic treatments of up to 3 weeks, with antibiotic treatment for 5 weeks required in order to fully resolve the symptoms and prevent relapsing infection (Griffin et al. 2011). The authors used in vivo luminescent imaging to detect emitted photons from *lux* expressing *Salmonella* in live anesthetized mice to follow infection and antibiotic treatment in various organs. In doing so, they confirmed that bacteria are largely undetectable within a few days of exposure to antibiotics, with MLNs being the final organ to display a detectable signal of infection (Griffin et al. 2011). Consistently, following antibiotic withdrawal, the earliest detection of bacteria also occurred in MLNs, with bacterial growth eventually progressing to include multiple systemic tissues, most notably the spleen and liver (Griffin et al. 2011). It should be noted in this context that bioluminescence approaches lack sensitivity, with a minimum of several hundred bacteria required for detectable signal even in vitro, without the added loss of signal due to skin and tissue (Avci et al. 2018); thus, the fate of individual antibiotic persisters cannot be tracked in this manner. Nonetheless, McSorley and colleages further confirmed their results by harvesting, homogenizing, and incubating whole organs from infected mice treated with enrofloxacin in overnight broth cultures (in order to amplify the very low numbers of bacteria prior to the plating these cultures onto MacConkey agar) (Griffin et al. 2011). Indeed, *Salmonella* could be cultured from the MLNs of all antibiotic-treated mice ($n = 15/15$) (Griffin et al. 2011). Altogether, these results suggested that MLNs represent a major site of bacterial persistence after antibiotic treatment of murine typhoid.

These observations were subsequently expanded on in an elegant study by Hardt and colleagues (Kaiser et al. 2014). In their model, mice were infected orally with *S.* Typhimurium and given a high dose of ciprofloxacin, which was administered twice daily by oral gavage starting 1 day post-infection (Kaiser et al. 2014); of note, starting antibiotic treatment this soon after infection inhibited pathogen spread to the spleen (a site of systemic infection). Tracking of *Salmonella* CFUs over time following administration of ciprofloxacin revealed a biphasic killing curve in the draining cecum lymph nodes (cLNs) of infected mice (Kaiser et al. 2014). Specifically, over a 90% decrease in CFUs was observed in the first 2 h of treatment, followed by only very limited further killing for the ensuing 10 days of treatment (Kaiser et al. 2014). It should be noted here that, in a separate study by Mastroeni and colleagues, no significant initial decrease in bacterial loads following antibiotic treatment was observed within MLNs of mice infected intravenously with *S.* Typhimurium for 3 days followed by intraperitoneal ciprofloxacin injection every 12 h (Rossi et al. 2017). This discrepancy may be due to the different infection routes used. Nonetheless, the fact that Hardt and colleagues, using the more physiologically relevant infection model, observed that cLN bacterial loads declined with fast kinetics by over tenfold during the first few hours of antibiotic treatment indicated that ciprofloxacin is bioactive at this site of infection (Kaiser et al. 2014). These observations were further supported by their pharmacokinetic analysis, which showed that ciprofloxacin concentration always remained >50× the MIC for inhibiting *Salmonella* growth ex vivo in the cLN (Kaiser et al. 2014); furthermore, their tissue culture experiments using labelled antibiotic further confirmed that ciprofloxacin efficiently penetrates into infected cells (Kaiser et al. 2014). Altogether, these results strongly argue for a role for antibiotic persisters in relapsing *Salmonella* infection, rather than relapse being due to insufficient antibiotic penetrance in the infected tissue/cells.

The capacity of antibiotic-tolerant bacteria within the cLN to cause a relapse-like infection was further supported by cell transfer experiments carried out by Hardt and colleagues, in which infected mice treated with antibiotics for 2 days were sacrificed and dissociated single cells of the cLN were prepared and injected into the peritoneal cavity of non-infected recipient mice currently undergoing prophylactic ciprofloxacin treatment (Kaiser et al. 2014). After the cell transfer, antibiotic treatment of the recipient mice was discontinued; 4 days later, recipient mice were sacrificed and pathogen loads were determined. Compared to recipient mice infected by intraperitoneal injection of *Salmonella* Typhimurium cultured in LB media, transfer of cLN cells led to high infection rates, especially in the spleen and liver (Kaiser et al. 2014). For a number of reasons, however, the observation that antibiotic-tolerant *Salmonella* found within the cLN can give rise to relapsing systemic infection (with high loads in spleen and liver) should be taken with a grain of salt. First, IP injection of antibiotic-tolerant *Salmonella* found within the cLN does not faithfully recapitulate normal relapsing infection (in which antibiotic treatment is simply stopped); specifically, in normal relapsing infection, high loads of bacteria are observed in the cLN and gut lumen as well (and not just in the spleen and liver) (Kaiser et al. 2014). Thus, as the authors themselves suggest, the site of reseeding (i.e., cLNs for normal relapse experiments vs. intraperitoneum for transfer experiments) likely affects the colonization patterns during relapse (Kaiser et al. 2014). Second, using isogenic tagged strains (ITS) of *Salmonella* Typhimurium, Mastroeni and colleagues monitored the population structure of *Salmonella* in a number of organs at various time points during infection and antibiotic treatment. This included: (1) after 3 days intravenous infection; (2) after 3 days intravenous infection and 4 days ciprofloxacin treatment; and (3) after 3 days intravenous infection, 4 days ciprofloxacin treatment, and 2 days of relapse (Rossi et al. 2017). They found that, within each mouse, the ITS population structure in MLNs was different from that of the spleen, liver, and blood, although the structure of the latter three were highly correlated (Rossi et al. 2017). Thus, it appears that the relapse of bacterial growth in sites of systemic infection are not necessarily being driven by migration of *Salmonella* from the MLNs. Rather, there is evidence to suggest that the spleen itself may also act as a preferred niche for antibiotic tolerant *Salmonella* during infection. For example, when McSorley and colleagues harvested, homogenized, and incubated whole organs from infected mice treated with enrofloxacin in overnight broth cultures (in order to amplify the very low numbers of bacteria prior to the plating these cultures onto MacConkey agar), they observed that *Salmonella* could be cultured from the spleen of a third of mice ($n = 5/15$) (Griffin et al. 2011). This suggests that the spleen represents a minor, but still significant, site of bacterial persistence after antibiotic treatment of murine typhoid. Moreover, these observations are further supported by Hardt and colleagues, who observed that, if ciprofloxacin treatment was started 2 or 3 days post-infection (rather than one day), *Salmonella* could be detected in the spleens of mice up to 10 days post-infection and antibiotic treatment (Kaiser et al. 2014). Furthermore, in an intravenous infection model in which they first let mice develop clear symptoms of *Salmonella* infection prior to daily administration of enrofloxacin, Bumann and colleagues were also clearly able to see antibiotic-tolerant bacteria in spleens even after 5 days of fluoroquinolone treatment (Claudi et al. 2014). Collectively, these results implicate the existence of *Salmonella* antibiotic persisters during mouse infection, with mesenteric lymph nodes and spleen, respectively, acting as a major and minor niches for these bacteria.

2.3.2.2 The Subpopulation of *S.* Typhimurium Capable of Surviving Antibiotic Treatment During Infection Are Slow or Non-Growing Bacteria Found Within Dendritic Cells and Macrophages

As described in the introduction, antibiotic persisters represent a subpopulation of bacteria within a clonal antibiotic-susceptible population that undergoes phenotypic switching to enter into a slow-growing or growth-arrested state (Fisher et al. 2017). Consistent with this definition, a number of studies tracking either the growth history or present growth rate of *S.* Typhimurium that survive antibiotic treatment during infection have revealed that these are indeed slow- or non-growing bacteria. Helaine and colleagues used a fluorescence dilution setup to analyze the growth history of *S.* Typhimurium in the MLNs of mice infected orally for 1 day followed by 5 days of enrofloxacin treatment (Helaine et al. 2014). With fluorescence dilution, the extent of bacterial proliferation at the single-cell level is monitored by dilution of a preformed pool of fluorescent protein after its induction has been stopped (Helaine et al. 2010). Bacteria with low and high fluorescence respectively represent cells that have undergone multiple or no rounds of cell division (Helaine et al. 2010). Indeed, following 5 days enrofloxacin treatment, all of the bacteria extracted from the

MLNs retained very high fluorescence levels, indicating that *Salmonella* capable of surviving antibiotic treatment in mice undergo no cell division (Helaine et al. 2014). Hardt and colleagues used an analogous plasmid dilution strategy, in which dilution of an IPTG-addicted plasmid is tracked followed removal of IPTG (Kaiser et al. 2014). Using this strategy, they showed that bacteria that survived ciprofloxacin treatment for 24 h in cLNs were highly over-represented for bacteria that retained the plasmid (compared with the relative proportion prior to antibiotic treatment) (Kaiser et al. 2014). Again, this suggested a highly reduced growth rate in the antibiotic-tolerant *Salmonella* population during infection.

Bumann and colleagues developed a fluorescent reporter system called TIMER to elucidate the present growth rate, rather than growth history, of *S.* Typhimurium at the single-cell level during mouse infection and enrofloxacin treatment (Claudi et al. 2014). TIMER refers to the DsRed S197T variant, which spontaneously changes fluorescence color from green to green/orange over time. In cells that have recently undergone cell division, the fast maturing green TIMER molecules are more concentrated compared to slowly maturing orange TIMER molecules, resulting in a dominant green fluorescence (Claudi et al. 2014). In contrast, in non-proliferating cells, the slowly maturing orange TIMER molecules accumulate, yielding a characteristic green/orange fluorescence (Claudi et al. 2014). Bumann and colleagues sorted *Salmonella* subsets with different ratios of green/orange isolated from infected spleen 1 h after initiating enrofloxacin treatment, and determined bacterial viability of the different subpopulations by comparing CFUs per sorted fluorescent *Salmonella*. They noticed that there was a correlation between killing and the pre-treatment growth rate, with fast-growing subsets extensively killed and slow-growing/non-dividing *Salmonella* much tolerated treatment better, resulting in their overrepresentation among survivors (Claudi et al. 2014). Their results suggested, however, that the largest number of survivors originated from an abundant *Salmonella* subset with moderate growth rates and partial tolerance, although this may be a result of the relatively lower doses of antibiotics used (Claudi et al. 2014). Intriguingly, the authors also showed that a surprisingly large proportion of TIMER-expressing *Salmonella* had low growth rates in the MLNs, but not the spleen, potentially explaining why these represent major and minor sites of relapse, respectively (Claudi et al. 2014). Collectively, the observations using reporters to track bacterial growth history and growth rates offer strong support for slow- or non-growing antibiotic persisters forming a reservoir for relapsing *Salmonella* infection in vivo.

Within the MLNs, antibiotic persistent *Salmonella* appear to reside within dendritic cells (DCs), with >80% of bacteria residing within CD11c$^+$ cells following ciprofloxacin treatment (compared with 53% in untreated MLNs) (Kaiser et al. 2014). Specifically, classical (CD103$^+$CX3CR1$^-$) dendritic cells rather than interstitial (CD103$^-$CX3CR1$^+$) DCs appear to be the preferred niche (Kaiser et al. 2014). Indeed, genetic or chemical manipulation of DC cell numbers revealed that survival of *S.* Typhimurium in MLNs following ciprofloxacin treatment correlated with the number of DCs (Kaiser et al. 2014). Moreover, in in vitro persister assays, bacteria residing within bone marrow-derived dendritic cells (BMDCs) displayed a 50-fold increase in ciprofloxacin survival compared with laboratory media (Kaiser et al. 2014). Within the spleen, non-growing antibiotic persistent *Salmonella* can be found within Cd11b$^+$F4/80$^+$ macrophages (Stapels et al. 2018), although it remains possible that other cell types may also act as a preferred niche. This is consistent with in vitro persister assays, in which bacteria residing within bone marrow-derived macrophages (BMMs) displayed a 100–1000× increase in survival to the cephalosporin cefotaxime (also gentamicin and cipro) compared with those in laboratory media (Helaine et al. 2014).

Collectively, the accumulated experimental evidence suggests that relapsing *S.* Typhimurium infection following antibiotic treatment in mice is due, in large part, to a reservoir or slow- or non-growing bacteria found within MLN dendritic cells and splenic macrophages.

2.4 Molecular Mechanisms: How to Cope with Combined Host and Antibiotic Challenges?

Successful antibiotic persistence during infection requires three steps (Fig. 2.3): (1) entry into a slow- or non-growing state (i.e., persister formation); (2) survival within the host environment in a slow- or non-growing state; and (3) persister reawakening following removal of the antibiotic, enabling bacterial proliferation and relapsing infection. Although very little is currently understood regarding the ability of *Salmonella* antibiotic persisters during infection to reawaken following antibiotic removal, the molecular mechanisms involved in the first two stages are beginning to emerge.

2.4.1 Formation of Salmonella Antibiotic Persisters During Infection

Persister formation, in which the bacteria enter into a slow- or non-growing state, represents perhaps the most important step enabling normally antibiotic-sensitive bacteria to evade killing by the antibiotic. In the case of antibiotic persistence by *S.* Typhimurium during infection, this step has best been studied following internalization of the bacteria by macrophages (Fig. 2.3). In one of the first studies to systematically track bacterial growth history during infection, Helaine and colleagues followed the fate of *S.* Typhimurium following internalization by bone marrow-derived macrophages using fluorescence dilution (see Sect. 2.3.2.2 for details) (Helaine et al. 2010). They observed numerous macrophages containing bacteria that had undergone different numbers of cell divisions over a 22-h period, revealing that bacteria can have different growth histories even within the same macrophage (Helaine et al. 2010). This suggests that heterogeneity with respect to

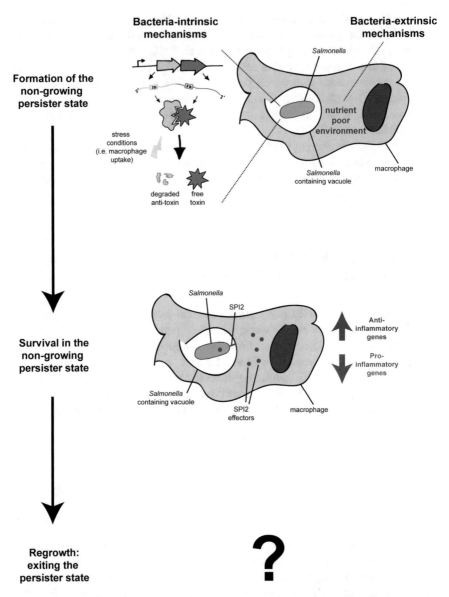

Fig. 2.3 Mechanisms involved in *Salmonella* antibiotic persistence during infection: formation; survival and regrowth. Successful antibiotic persistence during infection requires three steps: (1) entry into a slow or non-growing state (i.e., persister formation); (2) survival within the host environment in a slow- or non-growing state; and (3) persister reawakening following removal of the antibiotic (i.e., regrowth). Both bacteria intrinsic (e.g., toxin-antitoxin modules, stress responses) and extrinsic (e.g., host cell microenvironment, nutrient deprivation) mechanisms have been shown to be mechanistically involved in the formation of persisters. *Salmonella* antibiotic persisters, while in a non-growing state, still retain the ability to transcribe, translate and translocate SPI-2 effectors following internalization by macrophages. This enables the intracellular antibiotic

the ability of *S.* Typhimurium to grow within the immune cells relies, at least in part, on bacteria-intrinsic factors. On the other hand, using TIMER-expressing *Salmonella* (see Sect. 2.3.2.2 for details) to track growth rates of bacteria in vivo within spleen red pulp, Bumann and colleagues showed that bacteria within the same infected host cell were frequently observed to have similar growth rates, which often differed from those in neighboring infected cells (Claudi et al. 2014). This suggests, in addition to bacteria-intrinsic control, bacteria-extrinsic factors (e.g., the individual host cell microenvironment) also represent a major driver of growth heterogeneity.

Consistent with bacteria-intrinsic regulation, in a later study, Helaine and colleagues showed that the simple act of being internalized by macrophages for as little as 15 min is sufficient to dramatically increase the proportion of antibiotic persisters within a *S.* Typhimurium population (Helaine et al. 2014). In these experiments, *Salmonella* was phagocytosed by murine BMM; 15 min later, the macrophages were lysed and the internalized bacteria were placed in LB medium with high concentrations of cefotaxime, ciprofloxacin, or gentamicin (Helaine et al. 2014). After 24–72 h of treatment, the pre-internalized bacteria showed up to a 1000-fold increase in the level of antibiotic persisters compared to stationary phase *Salmonella* that had been directly subcultured into LB and antibiotics (Helaine et al. 2014). Similar results were also found following internalization by human monocyte-derived macrophages (Rycroft et al. 2018).

Using chemical perturbations, Helaine and colleagues were able to show that the stress of acidification and nutritional deprivation within the SCV were important contributors to this increase in persister levels (Helaine et al. 2014). They also showed that, following macrophage internalization, the expression of 14 type-II toxin-antitoxin (TA) modules were upregulated in the bacteria (Fig. 2.3). TA modules encode a stable toxin that may inhibit any one of a diverse set of metabolic processes in the bacterial cell, and an antitoxin that neutralizes the activity of the toxin when the cell is not under stress (Helaine et al. 2014). It is thought that, when stressed, the bacteria may degrade the antitoxin, enabling the toxin to inhibit the activity of its target and thus inhibit bacterial growth and division (Fisher et al. 2017). In support of a role for the upregulated *Salmonella* TA modules in increased antibiotic persistence following transient macrophage internalization, Helaine and colleagues showed that single genetic deletions of all 14 type-II TA modules dramatically decreased the ability of the bacteria to survive antibiotic treatment (Helaine et al. 2014). Consistently, the forced overexpression of a number of these toxins in *Salmonella* grown in laboratory medium has been shown to dramatically increase persister levels (Cheverton et al. 2016; Rycroft et al. 2018).

Fig. 2.3 (continued) persisters to reprogram the macrophage host cell from a pro-inflammatory (i.e., M1-like) bactericidal state to an anti-inflammatory (i.e., M2-like) permissive state, which is critical for the ability of the antibiotic persisters to survive long term in macrophages. Very little is currently understood regarding the ability of *Salmonella* antibiotic persisters during infection to reawaken following antibiotic removal

Helaine and colleagues went on to test the in vivo importance of the *shpAB* TA module (Helaine et al. 2014), which was previously shown to be involved in *Salmonella* antibiotic persistence in LB media (Slattery et al. 2013). They inoculated mice orally with an equal mixture of WT and *shpAB* mutant strains, and treated with or without enrofloxacin (Helaine et al. 2014). Consistent with a role in formation of nongrowing antibiotic persisters, the *shpAB* mutant showed a reduced survival compared with wild type upon antibiotic challenge, but enhanced net growth in the absence of fluoroquinolone treatment (Helaine et al. 2014). In contrast, using TIMER-expressing *Salmonella* Typhimurium depleted for three TA modules (*ecnB shpAB phD-doc*), Bumann and colleagues did not observe a significant change in mutant *Salmonella* growth rate or virulence 5 days post-oral infection when compared with wild type (Claudi et al. 2014). In view of these results, the extent to which TA modules contribute to the formation of non-growing antibiotic *Salmonella* persisters in vivo remains to be determined and represents an exciting future frontier in the field.

Bumann and colleagues also carried out proteomic analysis of antibiotic-tolerant slow-growing and antibiotic-sensitive fast-growing *Salmonella* Typhimurium isolated from infected mice and showed that slow-growing *Salmonella* were enriched for sigma factor- and CRP-dependent proteins (Claudi et al. 2014). This suggested that carbon limitation is an important factor contributing to slower growth in vivo (Claudi et al. 2014) (Fig. 2.3). Furthermore, the authors observed upregulation of proteins known to be involved in metabolism of the alarmome (p)ppGpp, suggesting elevated (p)ppGpp levels in response to amino acid starvation, other nutrient limitations, and/or heat and oxidative stress (Claudi et al. 2014).

Collectively, the aforementioned studies represent the first steps in trying to elucidate the molecular mechanism enabling the formation of *Salmonella* antibiotic persisters during infection. They outline the importance of host–pathogen interplay, with both bacteria intrinsic (e.g., TA modules, stress responses) and extrinsic (e.g., host cell microenvironment, nutrient deprivation) playing important, and potentially complementary, roles (Fig. 2.3).

2.4.2   Salmonella *Antibiotic Persisters Must Survive the Immune Response During Infection*

When *Salmonella* and other bacterial species are in laboratory culture media, antibiotic persisters are often observed to be inactive (i.e., dormant), which is thought to confer an advantage due to reduced target activity or low antibiotic uptake in the dormant cells (Conlon et al. 2016; Fisher et al. 2017; Shan et al. 2017). Consistent with this hypothesis, Helaine and colleagues showed that the artificial generation of a population of non-growing and translation incompetent *S.* Typhimurium through exposure to bacteriostatic concentrations of chloramphenicol resulted in increased survival upon exposure to high concentrations of the bactericidal cephalosporin cefotaxime in LB media (Stapels et al. 2018). However, when they tested whether a similar benefit was conferred to *Salmonella* cefotaxime persisters residing within BMM, the authors observed dramatically reduced survival of the chloramphenicol-treated population (Stapels et al. 2018). Furthermore, using *S.* Typhimurium carrying a reporter plasmid that allows for tracking of bacterial transcriptional/translational activity, Helaine and colleagues showed that a large proportion of non-growing bacteria found within antibiotic-treated BMM are not only active, but that only these active non-growing bacteria are capable of subsequent regrowth, and thus act as a reservoir for recrudescence (Stapels et al. 2018).

These seemingly contradictory results (that dormancy is beneficial to *Salmonella* antibiotic persisters in laboratory medium, but detrimental during infection) are explained in part by the fact that, unlike antibiotic persisters formed in laboratory media, those formed during infection have to not only withstand killing induced by the antibiotic but also killing induced by the immune system (Stapels et al. 2018). As discussed earlier, following entry into macrophages, *Salmonella* induces expression of the SPI-2 T3SS, through which it translocates approximately 30 effectors that inhibit host cell processes that are detrimental to the pathogen (Jennings et al. 2017). Helaine and colleagues showed that *Salmonella* antibiotic persisters, while in a non-growing state, still retain the ability to transcribe, translate, and translocate SPI-2 effectors following internalization by macrophages (Stapels et al. 2018) (Fig. 2.3). They showed that this strategy enables the intracellular antibiotic persisters to survive drug exposure (as they are non-growing) and also to reprogram the macrophage host cell from a pro-inflammatory (i.e., M1-like) bactericidal state to an anti-inflammatory (i.e., M2-like) permissive state (Stapels et al. 2018) (Fig. 2.3). This reprogramming is critical to the ability of the antibiotic persisters to survive long term in macrophages, and highlights the importance of *Salmonella* antibiotic persisters in retaining transcriptional/translational activity in the face of combined antibiotic and immune challenge (Stapels et al. 2018).

2.5 Going Forward: Future Directions and Challenges

In this chapter, we have outlined the clinical and experimental evidence for the existence and role of *Salmonella enterica* antibiotic persisters during infection. Although accumulating evidence supports a role for antibiotic persisters, we stress that it remains to be conclusively proven that this subpopulation of bacteria is directly responsible in relapsing *Salmonella* infection. Indeed, definitive proof will likely necessitate technological advances in in vivo imaging to track the complete life cycle of single bacteria in the host, including first entering into a non-growing, non-dividing state; then persisting in the face of both immune and antibiotic challenge; and ultimately resuming growth following antibiotic withdrawal to repopulate the infected host. This represents an exciting challenge going forward.

The field of antibiotic persistence has seen huge progress over the last decade. However, to date, most studies focused on the regulatory mechanisms governing antibiotic persistence have been carried out in vitro in laboratory medium (Fisher et al. 2017). While this has enabled many important advances, we are only just scraping the surface regarding physiologically relevant models of antibiotic persisters in vivo. Indeed, although in vitro studies can recapitulate certain aspects of infection-associated antibiotic persistence, models derived from persisters formed in laboratory medium may be misleading without taking into account the interaction with the host. This is most strikingly illustrated by the in vitro-derived paradigm that antibiotic persisters are metabolically inactive (i.e., dormant), which contrasts with in vivo data in which retention of metabolic activity appears to be highly beneficial (Stapels et al. 2018; Manina et al. 2015). Thus, the further development and use of in vivo models to tease apart the molecular mechanisms involved in antibiotic persistence represents a second exciting challenge going forward.

Finally, although this chapter has focused predominantly on pathogen-specific mechanisms involved in antibiotic persistence during infection, the interplay between host and persister represents an exciting new avenue in the investigation of persister biology. This includes both the influence of antibiotic persisters on the immune system phenotype, and, conversely, the impact of modulating the immune system on the ability of antibiotic persisters to survive. The former is highlighted by Helaine and colleagues who showed that *Salmonella* antibiotic persisters reprogram macrophages from a pro-inflammatory M1 to anti-inflammatory M2 phenotype (Stapels et al. 2018); the latter is illustrated by Hardt and colleagues who showed that triggering innate immune responses by injection of LPS or CpG into *Salmonella*-infected mice treated with ciprofloxacin significantly and dramatically reduced the number of antibiotic persisters (Kaiser et al. 2014). Thus, the further characterization of host–pathogen interactions in antibiotic persistence represents an exciting and largely unexplored field, with considerable therapeutic promise in our fight against relapsing *Salmonella* infections.

References

Avci, P., Karimi, M., Sadasivam, M., Antunes-Melo, W., Carrasco, E., & Hamblin, M. (2018). In-vivo monitoring of infectious diseases in living animals using bioluminescence imaging. *Virulence, 9*, 28–63.

Bhan, M., Bahl, R., & Bhatnagar, S. (2005). Typhoid and paratyphoid fever. *Lancet, 366*, 749–762.

Caron, J., Loredo-Osti, J., Laroche, L., Skamene, E., Morgan, K., & Malo, D. (2002). Identification of genetic loci controlling bacterial clearance in experimental *Salmonella enteritidis* infection: An unexpected role of Nramp1 (Slc11a1) in the persistence of infection in mice. *Genes and Immunity, 3*, 196–204.

Carter, P., & Collins, F. (1974). The route of enteric infection in normal mice. *The Journal of Experimental Medicine, 139*, 1189–1203.

Cellier, M., Courville, P., & Campion, C. (2007). Nramp1 phagocyte intracellular metal withdrawal defense. *Microbes and Infection, 9*, 1662–1670.

Cheverton, A., Gollan, B., Przydacz, M., Wong, C., Mylona, A., Hare, S., & Helaine, S. (2016). A Salmonella toxin promotes persister formation through acetylation of tRNA. *Molecular Cell, 63*, 86–96.

Cirillo, D., Valdivia, R., Monack, D., & Falkow, S. (1998). Macrophage-dependent induction of the Salmonella pathogenicity island 2 type III secretion system and its role in intracellular survival. *Molecular Microbiology, 30*, 175–188.

Claudi, B., Spröte, P., Chirkova, A., Personnic, N., Zankl, J., Schürmann, N., Schmidt, A., & Bumann, D. (2014). Phenotypic variation of Salmonella in host tissues delays eradication by antimicrobial chemotherapy. *Cell, 158*, 722–733.

Conlon, B., Rowe, S., Gandt, A., Nuxoll, A., Donegan, N., Zalis, E., Clair, G., Adkins, J., Cheung, A., & Lewis, K. (2016). Persister formation in *Staphylococcus aureus* is associated with ATP depletion. *Nature Microbiology, 1*, 16051.

Feasey, N., Dougan, G., Kingsley, R., Heyderman, R., & Gordon, M. (2012). Invasive non-typhoidal Salmonella disease: An emerging and neglected tropical disease in Africa. *Lancet, 379*, 2489–2499.

Fields, P., Swanson, R., Haidaris, C., & Heffron, F. (1986). Mutants of Salmonella typhimurium that cannot survive within the macrophage are avirulent. *Proceedings of the National Academy of Sciences of the United States of America, 83*, 5189–5193.

Figueira, R., & Holden, D. (2012). Functions of the Salmonella pathogenicity island 2 (SPI-2) type III secretion system effectors. *Microbiology, 158*, 1147–1161.

Fisher, R., Gollan, B., & Helaine, S. (2017). Persistent bacterial infections and persister cells. *Nature Reviews. Microbiology, 15*, 453–464.

Galán, J. (2001). Salmonella interactions with host cells: Type III secretion at work. *Annual Review of Cell and Developmental Biology, 17*, 53–86.

Galán, J., & Curtiss, R., 3rd. (1989). Cloning and molecular characterization of genes whose products allow *Salmonella typhimurium* to penetrate tissue culture cells. *Proceedings of the National Academy of Sciences of the United States of America, 86*, 6383–6387.

Griffin, A., Li, L., Voedisch, S., Pabst, O., & Mcsorley, S. (2011). Dissemination of persistent intestinal bacteria via the mesenteric lymph nodes causes typhoid relapse. *Infection and Immunity, 79*, 1479–1488.

Helaine, S., Thompson, J., Watson, K., Liu, M., Boyle, C., & Holden, D. (2010). Dynamics of intracellular bacterial replication at the single cell level. *Proceedings of the National Academy of Sciences of the United States of America, 107*, 3746–3751.

Helaine, S., Cheverton, A., Watson, K., Faure, L., Matthews, S., & Holden, D. (2014). Internalization of Salmonella by macrophages induces formation of nonreplicating persisters. *Science, 343*, 204–208.

Hensel, M., Shea, J., Gleeson, C., Jones, M., Dalton, E., & Holden, D. (1995). Simultaneous identification of bacterial virulence genes by negative selection. *Science, 269*, 400–403.

Hensel, M., Shea, J., Waterman, S., Mundy, R., Nikolaus, T., Banks, G., Vazquez-Torres, A., Gleeson, C., Fang, F., & Holden, D. (1998). Genes encoding putative effector proteins of the type III secretion system of Salmonella pathogenicity island 2 are required for bacterial virulence and proliferation in macrophages. *Molecular Microbiology, 30*, 163–174.

Jennings, E., Thurston, T., & Holden, D. (2017). Salmonella SPI-2 type III secretion system effectors: Molecular mechanisms and physiological consequences. *Cell Host and Microbe, 22*, 217–231.

Kaiser, P., Regoes, R., Dolowschiak, T., Wotzka, S., Lengefeld, J., Slack, E., Grant, A., Ackermann, M., & Hardt, W. (2014). Cecum lymph node dendritic cells harbor slow-growing bacteria phenotypically tolerant to antibiotic treatment. *PLoS Biology, 12*, e1001793.

Khan, S., Stratford, R., Wu, T., Mckelvie, N., Bellaby, T., Hindle, Z., Sinha, K., Eltze, S., Mastroeni, P., Pickard, D., Dougan, G., Chatfield, S., & Brennan, F. (2003). *Salmonella typhi* and *S. typhimurium* derivatives harbouring deletions in aromatic biosynthesis and Salmonella Pathogenicity Island-2 (SPI-2) genes as vaccines and vectors. *Vaccine, 21*, 538–548.

Klemm, E., Gkrania-Klotsas, E., Hadfield, J., Forbester, J., Harris, S., Hale, C., Heath, J., Wileman, T., Clare, S., Kane, L., Goulding, D., Otto, T., Kay, S., Doffinger, R., Cooke, F., Carmichael, A., Lever, A., Parkhill, J., Maclennan, C., Kumararatne, D., Dougan, G., & Kingsley, R. (2016). Emergence of host-adapted Salmonella Enteritidis through rapid evolution in an immunocompromised host. *Nature Microbiology, 1*, 15023.

Levine, M., Black, R., & Lanata, C. (1982). Precise estimation of the numbers of chronic carriers of *Salmonella typhi* in Santiago, Chile, an endemic area. *The Journal of Infectious Diseases, 146*, 724–726.

Manina, G., Dhar, N., & Mckinney, J. (2015). Stress and host immunity amplify *Mycobacterium tuberculosis* phenotypic heterogeneity and induce nongrowing metabolically active forms. *Cell Host and Microbe, 17*, 32–46.

Marzel, A., Desai, P., Goren, A., Schorr, Y., Nissan, I., Porwollik, S., Valinsky, L., Mcclelland, M., Rahav, G., & Gal-Mor, O. (2016). Persistent infections by nontyphoidal Salmonella in humans: Epidemiology and genetics. *Clinical Infectious Diseases, 62*, 879–886.

Monack, D. (2013). Helicobacter and salmonella persistent infection strategies. *Cold Spring Harbor Perspectives in Medicine, 3*, a010348.

Monack, D., Bouley, D., & Falkow, S. (2004). *Salmonella typhimurium* persists within macrophages in the mesenteric lymph nodes of chronically infected Nramp1+/+ mice and can be reactivated by IFNgamma neutralization. *The Journal of Experimental Medicine, 199*, 231–241.

Okoro, C., Kingsley, R., Quail, M., Kankwatira, A., Feasey, N., Parkhill, J., Dougan, G., & Gordon, M. (2012). High-resolution single nucleotide polymorphism analysis distinguishes recrudescence and reinfection in recurrent invasive nontyphoidal *Salmonella typhimurium* disease. *Clinical Infectious Diseases, 54*, 955–963.

Richter-Dahlfors, A., Buchan, A., & Finlay, B. (1997). Murine salmonellosis studied by confocal microscopy: *Salmonella typhimurium* resides intracellularly inside macrophages and exerts a cytotoxic effect on phagocytes in vivo. *The Journal of Experimental Medicine, 186*, 569–580.

Rossi, O., Dybowski, R., Maskell, D., Grant, A., Restif, O., & Mastroeni, P. (2017). Within-host spatiotemporal dynamics of systemic Salmonella infection during and after antimicrobial treatment. *The Journal of Antimicrobial Chemotherapy, 72*, 3390–3397.

Rycroft, J., Gollan, B., Grabe, G., Hall, A., Cheverton, A., Larrouy-Maumus, G., Hare, S., & Helaine, S. (2018). Activity of acetyltransferase toxins involved in Salmonella persister formation during macrophage infection. *Nature Communications, 9*, 1993.

Salcedo, S., Noursadeghi, M., Cohen, J., & Holden, D. (2001). Intracellular replication of *Salmonella typhimurium* strains in specific subsets of splenic macrophages in vivo. *Cellular Microbiology, 3*, 587–597.

Shan, Y., Brown Gandt, A., Rowe, S., Deisinger, J., Conlon, B., & Lewis, K. (2017). ATP-dependent persister formation in *Escherichia coli*. *MBio, 8*, e02267-16.

Shea, J., Hensel, M., Gleeson, C., & Holden, D. (1996). Identification of a virulence locus encoding a second type III secretion system in *Salmonella typhimurium*. *Proceedings of the National Academy of Sciences of the United States of America, 93*, 2593–2597.

Shpargel, J., Berardi, R., & Lenz, D. (1985). Salmonella Typhi carrier state 52 years after illness with typhoid fever: A case study. *American Journal of Infection Control, 13*, 122–123.

Sinnott, C., & Teall, A. (1987). Persistent gallbladder carriage of *Salmonella typhi*. *Lancet, 1*, 976.

Slattery, A., Victorsen, A., Brown, A., Hillman, K., & Phillips, G. (2013). Isolation of highly persistent mutants of *Salmonella enterica* serovar typhimurium reveals a new toxin-antitoxin module. *Journal of Bacteriology, 195*, 647–657.

Stapels, D., Hill, P., Westermann, A., Fisher, R., Thurston, T., Saliba, A., Blommestein, I., Vogel, J., & Helaine, S. (2018). Salmonella persisters undermine host immune defences during antibiotic treatment. *Science, 362*, 1156–1160.

Vogelsang, T., & Boe, J. (1948). Temporary and chronic carriers of *Salmonella typhi* and *Salmonella paratyphi* B. *The Journal of Hygiene (Lond), 46*, 252–261.

Wain, J., Hien, T., Connerton, P., Ali, T., Parry, C., Chinh, N., Vinh, H., Phuong, C., Ho, V., Diep, T., Farrar, J., White, N., & Dougan, G. (1999). Molecular typing of multiple-antibiotic-resistant *Salmonella enterica* serovar Typhi from Vietnam: Application to acute and relapse cases of typhoid fever. *Journal of Clinical Microbiology, 37*, 2466–2472.

Chapter 3
The Biology of Persister Cells in *Escherichia coli*

Alexander Harms

Abstract Bacterial persisters are dormant, antibiotic-tolerant cells that are phenotypic variants formed within a regularly growing, drug-susceptible population. They differ from genetically or phenotypically resistant cells in that their survival of antibiotic treatment is rooted in a dormant physiology and not in the obstruction of drug–target interactions. In this chapter, I assembled a concise overview of the formation, survival, and evolution of persisters formed by the model organism *Escherichia coli*. Though the formation of persister cells has stochastic aspects, it is often induced by starvation or stress as a specialized differentiation of part of the population (responsive diversification). Consequently, the phenotypic heterogeneity of persisters and regularly growing cells is commonly interpreted as a bet-hedging strategy that ensures population survival under the threat of catastrophic events and that at the same time optimizes the benefit from favorable conditions. Multiple different molecular mechanisms have been implicated in persister cell formation and can be grouped into two major classes. Non-specific mechanisms affect bacterial physiology on a global scale via, for example, alterations of energy metabolism, or are purely stochastic events that shut down cellular processes by an accidental malfunctioning (persistence as stuff happens). Conversely, specialized mechanisms directly inhibit antibiotic targets often through activation of fine-tuned molecular switches known as toxin-antitoxin modules. In addition, the repair of cellular damage caused by antibiotics is critical for the resuscitation of persister cells. A major obstacle to coherently interpreting these findings is the fragmented nature of the literature and several controversies that should be consolidated by future studies.

3.1 Basic Concepts of Persister Cell Biology

The prevailing crisis of antibiotic therapy is often seen as a consequence of rising antibiotic resistance (Laxminarayan et al. 2013). However, chronic and relapsing infections are often associated with genetically susceptible bacteria that survive even

A. Harms (✉)
Biozentrum, University of Basel, Basel, Switzerland
e-mail: alexander.harms@unibas.ch

© Springer Nature Switzerland AG 2019
K. Lewis (ed.), *Persister Cells and Infectious Disease*,
https://doi.org/10.1007/978-3-030-25241-0_3

massive and long-lasting antibiotic treatment (Levin and Rozen 2006; Fauvart et al. 2011; see also Chap. 4). This phenomenon is commonly linked to the formation of specialized "persister" cells that are transiently tolerant to nominally lethal doses of antibiotics. Traditionally, the tolerance of these cells is seen as rooted in a dormant physiological state in which the targets of antibiotic drugs are inactive and can thus not be poisoned or corrupted by the treatment, enabling bacterial survival (Harms et al. 2016; Lewis 2010; Wood et al. 2013). A major obstacle for the targeted development of effective treatment options against persister cells is the lack of a comprehensive understanding which molecular mechanisms and physiological changes truly underly their antibiotic tolerance. Furthermore, progress is hampered by the redundant and multifactorial nature of known persister mechanisms but also by the use of different model systems, methodologies, and definitions/understandings in the field (Balaban et al. 2013; Kaldalu et al. 2016).

In this chapter, I will focus on the by far most well-studied model organism for research on persister cells, *Escherichia coli*, and try to draw a comprehensive picture of the biology of persister cells of this organism. To this end, I will summarize the physiological concepts underlying the stress tolerance of persister cells, the different molecular pathways driving this phenomenon, and how these shape the survival and growth of a bacterial population. While most data have been generated with the laboratory strain *E. coli* K-12 MG165, I will also highlight insight from environmental and clinical strains like different isolates of uropathogenic *E. coli* (UPEC). Urinary tract infections are notorious for frequent relapse after treatment, which is often seen as a consequence of persister cell formation by UPECs (Blango and Mulvey 2010; Goneau et al. 2014). For a comprehensive view on persister cell biology involving other organisms or deeper insight into specific aspects, the reader is referred to the other chapters of this book or one of the recent review articles by different groups (Van Den Bergh et al. 2017; Harms et al. 2016; Fisher et al. 2017; Lewis 2010; Wood et al. 2013).

3.1.1 Persister Formation as a Phenotypic Switch into Dormancy

The general paradigm of bacterial persister formation in distinction from antibiotic resistance is that these cells attain transient antibiotic tolerance through a phenotypic switch into a dormant, slow- or non-growing state (Balaban et al. 2004). Put differently, the key difference between antibiotic resistance and drug tolerance is that resistance mechanisms impair the ability of the antibiotic to reach its target while persister cell formation comprises changes of bacterial physiology that interfere with the lethal effects of target poisoning (Keren et al. 2004b). Consistently, it is well established that the rate of antibiotic killing for a given set of bacteria is closely correlated to their growth rate and that the enforced shutdown of cellular activities through bacteriostatic drugs or ectopic expression of toxic proteins readily induces drug tolerance (Vazquez-Laslop et al. 2006; Claudi et al. 2014; Ocampo et al. 2014). Nevertheless, the majority of non-growing cells that arise without experimental intervention (e.g., in stationary phase) are not antibiotic tolerant (Orman and Brynildsen 2013; Dörr et al. 2009; Harms et al. 2017; Keren et al. 2004a), indicating that persisters "are not simply non-growing cells" but exhibit additional changes in their physiology that underly their survival and resuscitation (Lewis 2005).

The question of how persister cells can reversibly enter such a dormant state and survive lethal doses of antibiotics is intimately connected to the question of how antibiotics kill. Two major different views on this topic are prevalent in the field. One side understands antibiotics as drugs that poison or corrupt bacterial targets in a way that they "disrupt key functions of their target such that the activity of the crippled enzyme or multicomponent machine becomes toxic and reduces viability" (Cho et al. 2014). This view is commonly accepted by the majority of researchers and underlies the "dormancy model" of bacterial persistence in that persister formation involves the (selective of generalized) shutdown of cellular drug targets as the underlying reason of their tolerance as well as their lack of (significant) growth (Harms et al. 2016; Lewis 2010; Wood et al. 2013). An alternative, yet not inherently incompatible, view highlights that the actual killing of bacterial cells would not be caused by damage due to poisoned drug targets but due to their secondary induction of "active death processes" (Yang et al. 2017). More precisely, the killing activities of the various different classes of bactericidal antibiotics are proposed to converge in the production of reactive oxygen species (ROS) through metabolic perturbations (Kohanski et al. 2010). This idea has been repeatedly disputed (Renggli et al. 2013; Keren et al. 2013; Liu and Imlay 2013), but different variants of this theme are regularly invoked to explain phenotypes linked to bacterial persisters and drug tolerance.

3.1.2 Stochasticity and Heterogeneity of Persister Formation

Although persisters cells are often described to exhibit multidrug tolerance, multiple studies have shown that the far majority of persisters in a given experimental sample exhibit drug-specific tolerance (comprehensively reviewed by Van Den Bergh et al. 2017). As an example, studies exploring persister cells formed by various environmental, pathogenic, and laboratory strains of *E. coli* found that tolerance levels varied vastly between isolates and that tolerance to different antibiotics was not relevantly correlated (Wiuff and Andersson 2007; Hofsteenge et al. 2013; Stewart and Rozen 2012; Goneau et al. 2014; Luidalepp et al. 2011). Nevertheless, these studies also found a small proportion of multidrug-tolerant cells. Two relevant conclusions can be drawn from these findings: First, it is unlikely that global cellular dormancy causing multitarget inactivation and multidrug tolerance plays a major role in *E. coli* persister formation in nature, though this phenotype can readily be evoked by genetic screens or selection for high persister levels in diverse bacteria

(Michiels et al. 2016; Van Den Bergh et al. 2016; Fridman et al. 2014). The reason for this discrepancy might be the significant population-wide cost of persister cell formation that could be higher for multidrug tolerance (see below). Second, it is clear that any laboratory culture with a seemingly homogeneous population of clonal bacteria harbors a wide variety of phenotypically different types of persister cells. Consequently, batch culture experiments must be interpreted with caution, particularly also because mutant phenotypes can be highly sensitive to seemingly small changes in culture conditions (Luidalepp et al. 2011).

In laboratory experiments during unconstrained growth of *E. coli*, it is easily observed that tolerant persisters have formed prior to drug treatment as non- or slow-growing cells among an isogenic population of regularly growing cells (Balaban et al. 2004). From the view of the experimenter, these cells have emerged stochastically because they compose a seemingly stable subpopulation among identical peers. However, it is not clear to which extent persister cell formation is really induced by such a blind pacemaker. Repeated cycles of growth and dilution during exponential growth of *E. coli* progressively reduced the levels of persister cells, indicating that the majority of initially detected persisters had been carried over from stationary phase in the inoculum (Keren et al. 2004a; Orman and Brynildsen 2013). Consistently, the fraction of *E. coli* persisters in a classical exponential growth time–kill curve assay in LB medium is more or less proportional to the inoculum (Harms et al. 2017). These observations demonstrate that (1) the fraction of antibiotic-tolerant cells forming during exponential growth is very small and (2) actually too small to significantly affect the results of most studies, despite the common notion that experiments were performed in "exponential phase." According to the original definition of Balaban et al. (2004), most of the literature on stochastic persister formation, therefore, deals with "type I persisters" carried over from stationary phase and not with "type II persisters" forming during exponential growth. Knowledge about antibiotic-tolerant cells that form truly stochastically is therefore very limited. I speculate that many of them might arise accidentally by "persistence as stuff happens" (see below) or might not be persisters by common sense at all and instead exhibit phenotypic resistance (see below).

Conversely, it appears that persister cell formation has a significant deterministic component in the sense that various forms of sublethal stress induce the formation of these cells but without causing full conversion of population into persisters (Dörr et al. 2009; Goneau et al. 2014; Mordukhova and Pan 2014). Similarly, the level of persister cells generally increases in many bacteria throughout culture growth as nutrients become exhausted and the bacteria progressively enter stationary phase (Dörr et al. 2009; Harms et al. 2017; Keren et al. 2004a). These phenomena are best explained as "responsive diversification" in the sense that the diversification of the clonal population into different phenotypes is induced by environmental factors like stress and starvation (Kotte et al. 2014). The resulting phenotypic heterogeneity enables the population as a whole to be preadapted to different environmental conditions while at the same time maximizing the benefits from the currently encountered one.

3.1.3 Biological Functions of Persister Cells

The evolutionary success of a bacterial population is determined by its ability to reproduce. At first glance, it seems counter-intuitive that clonal bacterial populations would form persister cells that seem to be a drain of resources, which could better be invested in population growth. However, this kind of phenotypic heterogeneity is ubiquitous among bacteria and was also described in eukaryotes from yeast to humans (comprehensively described by Van Den Bergh et al. 2017). The phenomenon is commonly interpreted as a risk-spreading strategy that ensures the survival of the genotype in the face of unpredictable and lethal threats that would wipe out the fast-growing phenotype(s), a concept known as "bet hedging" (Veening et al. 2008). Consistently, the level of persister cells does not only differ significantly between different strains or isolates of an organism (see above) but can readily evolve and adapt to different treatment regimes in the laboratory with higher levels of persister formation being selected for under more narrow treatment regimens and duration of dormancy matching the treatment time (Fridman et al. 2014; Michiels et al. 2016; Van Den Bergh et al. 2016). These results are reminiscent of the observation that uropathogenic *E. coli* from recurrent infections display higher persister levels than other uropathogenic isolates and that *hipA7*, a known high-persister mutation, has been observed among uropathogenic *E. coli* (Goneau et al. 2014; Schumacher et al. 2015). Conversely, the formation of persister cells also seems to have fitness trade-offs with other bacterial traits (antagonistic pleiotropy) by compromising stationary phase survival and causing extended lag phases (Stepanyan et al. 2015). Beyond a baseline caused by cellular noise, it is therefore clear that the formation of antibiotic-tolerant persister cells is a genetically evolved trait of bacteria under strong selection by environmental conditions and physiological constraints (see also Chap. 8).

3.2 Unraveling the Genetic Basis of Persister Formation

3.2.1 Conceptual Overview

Since the first description of persister cells by J. Bigger in *Staphylococcus aureus* in 1944 (Bigger 1944) a lot of articles have been published on the molecular mechanisms of how they form and how they survive antibiotic treatment (comprehensively reviewed by Van Den Bergh et al. 2017). The key conclusions from multiple different classical genetic screens, candidate-based approaches, and physiological studies have been that these mechanisms are highly redundant on the population level but can be grouped into two major branches: While some mechanisms cause antibiotic tolerance by globally modulating bacterial physiology and/or through stochastic events (non-specific mechanisms; see Sect. 3.3), others shut down one or more cellular functions via dedicated mechanisms (specialized mechanisms; see Sect. 3.4). In addition, different damage repair pathways contribute to the survival of persister cells (Sect. 3.5). The line between these groups is often blurred because also very targeted, specialized mechanisms can have consequences for global physiology, by intimate links between different persister mechanisms, and because a shutdown of cellular processes generally favors the repair of damage.

As far as they are not just stochastic, these molecular mechanisms are not controlled by specific "persister regulators" but rather integrated into the regulons of different arms of bacterial stress signaling. Most importantly, the starvation-induced second messenger (p)ppGpp is a key factor in the induction of many different persister mechanisms (Hauryliuk et al. 2015). Beyond (p)ppGpp, other signals related to stress (via sigma factor RpoS), metabolism (via cAMP/CRP), or oxidative damage (via OxyR) contribute to the signaling underlying persister formation (Amato et al. 2013; Harms et al. 2016; Molina-Quiroz et al. 2016; Vega et al. 2012). Intriguingly, one dedicated study demonstrated that the type of persister cells formed during carbon source transitions of *E. coli* depends on the intracellular concentration of (p)ppGpp (Amato and Brynildsen 2015; see also Chap. 6). Another important signaling pathway is the SOS response, a transcriptional program controlling various DNA repair functions, that is activated by single-stranded DNA arising as a consequence of DNA damage (Baharoglu and Mazel 2014).

A major problem when summarizing the knowledge on different mechanisms of persister formation is that the methodologies used in the field to isolate and quantify persisters are highly variable and that the composition of the heterogeneous set of persisters is very sensitive to changes in experimental conditions. As an example, one article directly demonstrated that the qualitative observation and quantitative penetrance of different *E. coli* mutant phenotypes in persister formation were significantly influenced by the way of overnight culturing (Luidalepp et al. 2011). In consequence, the literature in the field can be described in the famous words of Fred Neidhardt as "apples, oranges, and unknown fruit" (Neidhardt 2006). Many articles with seemingly contradictory results have therefore been published and debates about the validity of different studies are commonplace (Kaldalu et al. 2016; Goormaghtigh et al. 2018a, b; Harms et al. 2017; Van Melderen and Wood 2017). It is therefore difficult to disentangle published results into a consistent picture of *E. coli* persister biology, so that in the following section I will merely summarize a number of important findings with the primary aim of illustrating key principles and concepts.

3.2.2   Distinguishing Persister Formation/Survival from Phenotypic Resistance

A critical aspect when summarizing pathways of persister formation is that widely different conceptual frameworks of the terms "persister," "tolerance," etc. are used in the field (Van Den Bergh et al. 2017; Balaban et al. 2013; Brauner et al. 2016). In this chapter, I adhere to the classical view that persister cells are transient, phenotypic variants which are drug tolerant in the sense that they survive nominally lethal antibiotic concentrations killing their clonal peers. This antibiotic tolerance is rooted in a shutdown of drug targets through some kind of dormancy, either globally or selectively (Lewis 2010; Harms et al. 2016; Wood et al. 2013). It is important to understand that this view does not comprise all imaginable mechanisms of how a cell can end up in the surviving subpopulation of a biphasic time–kill curve: Apart from classical persister cells, the survivors can merely exhibit phenotypic resistance (Corona and Martinez 2013; see also Figs. 3.1 and 3.2). Key examples of this phenomenon are heterogenic expression of drug efflux pumps (Pu et al. 2016) or fluctuations in the expression of the multiple antibiotic resistance activator MarA (El Meouche et al. 2016) that have both been described in *E. coli*. In addition, a well-known example in mycobacteria are cells that by chance have expressed only low levels of KatG, the enzyme that activates the prodrug isoniazid and can thus grow in presence of this antibiotic (Wakamoto et al. 2013). Consistently, a dedicated study using flow cytometry demonstrated that antibiotic survivors can form from regularly

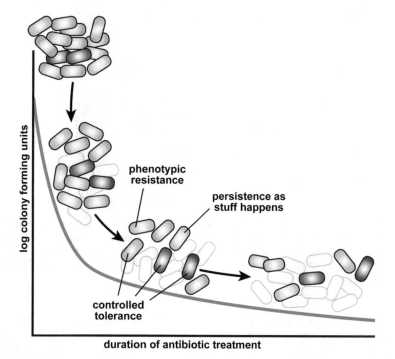

Fig 3.1 Heterogeneity of cells surviving antibiotic treatment. The illustration shows the typical biphasic appearance of a time kill curve with the rapid death of most regularly growing cells (grey, turning colorless) followed by a second phase of slower killing. Surviving cells can have a wide variety of physiological properties (colors). Drug tolerant, dormant persisters can arise either in a controlled manner via different molecular pathways (green/red/violet) or through cellular accidents ("persistence as stuff happens"; blue). Phenotypically resistant bacteria are not dormant and can divide in presence of the antibiotic (yellow). After treatment, surviving persisters can resuscitate and replenish the population

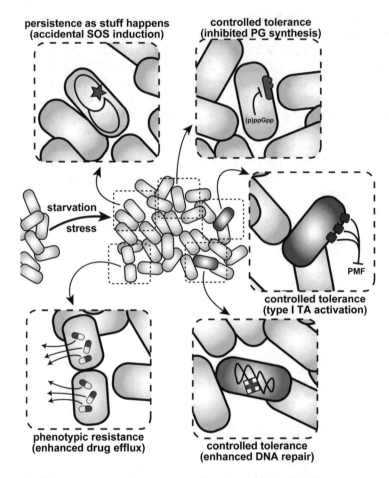

Fig 3.2 Multiple molecular mechanisms underlying the survival of antibiotic treatment. The illustration highlights how starvation or stress can induce the formation of antibiotic-tolerant cells (colored) among a population of susceptible peers (grey) through responsive diversification. Different molecular mechanisms enabling the survival of antibiotic treatment are highlighted schematically. *PG* peptidoglycan, *PMF* proton-motive force

replicating bacteria, though quite rarely (Orman and Brynildsen 2013). These different faces of single-cell phenotypic resistance are united in that they would, on the population level, increase the minimum inhibitory concentration (MIC) and enable bacterial growth in presence of the antibiotic. Phenotypic resistance is therefore fundamentally different from the tolerance exhibited by dormant, antibiotic-tolerant persister cells and requires different pharmacological strategies to be overcome. Consequently, I limit the content of this chapter to bacterial persister formation and survival in order to highlight the particular biology of this phenomenon.

3.3 Non-Specific Mechanisms of Persister Cell Formation

3.3.1 Energy Metabolism and Oxygen

Antibiotic tolerance and persister formation are intimately linked to cellular metabolism on multiple levels. Generally, it is commonly observed that the formation of persister cells is inversely correlated with metabolic activity and energy production, for example, when evaluating different bacterial mutants or growth conditions (Li and Zhang 2007; Orman and Brynildsen 2013; Shan et al. 2017). One core component of cellular energy metabolism is the electron transport chain (ETC), a series of protein complexes in the cytoplasmic membrane that transfers electrons from different donors like NADH or succinate onto receptors like oxygen. The energy generated along these electron transfers is used to pump protons out of the cytoplasm in order to create an electrochemical gradient known as the proton-motive force that fuels a variety of cellular processes including the synthesis of ATP. It is therefore unsurprising that *E. coli* strains carrying mutations in components of the ETC or its metabolic sources of electrons like GlpD or the TCA cycle displayed altered levels of persister formation (Ma et al. 2010; Spoering et al. 2006; Shan et al. 2015; Van Den Bergh et al. 2016; Luidalepp et al. 2011). Intriguingly, these mutants showed phenotypes of both increased and decreased persister formation depending on gene, particular mutation, and experimental conditions (see note in Harms et al. 2016, and literature cited therein).

The mechanism of how the electron transport chain is closely linked to persister formation or survival has remained elusive. Under some circumstances the link is trivial because, e.g., the proton-motive force is critical for the uptake of aminoglycoside antibiotics (Krause et al. 2016). Therefore, providing specific metabolic stimuli to activate the ETC can dramatically ramp up the intracellular drug concentration in some persisters and kill them (Allison et al. 2011). A similar approach was also effective against fluoroquinolone-tolerant persisters, yet required to provide carbon source and terminal electron acceptor in order to globally restart respiratory metabolism (Gutierrez et al. 2017). Similarly, it is tempting to speculate that the ETC might affect persister formation or survival through its role in ATP production. Different groups have reported links between the antibiotic tolerance of persisters and low cellular ATP levels that could be caused by a controlled shutdown or random malfunctioning of the ETC (Wilmaerts et al. 2018; Shan et al. 2017).

Apart from these aspects of cellular metabolism, the ETC plays also a major role in the idea that antibiotics would kill bacteria through production of ROS. In this view (see above), the cellular effects of different antibiotic classes converge in a hyperactivation of the ETC as a source of superoxide ions that finally result in the production of hydroxyl radicals damaging cellular macromolecules (Kohanski et al. 2010). From this perspective, drug tolerance is primarily seen as a matter of interfering with this secondary killing activity of antibiotics, and persister phenotypes of different mutants are generally interpreted in this context (Yang et al. 2017). Several articles have indeed reported key roles of reducing oxidant stress and increasing ROS detoxification in *E. coli* persister survival dependent on (p)ppGpp or (the absence of) cAMP/CRP signaling (Molina-Quiroz et al. 2016; Nguyen et al. 2011).

3.3.2 PASH: "Persistence as Stuff Happens"

One major alternative theory to concepts based on the various genetically encoded pathways covered in this book is "PASH" or "Persistence As Stuff Happens" (Levin et al. 2014; Johnson and Levin 2013; Vazquez-Laslop et al. 2006). In this view, the various types of heterogeneous persister cells primarily form more or less by chance as the "inadvertent consequence of different kinds of glitches and errors" in cellular metabolism and replication (Levin et al. 2014). It is largely undisputed that PASH exists and that it can well explain why the formation of persisters is ubiquitous among all organisms where it has been studied and why all attempts to create a mutant not forming persisters have failed (Johnson and Levin 2013). As an example for clear PASH, accidents during DNA replication and other DNA processing functions result in activation of the SOS response in almost 1% of *E. coli* during unconstrained exponential growth (Pennington and Rosenberg 2007). This phenomenon causes a heterogeneity of different states of SOS expression in the population and, in cells with very high SOS induction, will induce antibiotic tolerance through the different SOS-controlled pathways of persister formation or survival (see below and Fig. 3.2). It will be interesting to see future studies using single-cell approaches disentangling the molecular basis of different types of persister cells in a bacterial population and explore to what extent PASH is responsible for their formation and survival.

3.4 Specialized Mechanisms of Persister Cell Formation

Beyond broad changes in cellular physiology that interfere with antibiotic killing, persister cell formation has also been linked to a variety of more specific mechanisms that either shut down specific targets or are distinct from other more general mechanisms in that they act through fine-tuned molecular switches. Among these, toxin-antitoxin (TA) modules must be highlighted particularly. They are small genetic elements encoding a toxic protein and an antitoxin that can unleash this toxin's activity in response to cellular signaling (Harms et al. 2018). TA modules exhibit two features that make them well-suited as effectors of persister cell formation, the ability to shut down cellular processes through toxin activation and a multilayered autoregulation that can control the bistability of persister formation as well as the entry into and, equally important, exit from the persister state. The links between TA modules and persisters will be covered in detail in Chap. 8 but are shortly outlined below.

3.4.1   Type I Toxin-Antitoxin Modules

Type I TA modules are defined by the RNA nature of the antitoxin and its control of toxin activity by regulating toxin translation (Berghoff and Wagner 2017). They are the most well-established TA modules for persister formation of *E. coli* and two different representatives have been studied in details, the HokB/*sokB* system and the TisB/*istR* system (covered in detail in Chaps. 5 and 7). Both have toxins that are small membrane-targeting peptides, but while HokB/*sokB* is controlled by second messenger (p)ppGpp and the elusive GTPase Obg, TisB/*istR* is controlled by DNA damage signaling via the SOS response (Dörr et al. 2010; Verstraeten et al. 2015). For both it has been unraveled how the interaction of RNA antitoxin and toxin mRNA as well as RNA structures and regulatory elements can control the frequency, inducibility, and duration of persistence (Berghoff and Wagner 2017). The TisB and HokB toxins impair inner membrane integrity, causing membrane depolarization and shutting down many cellular processes either directly (if they are powered by the proton-motive force) or indirectly (through the resulting drop in ATP levels; see also Fig. 3.2). Consequently, persister cells forming through HokB/*sokB* or TisB/*istR* activation are multidrug tolerant (Dörr et al. 2010; Verstraeten et al. 2015; Berghoff et al. 2017).

3.4.2   Type II Toxin-Antitoxin Modules

Until recently, type II TA modules were central to many discussions about *E. coli* persister formation because of debates about a prominently published pathway linking the two. In brief, this pathway was based on stochastic peaks of (p)ppGpp that would activate a specific set of these TA modules through stimulation of polyphosphate production (Maisonneuve and Gerdes 2014; Van Melderen and Wood 2017). In a major paradigm shift, it was recently demonstrated that this pathway does not exist and that the original studies supporting it suffered from a number of biological and technical shortcomings (Goormaghtigh et al. 2018a; Harms et al. 2017). A few additional articles reporting links between type II TA modules and persister formation of *E. coli* K-12 have been published, but these could often not be reproduced in other laboratories and did not have any follow-up studies (see articles by Goormaghtigh et al. 2018b, Van Den Bergh et al. 2017, and literature cited therein). In the light of recent controversies, it seems therefore advisable to reserve a final conclusion on type II TA modules and persisters of *E. coli* K-12 for future studies that would approach the topic with an open mind and rigorous controls (see also Chap. 8). Regardless of the phenotypes of toxin-antitoxin deletions, gain-of-function mutants of type II TA modules have repeatedly been isolated in screens for bacterial mutants exhibiting high levels of persister formation (Moyed and Bertrand 1983; Fridman et al. 2014). The most well-studied of these, *hipA7*, was also found among uropathogenic *E. coli* isolates (Schumacher et al. 2015). If TA modules are so easily converted into genetically encoded switches controlling persister formation, then it seems reasonable to speculate that at least some of these loci might be involved in this phenotype also in *E. coli* K-12 wildtype.

While research so far has mostly focused on roles of *E. coli* type II TA modules in stochastic persister formation, it would be interesting to follow up on previous work that had studied the activation of these TA modules by different biologically relevant stresses (Shan et al. 2017). Intriguingly, type II TA modules of *Salmonella* Typhimurium are specifically essential for the strong induction of persister formation under starvation and acid stress after phagocytosis (Helaine et al. 2014).

3.4.3   Controlled Inhibition of Antibiotic Target Processes

β-lactam antibiotics cause futile cycles of the peptidoglycan biosynthesis machinery and thus poison cell wall formation (Cho et al. 2014). The killing rate of β-lactam treatment is therefore directly correlated with bacterial growth rate, and non-growing cells are inherently tolerant to these drugs (Lee et al. 2018). Consequently, any mechanism inhibiting bacterial growth will cause collateral tolerance specifically to β-lactam killing. In addition, a specific pathway has been described in which peaking (p)ppGpp levels shut down peptidoglycan biosynthesis in response to signaling involving ClpA and trans-translation (Amato and Brynildsen 2015; see also Fig. 3.2).

Fluoroquinolone antibiotics poison DNA gyrase and topoisomerase IV, causing the formation of covalent complexes in which the enzyme-drug complex bridges a DNA double-strand break. This is principally reversible, but open DNA breaks can form upon collision of these "roadblocks" with replication forks and other DNA tracking systems, requiring DNA double-strand break repair (see below). Lethality arises through chromosome fragmentation when this system is overwhelmed (Aldred et al. 2014; see also below). Consequently, direct mechanisms of FQ tolerance need to ramp down DNA tracking systems and/or ramp up DNA repair functions. One elegant study demonstrated that *E. coli* can become fluoroquinolone tolerant by modulating DNA gyrase activity through altered behavior of nucleoid-associated proteins in response to (p)ppGpp signaling (Amato et al. 2013; Amato and Brynildsen 2015).

Aminoglycoside antibiotics are commonly thought to poison ribosomal translation by impairing the fidelity of the process in a way that mis-translation produces aberrant polypeptides causing cell damage (Krause et al. 2016). Consequently, direct mechanisms of aminoglycoside tolerance need to reduce translation rates and/or upregulate relevant cellular repair pathways. One study indeed implicated the ribosome modulation factor Rmf in the survival of *E. coli* under prolonged aminoglycoside treatment, indicating a role in persister formation or survival (McKay and Portnoy 2015). Rmf is controlled by (p)ppGpp and can convert ribosomes into an inactive, dimeric conformation that has mostly been studied in the context of stationary phase biology (Gohara and Yap 2018).

3.5   Repair of Drug-Related Damage and Persister Resuscitation

Integral to an understanding of persister cell biology is not only the question how those bacteria enter a dormant, drug-tolerant state, but also how they can leave it again in a controlled manner. This ability distinguishes actual persister cell formation from laboratory models creating "persister-like" cells by transiently inhibiting cellular processes with bacteriostatic drugs or via the ectopic expression of toxic proteins. Though it is clear that at least some *E. coli* persisters can wake up in response to fresh nutrients, not much has been published about the seemingly stochastic resuscitation of persister cells under unchanged conditions (Allison et al. 2011; Joers et al. 2010; see also Chap. 9). Intimately connected to persister resuscitation is the repair of possible damage caused in the cell by antibiotic drugs during the period of dormancy. The role of cellular repair pathways in antibiotic tolerance has only emerged rather recently, and it is becoming clear that a simple view of persisters as hibernating cells that remain spotless upon antibiotic treatment is not true.

Cellular repair during drug tolerance has been best studied for fluoroquinolone antibiotics that cause DNA double-strand breaks by poisoning DNA processing. Not unexpectedly, fluoroquinolone tolerance of *E. coli* generally requires a functional SOS response including various SOS-controlled DNA repair functions, and pre-activating the SOS response can increase fluoroquinolone tolerance (Dörr et al. 2009; Theodore et al. 2013; see also Fig. 3.2; Goneau et al. 2014). The need for efficient DNA repair is clearly apparent from the facts that each poisoned topoisomerase complex can cause one double-strand break but that *E. coli* K-12 can only repair up to four such breaks per cell (see the article of Theodore et al. 2013, and literature cited therein). It is therefore critical that DNA lesions and poisoned topoisomerase complexes are removed from the chromosome before bacterial resuscitation (Völzing and Brynildsen 2015). Consistently, fluoroquinolone-tolerant persisters forming during exponential growth seem to experience only modest DNA damage compared to their dying peers (Dörr et al. 2009). Only under these conditions of growing populations and with high doses of fluoroquinolone treatment could a key role of the TisB/*istR* TA module be detected, probably because it shuts down cell division and DNA processing so that the number of active replication forks is reduced and the time available for DNA repair is extended (Dörr et al. 2010; Theodore et al. 2013). Stationary phase cells are inherently non-growing and, consistently, do not show a defect in persister formation or survival without TisB/*istR* (Dörr et al. 2010). Unlike during exponential growth, the DNA damage (measured as SOS induction) caused by fluoroquinolones in stationary phase persisters does not differ significantly from the rest of the population, but the persisters have a more abundant or proficient DNA repair machinery that can repair the damage before resuscitation (Völzing and Brynildsen 2015).

The repair of damage caused by other classes of antibiotics has been less well studied. A study performed in *Vibrio cholerae* described the WigKR two-component regulatory system as a key factor in the repair of cell wall damage caused by β-lactam antibiotics (Dörr et al. 2016). WigKR positively controls various genes involved in cell wall synthesis and remodeling, it is activated by antibiotic-induced cell wall damage, and mutants lacking this system had massively decreased levels of survivors of β-lactam treatment (Dörr et al. 2016). No comparable findings have been published for *E. coli*, but it was reported that the DpiBA two-component regulatory system would sense damage caused by β-lactam and consequently activate SOS signaling to inhibit cell division and induce drug tolerance (Miller et al. 2004). Analogous mechanisms of repair functions enabling persister survival have not been established for aminoglycoside antibiotics that poison ribosomal translation, and no obvious link to damage repair was found in a comprehensive transposon screen on aminoglycoside tolerance in *E. coli* (Shan et al. 2015). A recent study implicated trans-translation—a repair pathway rescuing stalled ribosomes—in the survival of aminoglycoside-tolerant persisters (Li et al. 2013). However, the knockout mutants deficient in trans-translation displayed lower MICs to aminoglycoside antibiotics and were also generally more sensitive to various stresses and also other classes of antibiotics, so that it is not clear whether there is a direct and specific link between cellular damage caused by aminoglycosides and trans-translation.

3.6 Discussion

This chapter summarized the classical views of persister cell biology by highlighting how *E. coli* populations use multiple molecular mechanisms to form a heterogeneous subset of persisters with a diverse profile of stress tolerance. A key conclusion is that some of these pathways are quite well understood on the molecular level but that a number of important questions remain unanswered.

For example, it is open for debate whether all the different molecular mechanisms are truly distinct or whether there is something like a "grand unified theory" of persister formation that links many or all of them. One obvious candidate for such an explanation would the drop in cellular ATP levels that different laboratories have observed for *E. coli* persisters formed by widely different mechanisms and that is driving persister formation also in *S. aureus* (Wilmaerts et al. 2018; Shan et al. 2017; Conlon et al. 2016; Dörr et al. 2010). This link would be intuitive because the processes poisoned by bactericidal antibiotics generally depend on ATP as an energy source, but a drop in cellular ATP levels among various types of persisters remains to be shown. Other researchers in the field are more skeptical about highlighting the role of specific molecular phenomena. Instead, they lean more or less strongly towards the idea that a significant proportion of persisters might just form through "PASH" (Goormaghtigh et al. 2018b; Kaldalu et al. 2016), though this view is not mutually exclusive with ATP depletion or other downstream phenomena as the actual cause of antibiotic tolerance. I believe that the continuous coexistence of these and many other very distinct views on antibiotic tolerance is primarily caused by the fragmented nature of the literature that makes it easy to cherry-pick studies supporting any imaginable viewpoint. Consequently, it would be useful to see future studies adopting some kind of standardized procedures regarding assay setups and culture media or the framework of classification and data quantification (Brauner et al. 2016; Balaban et al. 2013; Goormaghtigh et al. 2018b; Harms et al. 2017; Goormaghtigh and Van Melderen 2016).

In addition, any interpretation or conclusion of the persister phenomenon must continuously be probed against relevant controls and alternative hypotheses. A recent study provided an interesting null hypothesis for interpreting antibiotic tolerance by proposing that treatment failure might not be linked to biological phenomena like persisters but rather be due to population heterogeneity in the interaction of antibiotics and their targets (Abel Zur Wiesch et al. 2015). In this view, the biphasic appearance of time-kill curves could be explained without invoking biologically distinct bacterial subpopulations merely by cell-to-cell variability in drug susceptibility, i.e., phenotypic resistance alone. Examples would be population heterogeneity in drug target molecules and drug uptake or action that have all been previously described (see Sect. 3.2.2).

In order to resolve these debates, future work could focus on studying the physiological parameters of genetically susceptible bacteria that survive antibiotic treatment on the single cell level. Though technically challenging, such a single-cell view would enable the direct evaluation of the relative contributions of different routes to antibiotic tolerance or phenotypic resistance. Furthermore, I feel that it is important to rely less on test tube experiments and to make particular efforts to explore and possibly prove the role of persister cells in clinical infections in vivo.

Acknowledgements The author is grateful to Prof. Kenn Gerdes, Prof. Urs Jenal, Dr. Szabolcs Semsey, and Dr. Pablo Manfredi for stimulating discussions about the elusive nature of genetically encoded antibiotic tolerance. This work was supported by Swiss National Science Foundation (SNSF) Ambizione Fellowship PZ00P3_180085.

References

Abel Zur Wiesch, P., Abel, S., Gkotzis, S., Ocampo, P., Engelstadter, J., Hinkley, T., Magnus, C., Waldor, M. K., Udekwu, K., & Cohen, T. (2015). Classic reaction kinetics can explain complex patterns of antibiotic action. *Science Translational Medicine, 7*, 287ra73.

Aldred, K. J., Kerns, R. J., & Osheroff, N. (2014). Mechanism of quinolone action and resistance. *Biochemistry, 53*, 1565–1574.

Allison, K. R., Brynildsen, M. P., & Collins, J. J. (2011). Metabolite-enabled eradication of bacterial persisters by aminoglycosides. *Nature, 473*, 216–220.

Amato, S. M., & Brynildsen, M. P. (2015). Persister heterogeneity arising from a single metabolic stress. *Current Biology, 25*, 2090–2098.

Amato, S. M., Orman, M. A., & Brynildsen, M. P. (2013). Metabolic control of persister formation in *Escherichia coli*. *Molecular Cell, 50*, 475–487.

Baharoglu, Z., & Mazel, D. (2014). SOS, the formidable strategy of bacteria against aggressions. *FEMS Microbiology Reviews, 38*, 1126–1145.

Balaban, N. Q., Merrin, J., Chait, R., Kowalik, L., & Leibler, S. (2004). Bacterial persistence as a phenotypic switch. *Science, 305*, 1622–1625.

Balaban, N. Q., Gerdes, K., Lewis, K., & Mckinney, J. D. (2013). A problem of persistence: Still more questions than answers? *Nature Reviews. Microbiology, 11*, 587–591.

Berghoff, B. A., & Wagner, E. G. H. (2017). RNA-based regulation in type I toxin-antitoxin systems and its implication for bacterial persistence. *Current Genetics, 63*, 1011–1016.

Berghoff, B. A., Hoekzema, M., Aulbach, L., & Wagner, E. G. (2017). Two regulatory RNA elements affect TisB-dependent depolarization and persister formation. *Molecular Microbiology, 103*, 1020–1033.

Bigger, J. (1944). Treatment of staphylococcal infections with penicillin by intermittent sterilisation. *The Lancet, 244*, 497–500.

Blango, M. G., & Mulvey, M. A. (2010). Persistence of uropathogenic *Escherichia coli* in the face of multiple antibiotics. *Antimicrobial Agents and Chemotherapy, 54*, 1855–1863.

Brauner, A., Fridman, O., Gefen, O., & Balaban, N. Q. (2016). Distinguishing between resistance, tolerance and persistence to antibiotic treatment. *Nature Reviews. Microbiology, 14*, 320–330.

Cho, H., Uehara, T., & Bernhardt, T. G. (2014). Beta-lactam antibiotics induce a lethal malfunctioning of the bacterial cell wall synthesis machinery. *Cell, 159*, 1300–1311.

Claudi, B., Spröte, P., Chirkova, A., Personnic, N., Zankl, J., Schürmann, N., Schmidt, A., & Bumann, D. (2014). Phenotypic variation of *Salmonella* in host tissues delays eradication by antimicrobial chemotherapy. *Cell, 158*, 722–733.

Conlon, B. P., Rowe, S. E., Gandt, A. B., Nuxoll, A. S., Donegan, N. P., Zalis, E. A., Clair, G., Adkins, J. N., Cheung, A. L., & Lewis, K. (2016). Persister formation in *Staphylococcus aureus* is associated with ATP depletion. *Nature Microbiology, 1*, 16051.

Corona, F., & Martinez, J. L. (2013). Phenotypic resistance to antibiotics. *Antibiotics (Basel), 2*, 237–255.

Dörr, T., Lewis, K., & Vulić, M. (2009). SOS response induces persistence to fluoroquinolones in *Escherichia coli*. *PLoS Genetics, 5*, e1000760.

Dörr, T., Vulic, M., & Lewis, K. (2010). Ciprofloxacin causes persister formation by inducing the TisB toxin in *Escherichia coli*. *PLoS Biology, 8*, e1000317.

Dörr, T., Alvarez, L., Delgado, F., Davis, B. M., Cava, F., & Waldor, M. K. (2016). A cell wall damage response mediated by a sensor kinase/response regulator pair enables beta-lactam tolerance. *Proceedings of the National Academy of Sciences of the United States of America, 113*, 404–409.

El Meouche, I., Siu, Y., & Dunlop, M. J. (2016). Stochastic expression of a multiple antibiotic resistance activator confers transient resistance in single cells. *Scientific Reports, 6*, 19538.

Fauvart, M., De Groote, V. N., & Michiels, J. (2011). Role of persister cells in chronic infections: Clinical relevance and perspectives on anti-persister therapies. *Journal of Medical Microbiology, 60*, 699–709.

Fisher, R. A., Gollan, B., & Helaine, S. (2017). Persistent bacterial infections and persister cells. *Nature Reviews. Microbiology, 15*, 453–464.

Fridman, O., Goldberg, A., Ronin, I., Shoresh, N., & Balaban, N. Q. (2014). Optimization of lag time underlies antibiotic tolerance in evolved bacterial populations. *Nature, 513*, 418–421.

Gohara, D. W., & Yap, M. F. (2018). Survival of the drowsiest: The hibernating 100S ribosome in bacterial stress management. *Current Genetics, 64*, 753–760.

Goneau, L. W., Yeoh, N. S., Macdonald, K. W., Cadieux, P. A., Burton, J. P., Razvi, H., & Reid, G. (2014). Selective target inactivation rather than global metabolic dormancy causes antibiotic tolerance in uropathogens. *Antimicrobial Agents and Chemotherapy, 58*, 2089–2097.

Goormaghtigh, F., & Van Melderen, L. (2016). Optimized method for measuring persistence in *Escherichia coli* with improved reproducibility. *Methods in Molecular Biology, 1333*, 43–52.

Goormaghtigh, F., Fraikin, N., Putrins, M., Hallaert, T., Hauryliuk, V., Garcia-Pino, A., Sjodin, A., Kasvandik, S., Udekwu, K., Tenson, T., Kaldalu, N., & Van Melderen, L. (2018a). Reassessing the role of type II toxin-antitoxin systems in formation of *Escherichia coli* type II persister cells. *MBio, 9*, e00640-18.

Goormaghtigh, F., Fraikin, N., Putrins, M., Hauryliuk, V., Garcia-Pino, A., Udekwu, K., Tenson, T., Kaldalu, N., & Van Melderen, L. (2018b). Reply to holden and errington, "Type II toxin-antitoxin systems and persister cells". *MBio, 9*, e01838-18.

Gutierrez, A., Jain, S., Bhargava, P., Hamblin, M., Lobritz, M. A., & Collins, J. J. (2017). Understanding and sensitizing density-dependent persistence to quinolone antibiotics. *Molecular Cell, 68*, 1147–1154.e3.

Harms, A., Maisonneuve, E., & Gerdes, K. (2016). Mechanisms of bacterial persistence during stress and antibiotic exposure. *Science, 354*, aaf4268.

Harms, A., Fino, C., Sørensen, M. A., Semsey, S., & Gerdes, K. (2017). Prophages and growth dynamics confound experimental results with antibiotic-tolerant persister cells. *MBio, 8*, e01964-17.

Harms, A., Brodersen, D. E., Mitarai, N., & Gerdes, K. (2018). Toxins, targets, and triggers: An overview of toxin-antitoxin biology. *Molecular Cell, 70*, 768–784.

Hauryliuk, V., Atkinson, G. C., Murakami, K. S., Tenson, T., & Gerdes, K. (2015). Recent functional insights into the role of (p)ppGpp in bacterial physiology. *Nature Reviews. Microbiology, 13*, 298–309.

Helaine, S., Cheverton, A. M., Watson, K. G., Faure, L. M., Matthews, S. A., & Holden, D. W. (2014). Internalization of *Salmonella* by macrophages induces formation of nonreplicating persisters. *Science, 343*, 204–208.

Hofsteenge, N., Van Nimwegen, E., & Silander, O. K. (2013). Quantitative analysis of persister fractions suggests different mechanisms of formation among environmental isolates of *E. coli*. *BMC Microbiology, 13*, 25.

Joers, A., Kaldalu, N., & Tenson, T. (2010). The frequency of persisters in *Escherichia coli* reflects the kinetics of awakening from dormancy. *Journal of Bacteriology, 192*, 3379–3384.

Johnson, P. J., & Levin, B. R. (2013). Pharmacodynamics, population dynamics, and the evolution of persistence in *Staphylococcus aureus*. *PLoS Genetics, 9*, e1003123.

Kaldalu, N., Hauryliuk, V., & Tenson, T. (2016). Persisters-as elusive as ever. *Applied Microbiology and Biotechnology, 100*, 6545–6553.

Keren, I., Kaldalu, N., Spoering, A., Wang, Y., & Lewis, K. (2004a). Persister cells and tolerance to antimicrobials. *FEMS Microbiology Letters, 230*, 13–18.

Keren, I., Shah, D., Spoering, A., Kaldalu, N., & Lewis, K. (2004b). Specialized persister cells and the mechanism of multidrug tolerance in *Escherichia coli*. *Journal of Bacteriology, 186*, 8172–8180.

Keren, I., Wu, Y., Inocencio, J., Mulcahy, L. R., & Lewis, K. (2013). Killing by bactericidal antibiotics does not depend on reactive oxygen species. *Science, 339*, 1213–1216.

Kohanski, M. A., Dwyer, D. J., & Collins, J. J. (2010). How antibiotics kill bacteria: From targets to networks. *Nature Reviews. Microbiology, 8*, 423–435.

Kotte, O., Volkmer, B., Radzikowski, J. L., & Heinemann, M. (2014). Phenotypic bistability in *Escherichia coli*'s central carbon metabolism. *Molecular Systems Biology, 10*, 736.

Krause, K. M., Serio, A. W., Kane, T. R., & Connolly, L. E. (2016). Aminoglycosides: An overview. *Cold Spring Harbor Perspectives in Medicine, 6*, a027029.

Laxminarayan, R., Duse, A., Wattal, C., Zaidi, A. K., Wertheim, H. F., Sumpradit, N., Vlieghe, E., Hara, G. L., Gould, I. M., Goossens, H., Greko, C., SO, A. D., Bigdeli, M., Tomson, G., Woodhouse, W., Ombaka, E., Peralta, A. Q., Qamar, F. N., Mir, F., Kariuki, S., Bhutta, Z. A., Coates, A., Bergstrom, R., Wright, G. D., Brown, E. D., & Cars, O. (2013). Antibiotic resistance-the need for global solutions. *The Lancet Infectious Diseases, 13*, 1057–1098.

Lee, A. J., Wang, S., Meredith, H. R., Zhuang, B., Dai, Z., & You, L. (2018). Robust, linear correlations between growth rates and beta-lactam-mediated lysis rates. *Proceedings of the National Academy of Sciences of the United States of America, 115*, 4069–4074.

Levin, B. R., & Rozen, D. E. (2006). Non-inherited antibiotic resistance. *Nature Reviews. Microbiology, 4*, 556–562.

Levin, B. R., Concepcion-Acevedo, J., & Udekwu, K. I. (2014). Persistence: A copacetic and parsimonious hypothesis for the existence of non-inherited resistance to antibiotics. *Current Opinion in Microbiology, 21*, 18–21.

Lewis, K. (2005). Persister cells and the riddle of biofilm survival. *Biochemistry (Mosc), 70*, 267–274.

Lewis, K. (2010). Persister cells. *Annual Review of Microbiology, 64*, 357–372.

Li, Y., & Zhang, Y. (2007). PhoU is a persistence switch involved in persister formation and tolerance to multiple antibiotics and stresses in *Escherichia coli*. *Antimicrobial Agents and Chemotherapy, 51*, 2092–2099.

Li, J., Ji, L., Shi, W., Xie, J., & Zhang, Y. (2013). Trans-translation mediates tolerance to multiple antibiotics and stresses in *Escherichia coli*. *The Journal of Antimicrobial Chemotherapy, 68*, 2477–2481.

Liu, Y., & Imlay, J. A. (2013). Cell death from antibiotics without the involvement of reactive oxygen species. *Science, 339*, 1210–1213.

Luidalepp, H., Joers, A., Kaldalu, N., & Tenson, T. (2011). Age of inoculum strongly influences persister frequency and can mask effects of mutations implicated in altered persistence. *Journal of Bacteriology, 193*, 3598–3605.

Ma, C., Sim, S., Shi, W., Du, L., Xing, D., & Zhang, Y. (2010). Energy production genes *sucB* and *ubiF* are involved in persister survival and tolerance to multiple antibiotics and stresses in *Escherichia coli*. *FEMS Microbiology Letters, 303*, 33–40.

Maisonneuve, E., & Gerdes, K. (2014). Molecular mechanisms underlying bacterial persisters. *Cell, 157*, 539–548.

McKay, S. L., & Portnoy, D. A. (2015). Ribosome hibernation facilitates tolerance of stationary-phase bacteria to aminoglycosides. *Antimicrobial Agents and Chemotherapy, 59*, 6992–6999.

Michiels, J. E., Van Den Bergh, B., Verstraeten, N., Fauvart, M., & Michiels, J. (2016). In vitro emergence of high persistence upon periodic aminoglycoside challenge in the ESKAPE pathogens. *Antimicrobial Agents and Chemotherapy, 60*, 4630–4637.

Miller, C., Thomsen, L. E., Gaggero, C., Mosseri, R., Ingmer, H., & Cohen, S. N. (2004). SOS response induction by ß-lactams and bacterial defense against antibiotic lethality. *Science, 305*, 1629–1631.

Molina-Quiroz, R. C., Lazinski, D. W., Camilli, A., & Levy, S. B. (2016). Transposon-sequencing analysis unveils novel genes involved in the generation of persister cells in uropathogenic *Escherichia coli*. *Antimicrobial Agents and Chemotherapy, 60*, 6907–6910.

Mordukhova, E. A., & Pan, J. G. (2014). Stabilization of homoserine-O-succinyltransferase (MetA) decreases the frequency of persisters in *Escherichia coli* under stressful conditions. *PLoS One, 9*, e110504.

Moyed, H. S., & Bertrand, K. P. (1983). *hipA*, a newly recognized gene of *Escherichia coli* K-12 that affects frequency of persistence after inhibition of murein synthesis. *Journal of Bacteriology, 155*, 768–775.

Neidhardt, F. C. (2006). Apples, oranges and unknown fruit. *Nature Reviews. Microbiology, 4*, 876.

Nguyen, D., Joshi-Datar, A., Lepine, F., Bauerle, E., Olakanmi, O., Beer, K., Mckay, G., Siehnel, R., Schafhauser, J., Wang, Y., Britigan, B. E., & Singh, P. K. (2011). Active starvation responses mediate antibiotic tolerance in biofilms and nutrient-limited bacteria. *Science, 334*, 982–986.

Ocampo, P. S., Lazar, V., Papp, B., Arnoldini, M., Abel Zur Wiesch, P., Busa-Fekete, R., Fekete, G., Pal, C., Ackermann, M., & Bonhoeffer, S. (2014). Antagonism between bacteriostatic and bactericidal antibiotics is prevalent. *Antimicrobial Agents and Chemotherapy, 58*, 4573–4582.

Orman, M. A., & Brynildsen, M. P. (2013). Dormancy is not necessary or sufficient for bacterial persistence. *Antimicrobial Agents and Chemotherapy, 57*, 3230–3239.

Pennington, J. M., & Rosenberg, S. M. (2007). Spontaneous DNA breakage in single living *Escherichia coli* cells. *Nature Genetics, 39*, 797–802.

Pu, Y., Zhao, Z., Li, Y., Zou, J., Ma, Q., Zhao, Y., Ke, Y., Zhu, Y., Chen, H., Baker, M. A., Ge, H., Sun, Y., Xie, X. S., & BAI, F. (2016). Enhanced efflux activity facilitates drug tolerance in dormant bacterial cells. *Molecular Cell, 62*, 284–294.

Renggli, S., Keck, W., Jenal, U., & Ritz, D. (2013). Role of autofluorescence in flow cytometric analysis of *Escherichia coli* treated with bactericidal antibiotics. *Journal of Bacteriology, 195*, 4067–4073.

Schumacher, M. A., Balani, P., Min, J., Chinnam, N. B., Hansen, S., Vulic, M., Lewis, K., & Brennan, R. G. (2015). HipBA-promoter structures reveal the basis of heritable multidrug tolerance. *Nature, 524*, 59–64.

Shan, Y., Lazinski, D., Rowe, S., Camilli, A., & Lewis, K. (2015). Genetic basis of persister tolerance to aminoglycosides in *Escherichia coli*. *MBio, 6*, e00078-15.

Shan, Y., Brown Gandt, A., Rowe, S. E., Deisinger, J. P., Conlon, B. P., & Lewis, K. (2017). ATP-dependent persister formation in *Escherichia coli*. *MBio, 8*, e02267-16.

Spoering, A. L., Vulic, M., & Lewis, K. (2006). GlpD and PlsB participate in persister cell formation in *Escherichia coli*. *Journal of Bacteriology, 188*, 5136–5144.

Stepanyan, K., Wenseleers, T., Duenez-Guzman, E. A., Muratori, F., Van Den Bergh, B., Verstraeten, N., De Meester, L., Verstrepen, K. J., Fauvart, M., & Michiels, J. (2015). Fitness trade-offs explain low levels of persister cells in the opportunistic pathogen *Pseudomonas aeruginosa*. *Molecular Ecology, 24*, 1572–1583.

Stewart, B., & Rozen, D. E. (2012). Genetic variation for antibiotic persistence in *Escherichia coli*. *Evolution, 66*, 933–939.

Theodore, A., Lewis, K., & Vulic, M. (2013). Tolerance of *Escherichia coli* to fluoroquinolone antibiotics depends on specific components of the SOS response pathway. *Genetics, 195*, 1265–1276.

Van Den Bergh, B., Michiels, J. E., Wenseleers, T., Windels, E. M., Boer, P. V., Kestemont, D., De Meester, L., Verstrepen, K. J., Verstraeten, N., Fauvart, M., & Michiels, J. (2016). Frequency of antibiotic application drives rapid evolutionary adaptation of *Escherichia coli* persistence. *Nature Microbiology, 1*, 16020.

Van Den Bergh, B., Fauvart, M., & Michiels, J. (2017). Formation, physiology, ecology, evolution and clinical importance of bacterial persisters. *FEMS Microbiology Reviews, 41*, 219–251.

Van Melderen, L., & Wood, T. K. (2017). Commentary: What is the link between stringent response, endoribonuclease encoding type II toxin-antitoxin systems and persistence? *Frontiers in Microbiology, 8*, 191.

Vazquez-Laslop, N., Lee, H., & Neyfakh, A. A. (2006). Increased persistence in *Escherichia coli* caused by controlled expression of toxins or other unrelated proteins. *Journal of Bacteriology, 188*, 3494–3497.

Veening, J. W., Smits, W. K., & Kuipers, O. P. (2008). Bistability, epigenetics, and bet-hedging in bacteria. *Annual Review of Microbiology, 62*, 193–210.

Vega, N. M., Allison, K. R., Khalil, A. S., & Collins, J. J. (2012). Signaling-mediated bacterial persister formation. *Nature Chemical Biology, 8*, 431–433.

Verstraeten, N., Knapen, W. J., Kint, C. I., Liebens, V., Van Den Bergh, B., Dewachter, L., Michiels, J. E., Fu, Q., David, C. C., Fierro, A. C., Marchal, K., Beirlant, J., Versees, W., Hofkens, J., Jansen, M., Fauvart, M., & Michiels, J. (2015). Obg and membrane depolarization are part of a microbial bet-hedging strategy that leads to antibiotic tolerance. *Molecular Cell, 59*, 9–21.

Völzing, K. G., & Brynildsen, M. P. (2015). Stationary-phase persisters to ofloxacin sustain DNA damage and require repair systems only during recovery. *MBio, 6*, e00731–e00715.

Wakamoto, Y., Dhar, N., Chait, R., Schneider, K., Signorino-Gelo, F., Leibler, S., & Mckinney, J. D. (2013). Dynamic persistence of antibiotic-stressed mycobacteria. *Science, 339*, 91–95.

Wilmaerts, D., Bayoumi, M., Dewachter, L., Knapen, W., Mika, J. T., Hofkens, J., Dedecker, P., Maglia, G., Verstraeten, N., & Michiels, J. (2018). The persistence-inducing toxin HokB forms dynamic pores that cause ATP leakage. *MBio, 9*, e00744-18.

Wiuff, C., & Andersson, D. I. (2007). Antibiotic treatment in vitro of phenotypically tolerant bacterial populations. *The Journal of Antimicrobial Chemotherapy, 59*, 254–263.

Wood, T. K., Knabel, S. J., & Kwan, B. W. (2013). Bacterial persister cell formation and dormancy. *Applied and Environmental Microbiology, 79*, 7116–7121.

Yang, J. H., Bening, S. C., & Collins, J. J. (2017). Antibiotic efficacy-context matters. *Current Opinion in Microbiology, 39*, 73–80.

Chapter 4
Persister Formation and Antibiotic Tolerance of Chronic Infections

Kim Lewis and Sylvie Manuse

Abstract Two different types of mechanisms allow bacteria to evade killing by antibiotics—genetically encoded resistance and phenotypic tolerance conferred by persister cells. While our knowledge of resistance mechanisms is fairly sophisticated, understanding of tolerance is still fragmentary, partly because the phenomenon is only displayed by a few rare cells.

Treatment of acute infections has benefited substantially from our understanding of mechanisms of resistance. It is reasonable to expect that treatment of chronic infections will similarly benefit from deciphering the mechanisms that cause the formation of drug-tolerant persisters. In this chapter, we will discuss both the mechanism of persister formation and therapeutic approaches to eradicate these seemingly invincible cells.

4.1 Mechanism

4.1.1 Toxin-Antitoxins and Persisters

Tolerance was actually discovered prior to resistance—Josef Bigger described a small population of *Staphylococcus aureus* cells surviving treatment with penicillin, and showed that they are not mutants, in 1944 (Bigger 1944). Without a link to a clinical problem, the study of this curiosity was largely forgotten. Harris Moyed revisited this problem some 40 years later, and set out to find the mechanism by which persisters form, equipped with the tools of molecular genetics (Moyed and Bertrand 1983). A selection for *Escherichia coli* that survive (but do not grow in presence of) ampicillin produced mutants with a high level of persisters (Moyed and Bertrand 1983). The *hipA7* mutant carried a gain-of-function allele in the HipA toxin, belonging to a HipBA TA module. Overexpression of HipA causes an increase in persisters, however, deletion of either the operon, or *hipA* alone, had

K. Lewis (✉) · S. Manuse
Antimicrobial Discovery Center, Department of Biology, Northeastern University, Boston, MA, USA
e-mail: k.lewis@neu.edu

© Springer Nature Switzerland AG 2019   59
K. Lewis (ed.), *Persister Cells and Infectious Disease*,
https://doi.org/10.1007/978-3-030-25241-0_4

no phenotype, and this line of inquiry seemed to hit a dead end. Our group stumbled on persisters years later, while examining the puzzling properties of biofilms to resist killing by antibiotics (Spoering and Lewis 2001; Lewis 2001). We showed that persisters are largely responsible for biofilm tolerance, suggesting that this "curiosity" may be the long-sought culprit of recalcitrant chronic infections. Using microfluidics time-lapse tracking of *hipA7* cells, Nathalie Balaban showed that persisters form stochastically prior to antibiotic exposure, and this experiment attracted considerable attention to the field (Balaban et al. 2004). Genome sequencing showed that various TA modules are abundantly present in bacteria, and similarly to HipA, overexpression of toxins produced more persisters (Keren et al. 2004b; Shah et al. 2006). Also, similarly to HipA, knockouts had no phenotype, which was ascribed to their redundancy. We, therefore, searched for a toxin that can be highly expressed under natural conditions and zeroed in on TisB of *E. coli* (described in detail in Chap. 5). The TisB/IstR-1 module is induced by the SOS response, and IstR-1 is an antisense RNA antitoxin that inhibits translation of TisB (Vogel et al. 2004). Overexpression of TisB increased persister formation, similarly to other toxins, but a knockout also had a phenotype, decreasing persisters under conditions of SOS induction (Dorr et al. 2010, 2009; Berghoff et al. 2017). SOS response is induced by common fluoroquinolone antibiotics such as ciprofloxacin that target DNA gyrase and topoisomerase, converting them into DNA endonucleases. DNA damage induces the SOS response whose main function is to trigger expression of repair enzymes. It is interesting that the SOS response turns on two mechanistically distinct survival pathways—resistance through repair, and tolerance through the formation of persisters. While both pathways appear to be deterministic, only a small part of the population becomes persisters, primarily cells that happen to have a higher level of *tisB* expression (Dorr et al. 2010). Under these particular conditions—treatment of *E. coli* with fluoroquinolones—cells that attempt to repair are killed, and only persisters survive. This observation demonstrates the dramatic advantage of persisters confer to a population under attack by antibiotics.

TisB is an unusual protein—judging by its sequence, it is a typical antimicrobial peptide (AMP), cationic and hydrophobic. AMPs are the most common antimicrobials made by all plants and animals and by bacteria. It was surprising to see that *E. coli* protects itself from killing by antibiotics with an AMP. Most AMPs form ion channels in the membrane and kill by dissipating the pmf. Overexpression of TisB was shown to decrease ATP and kill cells as well (Unoson and Wagner 2008). We found that overexpression of TisB decreases the membrane potential (Dorr et al. 2010), and purified TisB forms voltage-gated ion channels in an artificial lipid bilayer (Gurnev et al. 2012), typical of AMPs. Apparently, mild expression of TisB in the course of the SOS response decreases the pmf, ATP, and as a result, shuts down the antibiotic targets. This mechanism of action provided a clear case for the mechanism of antibiotic tolerance we proposed some time ago—target inactivation (Keren et al. 2004b, 2013; Lewis 2010). Bactericidal antibiotics kill not by inhibiting targets, but by corrupting functions. Thus, aminoglycosides kill by causing mistranslation, which leads to the production of toxic peptides (Davis et al. 1986; Vakulenko and Mobashery 2003); fluoroquinolones inhibit the religation step of

DNA gyrase and topoisomerase, causing double-strand breaks (Hooper 2001; Malik et al. 2006), and β-lactams lead to a futile cycle of peptidoglycan synthesis and autolysis (Cho et al. 2014). If ATP level is low, targets are largely inactive and there is nothing to corrupt (Fig. 4.1).

Inactivation of targets is a straightforward way to cause tolerance, but could this be a general mechanism of persister formation? Specifically, does this apply to HipA? The HipA toxin is a protein kinase (Correia et al. 2006; Schumacher et al. 2009), and two groups determined that overexpression of HipA inhibits translation by phosphorylating the Glu-tRNA synthase (Kaspy et al. 2013; Germain et al. 2013). This observation agrees well with an empirical finding that bacteriostatic inhibitors of protein synthesis such as chloramphenicol and erythromycin antagonize cell wall acting antibiotics by causing drug tolerance (Robertson et al. 2002; Kwan et al. 2013). Blocking protein synthesis inhibits cell growth, which would account for tolerance to β-lactams and other cell wall acting antibiotics, and would similarly inhibit, through feedback control, synthesis of other biopolymers, RNA and DNA. This would fall under the general clause of the target shutdown. This is of course speculation; it would be interesting to know exactly how HipA, by inhibiting translation, causes multidrug tolerance. This is especially relevant in light of a recent report of the role of HipA in clinical manifestation of disease. We identified *hipA7* mutants among *E. coli* isolated from patients with relapsing UTI (Schumacher et al. 2015). Apparently, selection for high levels of tolerance helps the pathogen survive antibiotic treatment. We also determined the nature of the *hipA7* phenotype, and of another gain-of-function mutation we identified, P86L. Wild type HipA forms a dimer within a complex structure that includes the HipB antitoxin and the DNA operator regions upstream of the *hipBA* promoter. The dimer blocks ATP from entering the active sites of the kinase. The gain-of-function mutations occur at the

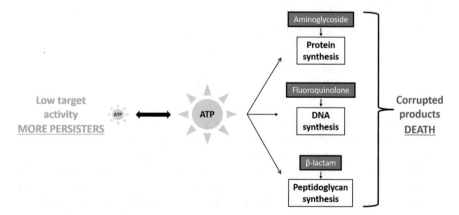

Fig. 4.1 A low-energy model of persister cell formation. In a regular growing cell, the energy level is high, which fuels the main antibiotic targets—translation, DNA synthesis, and cell wall synthesis. Corruption of these targets by antibiotics kills the cell. Random fluctuation in the expression of energy-producing components creates rare cells with low ATP, and low-target activity results in drug-tolerant persisters

interface of the dimer, loosening the connection and providing access to ATP. The active kinase then enables persister formation through translation inhibition.

While TisB and HipA present two firmly established cases for the mechanism of persister formation, they only explain how persister cells form under some special conditions—induction of the SOS response; or the acquisition of a gain-of-function mutation. The study of other TA modules in *E. coli*, specifically "interferases"—RNA endonucleases—produced a general paradigm for persister formation, which however did not hold up. This body of work, mainly from the Gerdes group, was based on a seemingly compelling observation—a knockout of 10 interferases TAs (Δ10) had almost no persisters (Maisonneuve and Gerdes 2014). Working with this Δ10 strain, we were able to see the same phenotype as reported with fluoroquinolone antibiotics, but not with other classes (Shan et al. 2017). It was subsequently reported that the phenotype of Δ10 was due to an insertion of a prophage into the strain during the construction of deletion mutants (Harms et al. 2017). Additional reevaluation of interferases (Goormaghtigh et al. 2018; Ramisetty et al. 2016) described in detail in Chap. 8, suggested that they are not linked to persisters in *E. coli*. Working with *S. aureus*, we showed that deletion of 3 TA modules present in that species has no effect on persister formation (Conlon et al. 2016). In the spirochete *Borrelia burgdorferi*, the causative agent of Lyme disease, there are no TAs (Pandey and Gerdes 2005), but there are persisters (Sharma et al. 2015). (p)ppGpp and stringent response have also been linked to persisters (Maisonneuve and Gerdes 2014). However, establishing such a link unambiguously in *E. coli* is challenging, since mutants disrupted in RelA and SpoT (p)ppGpp synthetases have growth defects and are generally pleiotropic. At the same time, we found that in *S. aureus*, knocking out all (p)ppGpp synthetases in the same strain has no obvious phenotype on growth, and the knockout had normal levels of persisters in both growing culture and stationary phase (Conlon et al. 2016). This tells us that neither TA modules nor the stringent response represent a general mechanism of persister formation.

4.1.2   The Search for a New Paradigm

The case of *S. aureus* seemed particularly challenging since everything we learned about persisters did not apply. There was, however, a potentially useful clue—stationary phase cells of *S. aureus* are almost fully tolerant to killing by antibiotics (Conlon et al. 2013, 2016); by contrast, persisters make about 1% of the stationary phase population in *E. coli* (Keren et al. 2004a). This suggested that stationary phase cells of *S. aureus* can be considered equivalent to persisters, resolving the main obstacle that has impeded progress in the field, the need to work with a small and temporary population of cells. In stationary *S. aureus*, the persister population is large and indeed stationary—permanent. The stationary phase is very complex, with multiple changes accompanying the shift to a non-growing state, but there is one factor that seemed particularly relevant to the acquisition of tolerance, the level of ATP. In the stationary state, ATP drops, and we indeed recorded a tenfold decrease by comparison to a growing culture of *S. aureus* (Conlon et al. 2016). A lower ATP level would lead to a decreased activity of targets and explain why persisters are tolerant to killing by antibiotics; this is indeed the mechanism by which TisB produces persisters (Dorr et al. 2010; Gurnev et al. 2012; Berghoff et al. 2017).

While low ATP level is a plausible explanation that accounts for the tolerance of stationary cells, it is not obvious that this would apply to cells in a growing population, where ATP levels are expected to be high. We nonetheless considered the possibility that rare cells in a growing population enter into the stationary state early, and set out to find them. We took advantage of two genes that are selectively expressed in stationary phase, *cap5A*, coding for capsular polysaccharide, and *arcA*, coding for arginine deiminase (Conlon et al. 2016). Using $P_{cap5A}::gfp$ and $P_{arcA}::gfp$ as transcriptional reporters, we analyzed their expression in single cells of a growing population by FACS. Interestingly, even in early exponential culture, some rare cells showed "stationary" levels of expression of these markers. As the culture progressed toward stationary phase, the proportion of cells expressing $P_{cap5A}::gfp$ and $P_{arcA}::gfp$ dramatically increased. Interestingly, this increase matches the pattern of the dramatic increase in persister levels as the culture deviates from strictly balanced growth (Keren et al. 2004a). We also found that $P_{cap5A}::gfp$ and $P_{arcA}::gfp$ are induced by addition of arsenate that specifically depletes ATP through a futile cycle of synthesis and hydrolysis: ADP-As $\leftrightarrow$ ADP + As (Moore et al. 1983). This suggests that these markers actually respond to ATP decrease, and the rare "stationary" cells in a growing population have low energy levels. Sorted out stationary cells in these growing cultures had a considerably higher antibiotic tolerance, showing that they are persisters. Importantly, dropping ATP to stationary levels with arsenate treatment in a growing culture recapitulates the persister level of a stationary population, showing that low energy is sufficient for tolerance. If low ATP results in tolerance, then high ATP should have the opposite effect. Indeed, supplementing TSB medium with glucose increased ATP significantly and resulted in a 100-fold reduction in persisters. We made similar observations linking ATP and persisters in a study of *E. coli* and in *Pseudomonas aeruginosa* (Shan et al. 2017; Cameron et al. 2018).

While tolerance due to low ATP/low target activity is the simplest interpretation of these findings, it is also possible that a decrease in ATP induces some pathway that leads to persisters. To test for this, we treated cells with rifampicin to inhibit transcription and then added arsenate. Rifampicin did not inhibit tolerance in this experiment, confirming that ATP decrease alone is responsible for persister formation.

Why would ATP drop in some cells of a growing population? One possibility is that expression of energy producing components is subject to stochastic fluctuation, and this would lead to a drop in the energy level. We tested this idea using GFP transcriptional fusions of Krebs cycle gene promoters in *S. aureus* (Zalis et al. 2019), and with YFP translational fusions in *E. coli* (manuscript in preparation). FACS analysis shows a wide distribution of expression in a population, and sorting out dim cells with low levels of expression (or low protein abundance) enriches in drug tolerant persisters. This observation provides a mechanistic basis for the low-energy hypothesis of persister formation. This hypothesis provides a satisfactory explanation for tolerance, immediately linking a drop in ATP to a decrease in target activity, and could represent a general mechanism of persister formation in bacteria (Fig. 4.1). Interestingly, this low-energy mechanism of tolerance is likely to operate in polymicrobial infections such as wounds or the CF lung, dominated by *P. aeruginosa* and *S. aureus*. *P. aeruginosa* produces 2-heptyl-4-hydroxyquinoline *N*-oxide (HQNO), which inhibits respiration in *S. aureus*, causing a reduction in ATP and multidrug tolerance (Radlinski et al. 2017). The low-energy hypothesis provides an explanation for other observations in the field as well.

One particular stubborn question is the nature of a dramatic increase in persister levels as the density of a culture increases (Keren et al. 2004a). Efforts to isolate a "persister-inducing" compound such as a quorum-sensing factor responsible for this have not been successful. Persister fraction increases as the culture deviates from strictly balanced growth, meaning at a point when nutrient depletion begins. A smaller drop in the expression of a Krebs cycle enzyme, for example, will be required for a cell to become a persister in a nutrient-poor medium as compared to nutrient rich (Fig. 4.2).

As we have mentioned, some specialized persister formation mechanisms such as TisB expression have been linked to a decrease in ATP as well (Dorr et al. 2010). Similarly, the pore-forming toxin HokB decreases ATP level through membrane depolarization and ATP leakage (Wilmaerts et al. 2018). Interestingly, protein aggregation and disaggregation have been shown to regulate persister dormancy

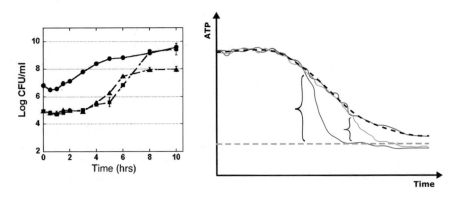

Fig. 4.2 Persister level increase in the course of growth. Left panel, as a culture of *E. coli* grows (circles), the level of persisters (tolerant to ampicillin; squares, or ofloxacin; triangles) dramatically increases (Keren et al. 2004a). Right panel, the hypothetical fate of cells in this population. The horizontal gray dotted line is the level of ATP beyond which target activity is low, and cells are tolerant to antibiotics. As the culture progresses toward the stationary phase, ATP gradually drops in a regular cell (blue) as the average population (black dotted line). At high-energy levels, a drop in ATP has to be significant in order for a cell (red) to become a persister. As the baseline ATP decreases, a smaller drop in ATP will lead to persister formation (orange)

depth and regrowth in an ATP-dependent manner, with ATP depletion being the main driver of protein aggresomes (Pu et al. 2019).

The low-energy hypothesis is satisfying, but also quite obvious; why was it not advanced two decades ago? For one, the field was following the lead produced by studies of HipA and then other toxins, which suggested the presence of specific, rather than a general mechanism for persister formation. Screens for persister genes (Hansen et al. 2008; Molina-Quiroz et al. 2016; Shan et al. 2015) discounted mutants with pleiotropic phenotypes, which knockouts in energy-generating compounds would have. Perhaps the most important consideration, at least for us, was the misconception about the nature of noise, that happens when a very small number of molecules is involved. In a classical example, *E. coli* only has about ten molecules of the *lac* repressor (LacI), and noise produces rare cells with no LacI that express the *lac* operon in the absence of an inducer. By contrast, energy-generating components such as Krebs cycle enzymes are abundant. However, our results clearly show that their expression is noisy. Interestingly, the Krebs cycle flux has been shown to be mainly controlled at the transcriptional level (Fong et al. 2006). One can hypothesize that fluctuations observed in the Krebs cycle enzyme expression could be the consequence of transcriptional noise, or possibly due to noise in an upstream regulator. For now, we can conclude that persisters are formed when ATP is low due to cell-to-cell variation in abundance of energy-producing components.

4.2 Persisters and Disease

4.2.1 Chronic Infections

Chronic infections are caused primarily by drug-susceptible pathogens, which are common; drug-resistant pathogens are in minority. The recalcitrance of biofilm infections caused by seemingly drug-susceptible pathogens has been known for a long time, and explanations to account for this paradox included poor penetration through the biofilm exopolymers (Gristina et al. 1987), or expression of resistance mechanisms that are silent in planktonic cells (Stewart and Costerton 2001). The finding of persisters in biofilms provided an explanation for the paradox—biofilms are not resistant but tolerant to killing by antibiotics. While the biofilm exopolymers are not a barrier for most antibiotics, they do restrict the penetration of the large components of the immune system such as lymphocytes (Jesaitis et al. 2003; Leid et al. 2002; Vuong et al. 2004). Antibiotics do not kill persisters that survive to live another day, fueling a chronic relapsing infection. In a way, the biofilm serves as a protective environment for persisters (Lewis 2001). Indeed, protection from the immune system is a general feature of all chronic infections. *Mycobacterium tuberculosis* hides from the immune system inside macrophages and granulomas; *Helicobacter pylori* lives in the stomach and *Neisseria meningitidis* in the cerebrospinal fluid where the presence of the immune components is limited. In all of these cases, the presence of persisters would account for the recalcitrant nature of chronic infections (Lewis 2010, 2007).

It is noteworthy that the prominence of chronic infections is a fairly recent phenomenon, and at least in the developed world, very much a side effect of otherwise successful clinical interventions. Biofilms form on indwelling devices, and cause serious problems for catheters, prosthetic joints, and heart valves. Replacement of the device requiring reoperation is a frequent solution to the problem of infection. Organ replacement requires immune suppression, as do therapies for autoimmune diseases such as IBD; anti-TNF antibody is currently the #1 drug by sales. Immunocompromised patients have a higher risk of infection, which are difficult to treat in the absence of a robust immune response. Perhaps the most telling example of the resilience of a pathogen population in the face of aggressive antibiotic therapy is that of cystic fibrosis. Formation of a thick mucus layer in the lungs provides a favorable environment for pathogens that cannot be eradicated. Cystic fibrosis (CF) is the only disease in the developed world that is untreatable by antibiotics, which only suppress, but not cure the infection, primarily by *P. aeruginosa*, to which patients eventually succumb.

Persisters provide a plausible explanation for the recalcitrance of chronic infections and hold the promise of developing cures based on agents that could target these resilient cells. This proposition, however, hinges on demonstrating directly the clinical relevance of persisters in disease.

4.2.2 Linking of Persisters to Disease

A thought experiment to test a link between persisters and disease, following the Koch postulates, seems straightforward: isolate persisters, introduce them into an animal, and then measure the ability of an antibiotic to eliminate this population by comparison to control with regular cells. This, however, is impractical. We do not have good methods to isolate persisters that would preserve them in their intact state. Even if we would, they will wake up upon introduction into an animal. Another standard approach could be borrowed from the field of resistance—introduce a mutant with a high or low level of antibiotic tolerance and measure the decrease of pathogen burden by antibiotic by comparison to the wild type. This will not work with a low-persister mutant, since we do not have such at the moment. This experiment can indeed be performed with a *hip* mutant, we just need to use one that is clinically relevant.

Periodic application of lethal doses of antibiotics to populations of *E. coli* or *P. aeruginosa* in vitro produces *hip* mutants (Moyed and Bertrand 1983; Fridman et al. 2014; Van Den Bergh et al. 2016; Michiels et al. 2016). We reasoned that this regimen emulates the clinical use of antibiotics, and if persisters help the pathogen survive, this will select for *hip* mutants in vivo. In a way, millions of people participated in this experiment and analyzing its results will provide a link between persisters and disease. We performed this analysis in isolates of *P. aeruginosa* obtained from patients with CF. As we have mentioned, this is the toughest chronic infection, and patients undergo treatment throughout their life. What we found is that a considerable proportion, 25–40% of all isolates are *hip* mutants, and many of them carry no mutations conferring resistance (Mulcahy et al. 2010). This strongly suggests causality between persisters and recalcitrance to antibiotics of the most difficult to treat chronic infection. Our initial attempts to find the mechanism leading to the *hip* phenotype were not successful, there were too many changes in the genome of isolates. Revisiting this problem when large cohorts of sequenced strains became available, but we did not find a distinct pattern of genetic changes in the *hip* isolates, suggesting many different paths leading to a similar phenotype (Mojsoska et al. 2019). One rather common theme was null mutations in the RpoN σ factor, and complementing it with an intact copy of the gene reduced the *hip* phenotype. However, knocking out *rpoN* in a lab strain *P. aeruginosa* PAO1 had no effect on persister levels, showing that this mutation required additional changes in the genome to manifest a phenotype. But this is a start, and as additional genomes of *P. aeruginosa* isolates from CF patients are sequenced, we are likely to get a better handle on the nature of *hip* mutations.

We had better luck in understanding the nature of high persistence with a similar study of *E. coli* isolates from patients with UTI, an infection characterized by frequent relapses. Knowing that in vitro selection for *hip* mutants often produces *hipA* isolates, we used PCR to screen for changes in the *hipA* gene of some 400 *E. coli* strains (Schumacher et al. 2015). About half of these strains carried some changes in *hipA*, suggesting a rapidly evolving locus, and 5% of these were *hipA7*, the mutation initially discovered by Harris Moyed. Introduction of *hipA7* UTI isolates into bladder cells showed that they have a higher tolerance to killing by antibiotics as compared to an isogenic wild type strain.

Screening clinical isolates of *M. tuberculosis* from patients treated with antibiotics showed the common occurrence of *hip* isolates as well (Torrey et al. 2016). It appears that unrelated, and perhaps all, pathogens produce *hip* isolates, and these are selected for during antibiotic treatment. We proposed the term "heritable tolerance" to name this phenomenon (Schumacher et al. 2015), similarly to the well-studied heritable resistance.

There are several additional lines of evidence linking persisters to disease. Entrance of *Salmonella* Typhimurium cells into macrophages sharply increases the level of persisters (discussed in Chap. 2); persisters are considered to be responsible for the very lengthy regimens of treatment in TB, and there is considerable evidence to support this (discussed in Chaps. 10 and 11); and finally, an anti-persister compound eradicates an otherwise untreatable biofilm infection of *S. aureus* (detailed in the next segment).

The challenge of combatting pathogens seems to be constantly increasing—from uncomplicated to multidrug resistant deadly acute infections, to chronic infections, to chronic multidrug-tolerant infections caused by *hip* pathogens. Clearly, the need is for new compounds acting against drug-resistant pathogens, and for antibiotics capable of killing persisters and eradicating a chronic infection.

4.2.3   Anti-persister Therapies

It is difficult to kill cells that evolved to survive. Most of our knowledge of persisters is based on the failure of clinically approved antibiotics to kill them. This phenomenon is universal—from Bigger's studies with penicillin, to the last approved drug, daptomycin—antibiotics do not sterilize a population. This varies depending on bacterial species, conditions, and antibiotics, and is relevant to both in vitro experiments and to develop treatment regimens. We already discussed the considerable difference in tolerance between a growing population and stationary phase cells. In publications describing new drug candidates, it is customary to show killing at low population density, around 10^6 cells/ml. In this population, there may be few if any persisters, and bactericidal antibiotics may achieve complete eradication. This, of course, will not happen with a stationary population. Unlike target-dependent antibiotics, daptomycin acts against the membrane and could eradicate persisters, but not at concentrations that are safe to use. Combinations of antibiotics have also been tested, and while some improvement of killing can be observed with growing populations, they do not eradicate stationary populations. There is however an exception—we found that stationary phase of *B. burgdorferi* is highly susceptible to killing by cell wall acting antibiotics (Wu et al. 2018). This was unexpected since this group of compounds has been known to only kill growing cells. In *B. burgdorferi*, cell wall remodeling occurs in stationary phase, and peptidoglycan continues to be synthesized (Wu et al. 2018); this explains susceptibility. Treatment with vancomycin leaves very few live cells, and the addition of gentamicin then eradicates cells of a stationary culture. But for other pathogens, we need to find a different solution to the problem.

Such a solution though is not at all obvious—we already know that existing antibiotics kill by corrupting targets, which are relatively inactive in persisters. An anti-persister compound will then have to corrupt a target that does not require energy. This proposition may seem far-fetched, but there is a compound that matches this requirement, acyldepsipeptide (ADEP). Discovered in the 1980s from *Streptomyces hawaiiensis* by a group from Eli Lilly (Michel and Kastner 1985), ADEP is only active against Gram-positive bacteria, and for this reason, was dropped. Twenty years later, drug-resistant Gram-positive pathogens such as *S. aureus* MRSA became a serious problem, and a group from Bayer took another look at ADEP, produced a more active analog ADEP4, and determined its mechanism of action (Brotz-Oesterhelt et al. 2005). Mutants resistant to ADEP all carried null mutations in the non-essential ClpP protease (Brotz-Oesterhelt et al. 2005). The ClpP protease recognizes misfolded proteins with the aid of ATP-dependent ClpX/C/A chaperones and degrades them (Lee et al. 2010). In the presence of ADEP, the pore of the protease keeps open, and the chaperones are no longer needed (Li et al. 2010; Lee et al. 2010). Because this proteolysis does not require energy (Kirstein et al. 2009), ADEP seemed like a great candidate for an anti-persister compound, but there were two studies that suggested otherwise. ADEP/ClpP was reported to only degrade nascent peptides coming off of the ribosome, which had not had a chance to properly fold (Kirstein et al. 2009), and a primary target, FtsZ, had been identified (Sass et al. 2011). Of course, nascent peptides require active translation, and FtsZ forms the septation ring during division. Both studies were pointing to activity against actively growing and dividing cells. However, the exposure time used was short, around 10 min, as is typical for biochemistry experiments. Antibiotics on the other hand act on a timescale of days to weeks. We decided to retest ADEP against stationary *S. aureus* over 24 h and found that this causes a dramatic hydrolysis of over 400 mature proteins (Conlon et al. 2013). It appeared that ADEP forces the cell to self-digest. In order to solve the problem with resistance, we paired it with another antibiotic. A combination of ADEP and rifampicin eradicated a stationary population of *S. aureus* as well as a biofilm. We then tested ADEP/rifampicin against an untreatable biofilm infection in the thigh of a neutropenic mouse. In this model, the immune system is abolished with cyclophosphamide, emulating the difficulty to treat infections in immunocompromised patients. While conventional antibiotics (vancomycin, rifampicin) had little effect, ADEP/rifampicin eradicated the infection. Currently, Arietis Pharma is producing additional analogs of ADEP with improved pharmacological properties with the aim of advancing ADEP/rifampicin into clinical trials.

Another compound with an ability to kill persisters was isolated from a soil *Lentzea kentuckiensis* sp. using in situ cultivation in a diffusion chamber (Gavrish et al. 2014). The screen was aimed to resolve the main bottleneck in natural product discovery—the enormous background of known and toxic compounds. We reasoned that for some pathogens such as *M. tuberculosis*, where the diagnosis is unambiguous, it is advantageous to have selective compounds rather than broad-spectrum that harm the microbiome. Then if nature evolved selective compounds, we could screen extracts against *M. tuberculosis*, and counter screen against a different species, such as *S. aureus*. Performing this screen indeed yielded specific hits, and one from *L. kentuckiensis* sp. yielded a novel antibiotic that we named lassomycin due to its fold (Gavrish et al. 2014). Lassomycin has excellent selectivity against mycobacteria and hits the C1 chaperone of the essential mycobacterial ClpP1P2C1 protease. This protease is only distantly related to the Clp of other bacteria, accounting for the selectivity. Interestingly, lassomycin was able to kill persisters in a stationary culture of *M. tuberculosis*, and in vitro, activated the ATPase of the C1 chaperone. Again, we see hydrolysis, in this case of ATP, as the target of an anti-persister compound. Degrading ATP beyond the point of no return will produce irreversibly dormant cells. Why the different parts of the Clp machinery are under attack by unrelated anti-persister compounds is an intriguing question for which we may never know the answer. Unfortunately, lassomycin is not orally available, an essential requirement for anti-TB treatments. The fact that we identified two natural products which evolved to kill persisters from a rather modest effort suggests that nature produced additional antimicrobials for eradicating competitor organisms, that we can borrow. A general theme for these compounds seems to be activating, or rather dysregulating hydrolytic enzymes. This is indeed an ideal anti-persister target, not requiring energy and good at killing cells. There are quite a few hydrolases in the cell that could be corrupted into killing machines, apart from various proteases—lipases, phosphatases, DNAses, RNAses, ATPases, and autolysins (the latter are activated by cell wall acting antibiotics, but only when peptidoglycan is synthesized).

Another potentially attractive target for anti-persister compounds is the membrane. As we have mentioned, daptomycin is unable to kill persisters at clinically achievable concentration; indeed, toxicity against mammalian cells is the obvious limitation for this group of compounds. At the same time, the membrane composition of bacterial and mammalian cells is quite different, and it should be possible to exploit this rationally to obtain anti-persister compounds. One recent advance in this direction was the identification of retinol analogs with anti-persister activity and a reasonable therapeutic index (Kim et al. 2018) (discussed in detail in Chap. 12).

Finally, there is an intriguing possibility of eradicating persisters with compounds that do not kill them. This was first proposed by Bigger in his 1944 Lancet paper (Bigger 1944). The rationale is to apply a bactericidal antibiotic, kill regular cells, then wash the antibiotic away, emulating the clearance in the course of therapy, and allow the persisters to wake up, but not regrow. Then apply antibiotic again, which in a simple scenario should sterilize the culture if all persisters woke up. We find that this works in vitro, and a biofilm of *S. aureus* can be eradicated with several pulse-doses of oxacillin (manuscript in preparation). The regimen we chose is based on the known pharmacokinetics of oxacillin. Introducing this approach in vivo may provide a useful method to clear chronic infections with currently available compounds.

4.3   Unanswered Questions

Is there a general mechanism of persister formation? As we noted, target inactivity is the likely cause of drug tolerance, and accounts for this principle feature of persisters. The problem then defaults to finding the main causes of antibiotic targets to decrease activity. Low ATP seems like a simple cause, and we have presented some evidence in support of this in the current chapter. There are probably a variety of ways a cell can lose ATP, apart from random noise in Krebs cycle enzyme expression. Low ATP is also unlikely to be the only cause of diminished target activity. Identifying the principal players leading to target inactivation that is shared by unrelated species will reveal the general mechanism(s) of persister formation.

Another question of principal importance is the role of persisters in the clinical manifestation of the disease. A growing body of evidence is consistent with these cells being responsible for the recalcitrance of chronic infections to antibiotics. However, direct evidence of the type we have for resistant bacteria is yet to be obtained. It seems though that establishing this connection is well within our reach.

Closely linked to their role in disease is the need to eradicate persisters, especially for Gram-negative bacteria. While we have some promising developments in identifying compounds acting against Gram-positive species, this is not the case for important pathogens such as *E. coli* and *P. aeruginosa*. This is not surprising, since Gram-negative bacteria have a highly restrictive permeability barrier, and the probability of finding a compound with any antimicrobial activity acting against these species is 100-fold lower as compared to Gram-positive bacteria (Lewis 2013). Apart from this simple consideration, the permeability barrier may present an even greater obstacle to anti-persister compounds. As we can see from ADEP and lassomycin, these are large molecules that perform sophisticated tasks, such as keeping a pore of a protease open. This is very different from a small molecule inhibiting an active site of an enzyme. The effective cutoff of molecular weight for a molecule to penetrate across the outer membrane is 600 Da (O'shea and Moser 2008). This means that an anti-persister compound that performs a complex task of corrupting a target has to be quite small; unclear how realistic this is. There is an alternative, however—small, well-penetrating prodrugs. Metronidazole provides a pertinent example, the small nitroaromatic antibiotic penetrates into the cell and is activated by microorganism-specific nitroreductases into a reactive, non-specific compound that hits a number of targets including DNA (Fleck et al. 2014). A more active nitrofurantoin ADC111 efficiently killed persisters in a stationary population of *E. coli*, decreasing the population by 7 log as compared to a 2 log killing by ciprofloxacin (Fleck et al. 2014). Nitroaromatic compounds have been associated with some toxicity, but a rational design of prodrugs holds the promise of producing anti-persister compounds acting against Gram-negative pathogens.

References

Balaban, N. Q., Merrin, J., Chait, R., Kowalik, L., & Leibler, S. (2004). Bacterial persistence as a phenotypic switch. *Science, 305*, 1622–1625.

Berghoff, B. A., Hoekzema, M., Aulbach, L., & Wagner, E. G. (2017). Two regulatory RNA elements affect TisB-dependent depolarization and persister formation. *Molecular Microbiology, 103*, 1020–1033.

Bigger, J. W. (1944). Treatment of staphylococcal infections with penicillin. *Lancet, 2*, 497–500.

Brotz-Oesterhelt, H., Beyer, D., Kroll, H. P., Endermann, R., Ladel, C., Schroeder, W., Hinzen, B., Raddatz, S., Paulsen, H., Henninger, K., Bandow, J. E., Sahl, H. G., & Labischinski, H. (2005). Dysregulation of bacterial proteolytic machinery by a new class of antibiotics. *Nature Medicine, 11*, 1082–1087.

Cameron, D. R., Shan, Y., Zalis, E. A., Isabella, V., & Lewis, K. (2018). A genetic determinant of persister cell formation in bacterial pathogens. *Journal of Bacteriology, 200*, e00303-18.

Cho, H., Uehara, T., & Bernhardt, T. G. (2014). Beta-lactam antibiotics induce a lethal malfunctioning of the bacterial cell wall synthesis machinery. *Cell, 159*, 1300–1311.

Conlon, B. P., Nakayasu, E. S., Fleck, L. E., Lafleur, M. D., Isabella, V. M., Coleman, K., Leonard, S. N., Smith, R. D., Adkins, J. N., & Lewis, K. (2013). Activated ClpP kills persisters and eradicates a chronic biofilm infection. *Nature, 503*, 365–370.

Conlon, B. P., Rowe, S. E., Gandt, A. B., Nuxoll, A. S., Donegan, N. P., Zalis, E. A., Clair, G., Adkins, J. N., Cheung, A. L., & Lewis, K. (2016). Persister formation in *Staphylococcus aureus* is associated with ATP depletion. *Nature Microbiology, 1*, 16051.

Correia, F. F., D'onofrio, A., Rejtar, T., Li, L., Karger, B. L., Makarova, K., Koonin, E. V., & Lewis, K. (2006). Kinase activity of overexpressed *HipA* is required for growth arrest and multidrug tolerance in *Escherichia coli*. *Journal of Bacteriology, 188*, 8360–8367.

Davis, B. D., Chen, L. L., & Tai, P. C. (1986). Misread protein creates membrane channels: An essential step in the bactericidal action of aminoglycosides. *Proceedings of the National Academy of Sciences of the United States of America, 83*, 6164–6168.

Dorr, T., Lewis, K., & Vulic, M. (2009). SOS response induces persistence to fluoroquinolones in *Escherichia coli. PLoS Genetics, 5*, E1000760.

Dorr, T., Vulic, M., & Lewis, K. (2010). Ciprofloxacin causes persister formation by inducing the TisB toxin in *Escherichia coli. PLoS Biology, 8*, E1000317.

Fleck, L. E., North, E. J., Lee, R. E., Mulcahy, L. R., Casadei, G., & Lewis, K. (2014). A screen for and validation of prodrug antimicrobials. *Antimicrobial Agents and Chemotherapy, 58*, 1410–1419.

Fong, S. S., Nanchen, A., Palsson, B. O., & Sauer, U. (2006). Latent pathway activation and increased pathway capacity enable *Escherichia coli* adaptation to loss of key metabolic enzymes. *The Journal of Biological Chemistry, 281*, 8024–8033.

Fridman, O., Goldberg, A., Ronin, I., Shoresh, N., & Balaban, N. Q. (2014). Optimization of lag time underlies antibiotic tolerance in evolved bacterial populations. *Nature, 513*, 418–421.

Gavrish, E., Sit, C. S., Cao, S., Kandror, O., Spoering, A., Peoples, A., Ling, L., Fetterman, A., Hughes, D., Bissell, A., Torrey, H., Akopian, T., Mueller, A., Epstein, S., Goldberg, A., Clardy, J., & Lewis, K. (2014). Lassomycin, a ribosomally synthesized cyclic peptide, kills *Mycobacterium tuberculosis* by targeting the ATP-dependent protease Clpc1p1p2. *Chemistry and Biology, 21*, 509–518.

Germain, E., Castro-Roa, D., Zenkin, N., & Gerdes, K. (2013). Molecular mechanism of bacterial persistence by HipA. *Molecular Cell, 52*, 248–254.

Goormaghtigh, F., Fraikin, N., Putrins, M., Hallaert, T., Hauryliuk, V., Garcia-Pino, A., Sjodin, A., Kasvandik, S., Udekwu, K., Tenson, T., Kaldalu, N., & Van Melderen, L. (2018). Reassessing the role of type II toxin-antitoxin systems in formation of *Escherichia coli* type II persister cells. *MBio, 9*, e00640.

Gristina, A. G., Hobgood, C. D., Webb, L. X., & Myrvik, Q. N. (1987). Adhesive colonization of biomaterials and antibiotic resistance. *Biomaterials, 8*, 423–426.

Gurnev, P. A., Ortenberg, R., Dorr, T., Lewis, K., & Bezrukov, S. M. (2012). Persister-promoting bacterial toxin TisB produces anion-selective pores in planar lipid bilayers. *FEBS Letters, 586*, 2529–2534.

Hansen, S., Lewis, K., & Vulić, M. (2008). The role of global regulators and nucleotide metabolism in antibiotic tolerance in *Escherichia coli. Antimicrobial Agents and Chemotherapy, 52*(8), 2718–2726.

Harms, A., Fino, C., Sorensen, M. A., Semsey, S., & Gerdes, K. (2017). Prophages and growth dynamics confound experimental results with antibiotic-tolerant persister cells. *MBio, 8*, e01964-17.

Hooper, D. (2001). Mechanism of action of antimicrobials: Focus on fluoroquinolones. *Clinical Infectious Diseases, 32*, S9–S15.

Jesaitis, A. J., Franklin, M. J., Berglund, D., Sasaki, M., Lord, C. I., Bleazard, J. B., Duffy, J. E., Beyenal, H., & Lewandowski, Z. (2003). Compromised host defense on *Pseudomonas aeruginosa* biofilms: Characterization of neutrophil and biofilm interactions. *Journal of Immunology, 171*, 4329–4339.

Kaspy, I., Rotem, E., Weiss, N., Ronin, I., Balaban, N. Q., & Glaser, G. (2013). Hipa-mediated antibiotic persistence via phosphorylation of the glutamyl-tRNA-synthetase. *Nature Communications, 4*, 3001.

Keren, I., Kaldalu, N., Spoering, A., Wang, Y., & Lewis, K. (2004a). Persister cells and tolerance to antimicrobials. *FEMS Microbiology Letters, 230*, 13–18.

Keren, I., Shah, D., Spoering, A., Kaldalu, N., & Lewis, K. (2004b). Specialized persister cells and the mechanism of multidrug tolerance in *Escherichia coli. Journal of Bacteriology, 186*, 8172–8180.

Keren, I., Wu, Y., Inocencio, J., Mulcahy, L. R., & Lewis, K. (2013). Killing by bactericidal antibiotics does not depend on reactive oxygen species. *Science, 339*, 1213–1216.

Kim, W., Zhu, W., Hendricks, G. L., Van Tyne, D., Steele, A. D., Keohane, C. E., Fricke, N., Conery, A. L., Shen, S., Pan, W., Lee, K., Rajamuthiah, R., Fuchs, B. B., Vlahovska, P. M., Wuest, W. M., Gilmore, M. S., Gao, H., Ausubel, F. M., & Mylonakis, E. (2018). A new class of synthetic retinoid antibiotics effective against bacterial persisters. *Nature, 556*, 103–107.

Kirstein, J., Hoffmann, A., Lilie, H., Schmidt, R., Rubsamen-Waigmann, H., Brotz-Oesterhelt, H., Mogk, A., & Turgay, K. (2009). The antibiotic ADEP reprogrammes ClpP, switching it from a regulated to an uncontrolled protease. *EMBO Molecular Medicine, 1*, 37–49.

Kwan, B. W., Valenta, J. A., Benedik, M. J., & Wood, T. K. (2013). Arrested protein synthesis increases persister-like cell formation. *Antimicrobial Agents and Chemotherapy, 57*, 1468–1473.

Lee, B. G., Park, E. Y., Lee, K. E., Jeon, H., Sung, K. H., Paulsen, H., Rubsamen-Schaeff, H., Brotz-Oesterhelt, H., & Song, H. K. (2010). Structures of ClpP in complex with acyldepsipeptide antibiotics reveal its activation mechanism. *Nature Structural and Molecular Biology, 17*, 471–478.

Leid, J. G., Shirtliff, M. E., Costerton, J. W., & Stoodley, P. (2002). Human leukocytes adhere to, penetrate, and respond to *Staphylococcus aureus* biofilms. *Infection and Immunity, 70*, 6339–6345.

Lewis, K. (2001). Riddle of biofilm resistance. *Antimicrobial Agents and Chemotherapy, 45*, 999–1007.

Lewis, K. (2007). Persister cells, dormancy and infectious disease. *Nature Reviews. Microbiology, 5*, 48–56.

Lewis, K. (2010). Persister cells. *Annual Review of Microbiology, 64*, 357–372.

Lewis, K. (2013). Platforms for antibiotic discovery. *Nature Reviews. Drug Discovery, 12*, 371–387.

Li, D. H., Chung, Y. S., Gloyd, M., Joseph, E., Ghirlando, R., Wright, G. D., Cheng, Y. Q., Maurizi, M. R., Guarne, A., & Ortega, J. (2010). Acyldepsipeptide antibiotics induce the formation of a structured axial channel in ClpP: A model for the ClpX/ClpA-bound state of ClpP. *Chemistry and Biology, 17*, 959–969.

Maisonneuve, E., & Gerdes, K. (2014). Molecular mechanisms underlying bacterial persisters. *Cell, 157*, 539–548.

Malik, M., Zhao, X., & Drlica, K. (2006). Lethal fragmentation of bacterial chromosomes mediated by DNA gyrase and quinolones. *Molecular Microbiology, 61*, 810–825.

Michel, K. H., & Kastner, R. E. (Eli Lilly and Company). (1985). *A54556 antibiotics and process for production thereof. US Patent 4492650*.

Michiels, J. E., Van Den Bergh, B., Verstraeten, N., Fauvart, M., & Michiels, J. (2016). In vitro emergence of high persistence upon periodic aminoglycoside challenge in the ESKAPE pathogens. *Antimicrobial Agents and Chemotherapy, 60*, 4630–4637.

Mojsoska, B., Cameron, D. R., Bartell, J. A., Haagensen, J. A. J., Sommer, L. M., Lewis, K., Molin, S., & Johansen, H. K. (2019). The high persister phenotype of *Pseudomonas aeruginosa* is associated with increased fitness and persistence in cystic fibrosis airways. bioRxiv, 561589.

Molina-Quiroz, R. C., Lazinski, D. W., Camilli, A., & Levy, S. B. (2016). Transposon-sequencing analysis unveils novel genes involved in the generation of persister cells in uropathogenic *Escherichia coli*. *Antimicrobial Agents and Chemotherapy, 60*, 6907–6910.

Moore, S. A., Moennich, D. M., & Gresser, M. J. (1983). Synthesis and hydrolysis of ADP-arsenate By beef heart submitochondrial particles. *The Journal of Biological Chemistry, 258*, 6266–6271.

Moyed, H. S., & Bertrand, K. P. (1983). *hipA*, a newly recognized gene of *Escherichia coli* K-12 that affects frequency of persistence after inhibition of murein synthesis. *Journal of Bacteriology, 155*, 768–775.

Mulcahy, L. R., Burns, J. L., Lory, S., & Lewis, K. (2010). Emergence of *Pseudomonas aeruginosa* strains producing high levels of persister cells in patients with cystic fibrosis. *Journal of Bacteriology, 192*, 6191–6199.

O'shea, R., & Moser, H. E. (2008). Physicochemical properties of antibacterial compounds: Implications for drug discovery. *Journal of Medicinal Chemistry, 51*(10), 2871–2878.

Pandey, D. P., & Gerdes, K. (2005). Toxin-antitoxin loci are highly abundant in free-living but lost from host-associated prokaryotes. *Nucleic Acids Research, 33*, 966–976.

Pu, Y., Li, Y., Jin, X., Tian, T., Ma, Q., Zhao, Z., Lin, S. Y., Chen, Z., Li, B., Yao, G., Leake, M. C., Lo, C. J., & Bai, F. (2019). ATP-dependent dynamic protein aggregation regulates bacterial dormancy depth critical for antibiotic tolerance. *Molecular Cell, 73*, 143–156. e4.

Radlinski, L., Rowe, S. E., Kartchner, L. B., Maile, R., Cairns, B. A., Vitko, N. P., Gode, C. J., Lachiewicz, A. M., Wolfgang, M. C., & Conlon, B. P. (2017). *Pseudomonas aeruginosa* exoproducts determine antibiotic efficacy against *Staphylococcus aureus*. *PLoS Biology, 15*, e2003981.

Ramisetty, B. C., Ghosh, D., Roy Chowdhury, M., & Santhosh, R. S. (2016). What is the link between stringent response, endoribonuclease encoding type II toxin-antitoxin systems and persistence? *Frontiers in Microbiology, 7*, 1882.

Robertson, G. T., Zhao, J., Desai, B. V., Coleman, W. H., Nicas, T. I., Gilmour, R., Grinius, L., Morrison, D. A., & Winkler, M. E. (2002). Vancomycin tolerance induced by erythromycin but not by loss of *vncrs, vex3*, or *pep27* function in *Streptococcus pneumoniae*. *Journal of Bacteriology, 184*, 6987–7000.

Sass, P., Josten, M., Famulla, K., Schiffer, G., Sahl, H. G., Hamoen, L., & Brotz-Oesterhelt, H. (2011). Antibiotic acyldepsipeptides activate ClpP peptidase to degrade the cell division protein FtsZ. *Proceedings of the National Academy of Sciences of the United States of America, 108*, 17474–17479.

Schumacher, M. A., Piro, K. M., Xu, W., Hansen, S., Lewis, K., & Brennan, R. G. (2009). Molecular mechanisms of HipA-mediated multidrug tolerance and its neutralization by HipB. *Science, 323*, 396–401.

Schumacher, M. A., Balani, P., Min, J., Chinnam, N. B., Hansen, S., Vulic, M., Lewis, K., & Brennan, R. G. (2015). Hipba-promoter structures reveal the basis of heritable multidrug tolerance. *Nature, 524*, 59–64.

Shah, D., Zhang, Z., Khodursky, A., Kaldalu, N., Kurg, K., & Lewis, K. (2006). Persisters: A distinct physiological state of *E. coli*. *BMC Microbiology, 6*, 53.

Shan, Y., Lazinski, D., Rowe, S., Camilli, A., & Lewis, K. (2015). Genetic basis of persister tolerance to aminoglycosides in *Escherichia coli*. *MBio, 6*, e00078-15.

Shan, Y., Brown Gandt, A., Rowe, S. E., Deisinger, J. P., Conlon, B. P., & Lewis, K. (2017). ATP-dependent persister formation in *Escherichia coli*. *MBio, 8*, e02267-16.

Sharma, B., Brown, A. V., Matluck, N. E., Hu, L. T., & Lewis, K. (2015). Borrelia burgdorferi, the causative agent of Lyme disease, forms drug-tolerant persister cells. *Antimicrobial Agents and Chemotherapy, 59*, 4616–4624.

Spoering, A. L., & Lewis, K. (2001). Biofilms and planktonic cells of *Pseudomonas aeruginosa* have similar resistance to killing by antimicrobials. *Journal of Bacteriology, 183*, 6746–6751.

Stewart, P. S., & Costerton, J. W. (2001). Antibiotic resistance of bacteria in biofilms. *Lancet, 358*, 135–138.

Torrey, H. L., Keren, I., Via, L. E., Lee, J. S., & Lewis, K. (2016). High persister mutants in *Mycobacterium tuberculosis*. *PLos One, 11*, e0155127.

Unoson, C., & Wagner, E. (2008). A small SOS-induced toxin is targeted against the inner membrane in *Escherichia coli*. *Molecular Microbiology, 70*, 258–270.

Vakulenko, S. B., & Mobashery, S. (2003). Versatility of aminoglycosides and prospects for their future. *Clinical Microbiology Reviews, 16*, 430–450.

Van Den Bergh, B., Michiels, J. E., Wenseleers, T., Windels, E. M., Boer, P. V., Kestemont, D., De Meester, L., Verstrepen, K. J., Verstraeten, N., Fauvart, M., & Michiels, J. (2016). Frequency of antibiotic application drives rapid evolutionary adaptation of *Escherichia coli* persistence. *Nature Microbiology, 1*, 16020.

Vogel, J., Argaman, L., Wagner, E. G., & Altuvia, S. (2004). The small RNA IstR inhibits synthesis of an SOS-induced toxic peptide. *Current Biology, 14*, 2271–2276.

Vuong, C., Voyich, J. M., Fischer, E. R., Braughton, K. R., Whitney, A. R., Deleo, F. R., & Otto, M. (2004). Polysaccharide intercellular adhesin (PIA) protects *Staphylococcus epidermidis* against major components of the human innate immune system. *Cellular Microbiology, 6,* 269–275.

Wilmaerts, D., Bayoumi, M., Dewachter, L., Knapen, W., Mika, J. T., Hofkens, J., Dedecker, P., Maglia, G., Verstraeten, N., & Michiels, J. (2018). The persistence-inducing toxin HokB forms dynamic pores that cause ATP leakage. *MBio, 9,* e00744-18.

Wu, X., Sharma, B., Niles, S., O'connor, K., Schilling, R., Matluck, N., D'onofrio, A., Hu, L. T., & Lewis, K. (2018). Identifying vancomycin as an effective antibiotic for killing *Borrelia burgdorferi*. *Antimicrobial Agents and Chemotherapy, 62,* e01201-18.

Zalis, E. A., Nuxoll, A. S., Manuse, S., Clair, G., Radlinski, L. C., Conlon, B. P., Adkins, J., & Lewis, K. (2019). Stochastic variation in expression of the tricarboxylic acid cycle produces persister cells. *MBio, 10,* e01930–19.

Chapter 5
Persister Formation Driven by TisB-Dependent Membrane Depolarization

Bork A. Berghoff and E. Gerhart H. Wagner

Abstract The membrane-depolarizing toxin TisB encoded by the chromosomal type I toxin-antitoxin (TA) locus *tisB/istR-1* can induce a persister state in *Escherichia coli*. While transcription of *tisB* is effectively induced by DNA damage as part of the SOS response, efficient TisB translation requires processing of the mRNA to an active species that works through ribosome standby. This latter step is inhibited by the RNA antitoxin, IstR-1. This regulatory complexity contributes to a delay in toxin production under stress conditions and favors phenotypic heterogeneity in terms of membrane depolarization. Removing the layer of translational inhibition by *cis-* and *trans*-regulatory RNA elements increases the likelihood of depolarization and, as a consequence, triggers higher levels of persisters. The *tisB/istR-1* locus represents a useful model system for "persistence by depolarization" and considerably contributes to our understanding of how bacteria control persistence as a strategy to encounter stress and maintain survival on the population level.

5.1 Introduction

Bacterial populations typically display some degree of cell-to-cell variation, either manifested genetically through mutagenic events or phenotypically through fluctuations in protein expression. Cell-to-cell variations on the protein level can cause different phenotypes and, consequently, the formation of distinct subpopulations within isogenic cultures. This is referred to as phenotypic heterogeneity. Since the occurrence of environmental stress is generally unpredictable, phenotypic

B. A. Berghoff
Institute for Microbiology and Molecular Biology, Justus Liebig University Giessen, Giessen, Germany
e-mail: bork.a.berghoff@mikro.bio.uni-giessen.de

E. G. H. Wagner (✉)
Department of Cell and Molecular Biology, Biomedical Center, Uppsala University, Uppsala, Sweden
e-mail: gerhart.wagner@icm.uu.se

© Springer Nature Switzerland AG 2019
K. Lewis (ed.), *Persister Cells and Infectious Disease*,
https://doi.org/10.1007/978-3-030-25241-0_5

heterogeneity provides a valuable survival strategy on the population level (Veening et al. 2008). If a sudden threat can be tolerated by a subpopulation, it may eventually repopulate the environment after the harmful situation has been overcome. Persister cells represent a prominent example of phenotypic variants that tolerate environmental stress and antibiotic treatments to maintain survival and have been found in almost every bacterial species examined so far (Van den Bergh et al. 2017). The presence of persister cells is typically revealed in killing curve experiments. Cultures are treated with high concentrations of bactericidal antibiotics, and colony counts are determined before, and at several time-points during, the treatment. Early on, non-persister cells are rapidly killed, seen as a steep slope in a colony count curve. Later on, only persister cells remain and, hence, viable counts now show a shallow slope or no decrease at all. This characteristic biphasic curve is regarded a hallmark for the presence of persisters in a laboratory setting, and by definition, bacteria surviving during the second phase of the curve represent the persister fraction (Brauner et al. 2016). For the same bacterial strain, persister levels are often highly variable between experimental conditions. For example, persister levels are typically high in stationary phase and comparably low in exponential phase. Furthermore, different classes of antibiotics give different results in persister assays dependent on their particular mode of action. In *Escherichia coli*, for instance, the β-lactam antibiotic ampicillin, which is an inhibitor of cell wall synthesis, is ineffective in stationary phase cultures (Tuomanen et al. 1986; Bayles 2000). By contrast, the quinolone antibiotic ciprofloxacin damages DNA and kills >90% of stationary phase cells (Harms et al. 2017). Accumulation of persister cells during the stationary phase ultimately links the persister phenotype to growth stasis (Balaban et al. 2004). Non-growing or slowly growing bacteria are more likely to become persisters and survive an antibiotic treatment. This is further underscored by increased persister levels upon bacteriostatic drug-induced growth arrest in exponential phase (Kwan et al. 2013). At this point, it is not clear whether persisters are entirely dormant or retain metabolic activity in the persistent state. The latter has been supported by several studies (Orman and Brynildsen 2013; Pu et al. 2016; Radzikowski et al. 2016), but is still subject to scientific debate (Kim and Wood 2016). Recently, studies showed that *Salmonella* Typhimurium enters a persister state in macrophages (Rycroft et al. 2018), which is associated with the detectable metabolic activity (Helaine et al. 2014). Dual-RNAseq experiments indicated that effectors produced by these persisters reprogram the macrophage to the advantage of the pathogen (Stapels et al. 2018). Nevertheless, it seems that in general the physiological state of persister cells remains poorly defined (Ronneau and Helaine 2019).

How do bacteria enter the persistent state? There may be no single answer, since mechanisms for persister generation appear diverse, and universal "persistence factors" are yet to be defined. Early work on persister cells suggested toxins from chromosomal toxin-antitoxin (TA) systems to be involved in persister generation (Moyed and Bertrand 1983; Keren et al. 2004; Shah et al. 2006), which was later corroborated for several toxins. For example, deletion of toxin gene *tisB* in *E. coli* decreases persister levels upon ciprofloxacin treatment (Dörr et al. 2010), and toxin gene *yafQ* mediates tolerance to cefazolin or tobramycin in *E. coli* biofilms (Harrison et al. 2009). When expressed at moderate levels, toxins have the potential to corrupt essential cellular processes without killing the cell, thereby inducing growth stasis and persistence. For mRNA interferase-like toxins from type II TA systems, how-ever, there is an ongoing debate about their importance for persistence in general, and their activation pathway in particular (Van Melderen and Wood 2017; Shan et al. 2017; Harms et al. 2017; Goormaghtigh et al. 2018). It seems likely that some bacterial toxins are primarily modulators of cell physiology with the potential to counteract stress or stabilize the persistent state, rather than being sole causative agents for persister formation. This might explain why most single toxin gene deletions fail to produce clear persister phenotypes. Also, if TA systems are func-tionally redundant, phenotypes will be negligible upon deletion of single toxin genes. There are, however, cases where these limitations are partly eliminated. For example, internalization of *Salmonella* Typhimurium by bone marrow-derived murine macrophages triggered persistence by 100–1000-fold, demonstrating that persistence is an inducible trait. Interestingly, in the *Salmonella* macrophage model, several single toxin gene deletions (including mRNA interferase genes) caused a reduction in persister levels (Helaine et al. 2014). Reliably identifying true causative links between toxins and persister formation may require finding a set of standard-ized appropriate growth conditions.

A system for which the inducing condition and mode of action are quite well understood is the type I TA system *tisB/istR-1* from *E. coli*. The toxin TisB is induced upon DNA damage and localizes to the inner membrane, leading to depo-larization and ATP depletion in a subset of cells. TisB has been shown to favor persistence under SOS conditions. In the following sections, we will focus on how *tisB* expression is regulated on the transcriptional level upon DNA damage stress and on the post-transcriptional level by regulatory RNA elements, and how this regula-tion affects subpopulation dynamics with regard to persister formation. Furthermore, we will discuss current models of how TisB might cause depolarization of the inner membrane.

5.2 Toxin-Antitoxin Systems

Subsequent to the discovery of the *hok/sok* system on the enterobacterial plasmid R1, which promotes post-segregational killing of plasmid-free segregants (Gerdes et al. 1986a, b), numerous TA systems have been found to be encoded by bacterial chromosomes in bacteria (Gotfredsen and Gerdes 1998). Since other chapters cover some of these in great detail, a short summary will suffice. TA loci encode stable toxins, which are subject to inhibition by their specific antitoxins. In type I systems, an antisense RNA (antitoxin) base pairs with, and inhibits, toxin mRNA translation (Gerdes and Wagner 2007). Type II systems encode unstable antitoxin proteins that form complexes with the toxin to inhibit its function (Harms et al. 2018). Several other TA systems (types III–VI) have been identified (Hayes and Van Melderen 2011; Page and Peti 2016; Harms et al. 2018), but are less prevalent and not well characterized with respect to the present topic. Toxins act on specific intracellular targets to affect central functions that, in almost all cases, suggest severe growth/ replication/ cell division retardation or arrest. Many toxins that ultimately affect protein synthesis are (m)RNAses [e.g., RelE (Neubauer et al. 2009), MazF (Zhang et al. 2003), MqsR (Yamaguchi et al. 2009), YafQ], others target tRNAs or aminoacyl-tRNA synthetases [e.g., TacT (Cheverton et al. 2016), HipA (Germain et al. 2013)]. Yet others compromise inner membrane integrity [e.g., TisB (Unoson and Wagner 2008), DinQ (Weel-Sneve et al. 2013), HokB (Wilmaerts et al. 2018)] or affect DNA replication via targeting of topoisomerases.

The question whether all or most of these various toxins—under relevant physiological conditions and without overexpression from plasmid-borne genes—slow down/arrest cell growth or instead kill cells (altruistic suicide) (Amitai et al. 2004) has been a long-standing debate. As it stands, most labs come down on the former side (e.g., Song and Wood 2018). Clearly, a toxin-dependent induction of a dormant/ slow-growing state is more congruent with a persister state.

5.3   Transcriptional Regulation of the *tisB/istR* Locus

We will first briefly summarize what is known about transcriptional regulation in type II TA systems to facilitate a comparison to the different characteristics of type I systems. Type II toxin and antitoxin genes are organized in operons and co-transcribed from the same promoter. Transcriptional autoregulation is a typical feature. Antitoxins have two domains, one interacting with the toxin and one (DNA-binding domain) active in the repression of the TA promoter. The toxin can either act as corepressor or de-repressor, depending on the toxin: antitoxin ratio (Overgaard et al. 2008; Garcia-Pino et al. 2016). The term "conditional cooperativity" refers to the ratio-dependent interplay between toxins and antitoxins (Chan et al. 2016; Page and Peti 2016). While toxins are relatively stable, antitoxins are prone to degradation by cellular proteases (Lon, Clp). Upon degradation of the antitoxin, the toxin level exceeds that of the antitoxin, a situation in which the toxin acts as de-repressor. Consequently, transcription is stimulated, leading to the replenishment of antitoxin levels and neutralization of toxin activity.

Transcriptional regulation in type I TA systems is strikingly different. Toxin and antitoxin genes are divergently transcribed from individual promoters (in some cases generating overlapping transcripts, in some cases not). The RNA antitoxins are usually constitutively expressed, as shown for Sib RNAs (Fozo et al. 2008), AgrAB (Weel-Sneve et al. 2013), and IstR-1 (Vogel et al. 2004). Constitutive expression of RNA antitoxins ensures sufficiently high antitoxin to toxin mRNA ratios under non-stress growth conditions to suppress toxin synthesis. In *Bacillus subtilis*, for instance, the antitoxin RNA SR4 is in 12–48-fold excess over *bsrG* mRNA in exponential growth (Jahn and Brantl 2016). Since transcriptional bursts can be expected in individual cells at any time (Golding et al. 2005), the excess of RNA antitoxins provides a suitable buffer for variations in toxin mRNA levels, thereby efficiently preventing inadvertent toxin synthesis. In contrast to their anti-toxin counterparts, toxin genes are often preceded by stress-inducible promoter sequences and are therefore transcribed only under certain conditions. In the case of *bsrG/SR4* of *B. subtilis*, an increase of *bsrG* mRNA was monitored upon transition into stationary phase, resulting in excess *bsrG* levels, likely favoring toxin synthesis (Jahn and Brantl 2016).

In *E. coli*, several type I toxin genes, for example, *tisB* (Vogel et al. 2004), *symE* (Kawano et al. 2007), and *dinQ* (Weel-Sneve et al. 2013), are under control of the LexA repressor. LexA is the master regulator of the response to DNA damage (SOS response) and represses transcription of genes preceded by so-called LexA box sequences during normal growth (Lewis et al. 1994; Fernandez De Henestrosa et al. 2000; Courcelle et al. 2001). Upon DNA damage, auto-cleavage of LexA is stimulated by the formation of RecA nucleoprotein filaments (Little 1991), and LexA-dependent genes are de-repressed. The LexA regulon in *E. coli* comprises more than 50 genes, many of which are implicated in cell cycle arrest and DNA repair. Expression of toxins as part of the SOS response is considered a strategy to maintain survival. SymE might be involved in recycling of mRNAs (Kawano et al. 2007), DinQ seems to be important for nucleoid compaction during DNA repair (Weel-Sneve et al. 2013), and TisB induces growth arrest and eventually promotes persister formation (Dörr et al. 2010; Berghoff et al. 2017a). The *tisB* gene is preceded by a typical LexA box of 20 bp. De-repression by LexA cleavage produces two transcripts: the *tisB* primary transcript (+1) with an unusually long 5′ UTR and the divergently transcribed, 140-nt long IstR-2 RNA (Fig. 5.1). The function of IstR-2 remains unclear, but it is not involved in the control of TisB toxicity (Vogel et al. 2004). The 75-nt long IstR-1 RNA is transcribed from a constitutive σ^{70} promoter internal to *istR-2* and is identical to the 3′ segment of IstR-2 (shared terminator; Fig. 5.1). IstR-1 is the cognate antitoxin of *tisB* and controls its translation (Vogel et al. 2004; Darfeuille et al. 2007). Under non-stress growth conditions, IstR-1 levels exceed *tisB* mRNA levels by ~15-fold (B.A. Berghoff, unpublished). Upon treatment with the DNA-damaging agent mitomycin C (MMC) for 1 h, *tisB* transcription rates are strongly increased, and *tisB* +1 transcript levels consequently exceed IstR-1 levels by ~6-fold (B.A. Berghoff, unpublished). LexA-dependent genes are ranked according to the "heterology index" (HI) value of their LexA box sequences. The LexA box preceding *tisB* has the lowest reported HI value (1.81) and indeed exhibits the strongest induction of all SOS genes upon MMC treatment (Berghoff et al. 2017b). Interestingly, *tisB* transcript levels further increase upon prolonged MMC treatment, when those of other SOS genes decline. Transcriptional regulation within the *tisB/istR-1* TA system conforms to the concept that toxin expression is only favored upon enduring environmental stress, while short periods of cellular perturbations are likely buffered by excess antitoxin.

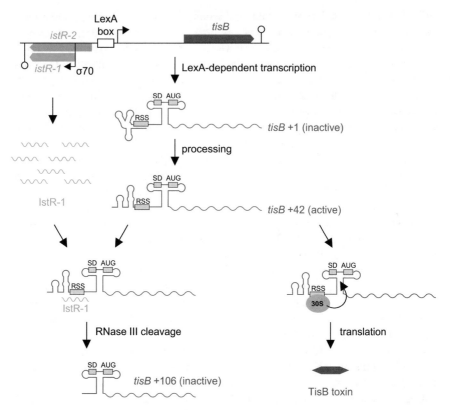

Fig. 5.1 Organization and RNA-based regulation of the *tisB/istR* locus. Toxin gene *tisB* and the 140-nt long IstR-2 RNA are divergently transcribed and controlled by a LexA box. The antitoxin IstR-1 is transcribed by Sigma70 (σ^{70}). Lollipop structures: Rho-independent transcription terminators. Upon LexA cleavage, the translationally inactive *tisB* primary transcript (+1 mRNA) is produced. Both the ribosome binding site (RBS) and ribosome standby site (RSS) are sequestered in stable structures. Processing near the 5′ end produces the translationally active +42 mRNA, which has an accessible RSS. The +42 mRNA is either bound by antitoxin IstR-1 (left) or translated into TisB toxin (right). IstR-1 binding blocks the RSS and triggers cleavage by RNase III, resulting in the translationally inactive +106 mRNA. Translation of +42 mRNA is initiated by 30S binding to the RSS, followed by sliding/jumping into the transiently open RBS (breathing). *SD* Shine-Dalgarno sequence, *AUG* start codon

5.4   Tight Regulation of Toxin Synthesis: RNA Structure Is the Key

As described above, induction of *tisB* transcription upon MMC treatment leads to a ~sixfold excess of *tisB* +1 transcript over antitoxin IstR-1. However, it was shown that sequestration of the ribosome binding site (RBS) within a stem-loop structure prevents immediate access to the 30S ribosomal subunit, and that translation initiation depends on 30S preloading at a so-called ribosome standby site (RSS) far upstream of the RBS (Darfeuille et al. 2007). The concept of "ribosome standby" was introduced by de Smit and van Duin to explain the translation efficiency observed for the coat protein of RNA bacteriophage MS2 (de Smit and van Duin 1993, 2003). The canonical RBS for coat protein translation is sequestered in a stable stem-loop structure (ΔG^0-value of -11 kcal/mol) (de Smit and van Duin 1994), similar to what is observed for *tisB* mRNA (ΔG^0-value of -16 kcal/mol) (Darfeuille et al. 2007). In the case of MS2, the stem-loop structure is flanked by short single-stranded regions, which serve as RSS. In this model, "standby" involves the transient and sequence-independent association of a 30S subunit. A recent study demonstrated the importance of a $5'$ single-stranded region for translation initiation, and that artificial, unstructured CA- and AU-rich tails of at least six repeats create a functional RSS (Sterk et al. 2018). In the primary *tisB* +1 transcript (354 nt), the RSS is structurally sequestered in a stem, rendering it translationally inactive (Fig. 5.1). A processing event by an unknown ribonuclease removes the first 41 nucleotides, producing the +42 mRNA variant (313 nt) with an accessible, single-stranded RSS which can undergo two fates: the RSS is either bound by antitoxin IstR-1 or preloaded with a 30S subunit (Fig. 5.1). Binding of IstR-1 forms a 22-bp double-stranded RNA duplex which is cleaved by RNase III (Vogel et al. 2004; Darfeuille et al. 2007). The resulting +106 mRNA lacks the RSS and is translationally inert. If the RSS in the +42 mRNA is preloaded with a 30S subunit, translation can be initiated by 30S sliding/ jumping into the RBS whenever the inhibitory stem-loop transiently opens ("breathing"; Fig. 5.1). A recent study shed more light on the anatomy of the *tisB* RSS. In addition to the single-stranded region, a structure element at the $5'$ end of the active +42 mRNA is strictly required for standby, and S1 was identified as the ribosomal protein that mediates 30S-RSS association. This entails lateral movement throughout downstream structures towards the *tisB* RBS (Romilly et al. 2019). In summary, *tisB* expression requires at least three subsequent events. Firstly, transcription is dependent on SOS induction (LexA cleavage). Following transcription, the *tisB* +1 mRNA needs to become processed to generate the translationally active +42 mRNA. Finally, the RSS has to be unbound by IstR-1 to enable 30S preloading. Since the last step determines whether or not TisB is produced, the +42/IstR-1 ratio affects the probability of TisB synthesis in individual cells. Interestingly, we obtained a ~1:1 ratio in bulk measurements after 1 h of MMC treatment (B.A. Berghoff, unpublished). The implications for depolarization and persister formation will be discussed below.

Tight regulation of toxin expression at the post-transcriptional level, as observed for *tisB*, rather seems to be the rule than the exception within type I TA systems. Several examples conform to a common scheme: the primary transcript of the toxin gene is translationally inert due to 30S exclusion, and a processing step produces a translationally active transcript that is either translated or bound by the RNA antitoxin to inhibit 30S binding (Table 5.1). The first, classical example of such an RNA-based regulatory cascade was described for the *hok/sok* system of plasmid R1 (Gerdes et al. 1986a, b; Gerdes and Wagner 2007). In contrast to *tisB*, *hok* is translationally coupled to an overlapping upstream open reading frame (ORF),

Table 5.1 Regulatory features of selected type I TA systems in *E. coli*

TA system	Stress response	RNA-based regulation		Translation
		Transcript	Feature	
tisB/istR-1	SOS	*tisB* +1	RBS and RSS structurally sequestered	No
		tisB +42	RBS sequestered; RSS accessible to 30S preloading	Yes
		IstR-1	Blocks RSS in *tisB* +42 and triggers RNase III cleavage	
dinQ/agrB	SOS	*dinQ* +1	RBS structurally sequestered	No
		dinQ +44	RBS accessible	Yes
		AgrB	Induces structural rearrangements and triggers RNase III cleavage	
hok/sok	Starvation[a]	*mok-hok* (full-length)	Translational coupling of *mok* and *hok*; 3′ end fold-back structure sequesters *mok* RBS	No
		mok-hok (processed)	Truncated 3′ end after processing by RNase II and PNPase; *mok* RBS accessible	Yes
		Sok	Blocks *mok* RBS and triggers RNase III cleavage	
zorO/orzO	Not known	*zorO* (full-length)	RBS and EAP region structurally sequestered	No
		zorO Δ28	RBS sequestered; EAP region accessible to 30S preloading	Yes
		OrzO	Blocks EAP region in *zorO* Δ28 (and triggers RNase III cleavage)	

[a]The chromosomal *hokB/sokB* system is triggered by the stringent response alarmone (p)ppGpp in an Obg-dependent manner (Verstraeten et al. 2015)
RBS ribosome binding site, *RSS* ribosome standby site, *EAP* exposure after processing

denoted *mok* (Thisted and Gerdes 1992). In the primary *mok-hok* transcript (398 nt), the *mok* RBS is sequestered due to a 3′ end fold-back structure, which efficiently represses translation (Thisted et al. 1995). Processing by RNase II and PNPase removes 39 nt from the 3′ end and induces structural rearrangements that render the *mok* RBS free, which then entails translation of Mok and, by coupling, Hok (Gerdes and Wagner 2007). If the 67-nt long RNA antitoxin Sok is abundant, coupled *mok-hok* translation is repressed at the *mok* RBS (Thisted and Gerdes 1992; Franch et al. 1999).

In the SOS-responsive TA system *dinQ/agrB* from *E. coli*, the primary *dinQ* transcript (331 nt) is translationally inactive due to structural sequestration of the RBS. 5′ processing removes 43 nt to produce the +44 mRNA (288 nt), which—after structural rearrangements—is compatible with 30S binding to the RBS of the *dinQ* ORF (Kristiansen et al. 2016). The 84-nt long RNA antitoxin AgrB, when abundant, acts differently from the otherwise similarly organized *tisB/istR-1* system: rather than interfering with "standby," it binds far upstream of the *dinQ* RBS to induce structural rearrangements. This refolding restores the inhibitory elements that were present in the *dinQ* primary transcript and that efficiently repressed toxin translation (Kristiansen et al. 2016).

The *zorO/orzO* system from enterohemorrhagic *E. coli* (EHEC) strain O157:H7 appears to be very similar to *tisB/istR-1* in terms of RNA-based regulation. Full-length *zorO* mRNA is translationally inactive due to sequestration of both the RBS and a so-called EAP (exposure after processing) region, located ~100 nt upstream of the RBS. The EAP region likely represents an RSS that is needed for efficient translation of *zorO* (Wen et al. 2016). Primer extension revealed a 5' processing product of *zorO* mRNA that lacks the first 28 nt (Wen et al. 2014). The corresponding mRNA (Δ28) was efficiently translated, likely due to opening of the structure that occludes the EAP region in the full-length mRNA. Akin to *tisB* +42, translation is inhibited by binding of the RNA antitoxin OrzO to the EAP region (Wen et al. 2016).

A final example is from the Epsilonproteobacterium *Helicobacter pylori*, the causative agent of stomach-related diseases like gastritis, peptic ulcer, and cancer. *H. pylori* encodes several type I TA systems (Sharma et al. 2010), among them *aapA1/isoA1*. The full-length transcript of toxin *aapA1* is translationally inert due to a 3' fold-back structure that blocks the SD sequence (Arnion et al. 2017). 3' end processing produces a truncated transcript with an accessible SD sequence. The truncated *aapA1* transcript has two 5' apical loops, to which the RNA antitoxin IsoA1 can bind to form a kissing-loop complex, followed by an extension to a 76-bp long IsoA1-*aapA1* RNA duplex. This causes structural sequestration of the SD sequence and efficient repression of translation (Arnion et al. 2017). Recent results additionally identified several anti-SD elements that, in a temporal fashion, act to maintain a translationally silent state of the toxin mRNA during ongoing transcription (Masachis and Darfeuille, in preparation).

The examples listed above, and additional type I TA system variants not covered here, demonstrate that primary transcripts of toxin genes employ intrinsic RNA structures (e.g., 5' stem-loops or 3' fold-back structures) that block 30S binding sites (canonical and non-canonical/standby). Initially, inactive toxin mRNAs, thus, generate a delay in toxin translation and ensure that transcription and translation become strictly uncoupled. The translationally active transcripts, generated by processing, are then inhibited by the cognate RNA antitoxin. This two-layer control avoids inadvertent toxin production under non-stress conditions and provides suitable thresholds for decision-making during persister cell formation upon stress (Berghoff and Wagner 2017).

5.5 Regulation of the IstR-1 Antitoxin Pool

The RNA-RNA duplexes formed by antitoxin RNA binding to toxin mRNAs are often cleaved by RNase III (Gerdes et al. 1992; Vogel et al. 2004; Wen et al. 2014; Kristiansen et al. 2016; Arnion et al. 2017). Co-degradation by RNase III, therefore, plays an important role in irreversibly destroying the toxin mRNA, and in simultaneously depleting the antitoxin pool. Upon treatment of *E. coli* wild-type cells with the DNA-damaging antibiotic ciprofloxacin, IstR-1 levels drop to ~15% after 2 h, which is accompanied by an increase in an RNase III-dependent IstR-1 cleavage product (Berghoff et al. 2017a). In a Δ*tisB* background, IstR-1 levels remain high (~80% of the level before ciprofloxacin treatment), suggesting that the antitoxin level is strongly affected by co-degradation with the toxin mRNA. Nevertheless, IstR-1 drops to ~3% in the wild type, and ~12% in the Δ*tisB* strain, after prolonged ciprofloxacin treatment (Berghoff et al. 2017a). This indicates that depletion of the IstR-1 pool at later stages depends on additional, so far unknown, factors. One unexplored possibility is inhibition of *istR-1* transcription. In *E. coli*, the rate-limiting step for transcription initiation of rRNA operons is the lifetime of the open complex intermediate of RNA polymerase (RNAP) on the *rrn* promoter sequences (Barker et al. 2001). The lifetime of open complexes is reduced by the stringent response alarmone ppGpp and the RNAP-binding protein DksA (Paul et al. 2004), adjusting the rate of rRNA transcription to growth rate and amino acid availability. Additionally, *rrn* P1 promoters are sensitive to NTP concentrations (Schneider et al. 2002). It was recently shown that the *rrnB* P1 promoter activity is positively correlated with ATP levels, and its use as an ATP sensor has been suggested (Shan et al. 2017). Assuming that the σ^{70} promoter of *istR-1* is an ATP sensor as well, *istR-1* transcription would decrease after high TisB production and concomitant ATP depletion. The resulting positive feedback on TisB expression is tempting but remains speculative. Alternatively, IstR-1 might be destabilized by the action of ribonucleases different from RNase III.

5.6 TisB Expression as a Phenotypic Switch that Triggers Persister Formation

Quinolone antibiotics kill bacteria by converting gyrase and topoisomerase IV into toxic enzymes that cause double-strand breaks (DSBs) (Aldred et al. 2014). DSBs are bound by the RecBCD complex that subsequently generates 3′ overhangs of single-stranded DNA (ssDNA). Binding of RecA to ssDNA leads to the formation of nucleoprotein filaments, a crucial event for initiation of DNA repair by homologous recombination, and for stimulation of LexA auto-cleavage and subsequent activation of the SOS response (Kreuzer 2013). In *E. coli*, a functional SOS response supports persister formation upon ciprofloxacin treatment, as demonstrated by decreased persister levels in *recA* and *recB* deletion strains, and in a strain harboring a non-inducible SOS repressor (*lexA3*). This phenotype was, however, specific to ciprofloxacin and SOS induction, since neither of these strains was affected by ampicillin or streptomycin (Dörr et al. 2009). Importantly, deletion of *tisB* reduced the fraction of persisters by ~tenfold when cells were treated with ciprofloxacin. This represents a rare example of a single toxin gene deletion with a clear persister phenotype (Dörr et al. 2010). Moreover, a Δ*istR-1* strain exhibited ~tenfold higher persister levels, and plasmid-borne overexpression of TisB caused increased persistence to ciprofloxacin, ampicillin, and streptomycin (Dörr et al. 2010). These findings indicate that increased TisB synthesis induces the persister state and renders cells tolerant to different classes of antibiotics. TisB is a small protein (29 amino acids) that is targeted to the inner membrane, where it compromises the proton motive force (PMF) and, thereby, causes depolarization of the inner membrane (Gurnev et al. 2012). Subsequent ATP depletion is believed to favor the persister state (Unoson and Wagner 2008; Wagner and Unoson 2012). Along the same lines, ATP depletion in the human pathogen *Staphylococcus aureus* seemingly explains high persister levels during stationary phase (Conlon et al. 2016). Furthermore, artificial depletion of ATP by the addition of arsenate to exponential cultures increases the number of persister cells to levels comparable to stationary phase in both *S. aureus* and *E. coli* (Conlon et al. 2016; Shan et al. 2017). Importantly, the number of DSBs upon ciprofloxacin treatment is clearly reduced in ATP-depleted cells, pointing to a direct link between ATP levels and protection against antibiotics (Shan et al. 2017). It is, therefore, reasonable to assume that ATP depletion by TisB-dependent depolarization is a direct cause of persister formation.

How does the RNA-based regulation of *tisB* affect persister formation on the single-cell level? Since reporter gene fusions to *tisB* have been difficult to achieve, depolarization of the inner membrane can be used as a proxy for TisB production in individual cells. Depolarization can be measured by the use of DiBAC (bis-oxonol) dyes, which enter depolarized cells and exhibit enhanced fluorescence after binding to intracellular proteins or membranes. When the potential-sensitive probe $DiBAC_4(3)$ was applied in flow cytometry experiments with *E. coli*, depolarization was undetectable in a $\Delta tisB$ strain upon 6 h of ciprofloxacin treatment, demonstrating that TisB was the main factor for depolarization in this experimental setup (Berghoff et al. 2017a). In wild-type cultures, treatment generated two subpopulations, one composed of brightly fluorescent (depolarized) cells and one of dim (normal) cells; their ratio was ~1:1, that is, ~50% of the cells were depolarized by the action of TisB. The depolarized subpopulation was not observed upon IstR-1 overexpression, strengthening the conclusion that depolarized wild-type cells were associated with TisB production (Berghoff et al. 2017a). The ~1:1 ratio of depolarized vs. polarized cells is reminiscent of the ~1:1 ratio of IstR-1 antitoxin vs. translationally active *tisB* +42 mRNA upon DNA damage (see above). Though this similarity in numbers might be purely coincidental, a link between these two ratios could be tentatively explained as follows. Due to stochastic cell-to-cell variations at the transcript level, some cells will have a slight excess of IstR-1 and likely not produce TisB. These cells would remain normal (polarized). Other cells, however, will have an excess of +42 mRNA and produce TisB at levels sufficiently high to cause depolarization. The RNA-based regulation of *tisB*, therefore, sets a threshold for TisB production in individual cells, which is displayed by ON-OFF phenotypic characteristics on the population level. If depolarization and concomitant ATP depletion favor the persistent state, deletion of both the inhibitory *tisB* 5′ UTR structure and *istR-1* is expected to increase the likelihood of persister formation. Indeed, deletion of both regulatory RNA elements in *E. coli* (strain Δ1-41 Δ*istR*)

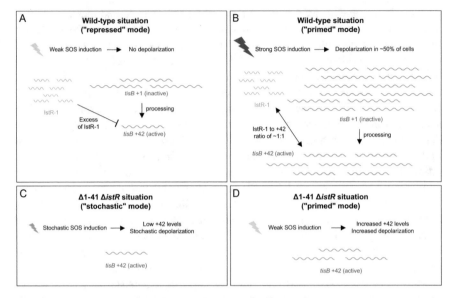

Fig. 5.2 Effects of regulatory RNA elements on TisB expression and depolarization. Different stress scenarios are illustrated for (**a, b**) wild type and (**c, d**) a strain devoid of both regulatory RNA elements (Δ1-41 Δ*istR*) (Berghoff et al. 2017a). Colored flashes indicate the strength of SOS induction. (**a**) Constitutive IstR-1 expression prevents TisB-dependent depolarization upon weak SOS induction ("repressed" mode). (**b**) Strong SOS induction leads to increased amounts of translationally active *tisB* +42 mRNA, eventually causing depolarization in ~50% of the cells. Depolarization favors persister cell formation ("primed" mode). (**c**) Due to the deletion of both regulatory RNA elements, stochastic SOS induction is sufficient to produce depolarized cells ("stochastic" mode). (**d**) Weak SOS induction strongly triggers depolarization in strain Δ1-41 Δ*istR* and favors persister cell formation ("primed" mode)

gave ~100-fold increased persister levels compared to the wild type (Berghoff et al. 2017a).

Figure 5.2 illustrates how the original *tisB/istR-1* system (wild-type situation) responds to SOS induction compared to the system devoid of both negative regulatory RNA elements (Δ1-41 Δ*istR* situation). Due to tight repression of *tisB* by the inhibitory RNA elements in wild-type cells, weak SOS induction is not sufficient to cause depolarization (Fig. 5.2a). Upon strong SOS induction, ~50% of cells escape RNA-based inhibition and depolarize their membrane (Fig. 5.2b). Since depolarization causes ATP depletion, wild-type cells are now primed for persister formation. In the double deletion strain, the situation is different. Depolarization and persister formation are elevated even without strong SOS induction (Berghoff et al. 2017a). Since stochastic induction of the SOS response occurs in some cells at any time during exponential phase (Pennington and Rosenberg 2007), the double deletion strain is prone to stochastic TisB-dependent depolarization (Fig. 5.2c). Weak SOS induction, by low concentrations of ciprofloxacin (Berghoff et al. 2017a) or by ampicillin (Miller et al. 2004), leads to elevated +42 levels and to an increased number of depolarized cells (Fig. 5.2d). In contrast to the wild type, weak SOS induction is sufficient to prime the double deletion strain for persister formation. Since the wild-type situation is expected to represent the "optimal" solution to control TisB production, the *tisB/istR-1* system appears to have evolved to be silent under conditions of minor environmental stress, whereas TisB-dependent depolarization and persister formation are favored upon strong and enduring stress (Berghoff and Wagner 2017). The same rationale likely applies to many other type I TA systems.

We intend to use the term "primed" for TisB-dependent persister formation because clearly not every depolarized cell turns into a persister. In wild-type cultures, only 0.01–0.02% of the population become TisB-dependent persisters after 6 h of ciprofloxacin treatment, even though ~50% of the cells are depolarized (Berghoff et al. 2017a). Clearly, there are further events that shape the fate of a depolarized cell. Many, if not most, depolarized cells are expected to be killed by the antibiotic before being able to fully pass on to the persistent state. Additionally, many cells might fail to activate further cellular factors that are needed to fully establish the persistent state. As a conclusion, induction of TisB by SOS increases the likelihood of persister formation but does not ultimately determine the fate of the individual cells.

5.7 Possible Mechanisms for Membrane Depolarization by TisB

TisB-dependent persister formation is initiated by depolarization of the inner membrane. A central question concerns the mechanism by which TisB proteins cause collapse of the PMF. TisB is a small amphiphilic protein of 29 amino acids. Circular dichroism experiments and secondary structure predictions suggested that ~22 of the 29 amino acids form a transmembrane α-helix (Steinbrecher et al. 2012). Since the five charged amino acids Asp^5, Lys^{12}, Asp^{22}, Lys^{26}, and Lys^{29} form a polar face (Fig. 5.3a), insertion of TisB into the hydrophobic environment of lipid bilayers would be strongly favored by some kind of oligomeric structure after initial contact of monomers with the inner membrane via hydrophobic interactions (Fig. 5.3b, c). The "charge zipper" model predicts the formation of antiparallel dimers, stabilized by electrostatic interactions between negatively charged aspartate (Asp^5 and Asp^{22}) and positively charged lysine residues (Lys^{12} and Lys^{26}), giving rise to four salt bridges (Fig. 5.3b). Experimental support for the "charge zipper" model comes from dye leakage experiments and coarse-grained molecular dynamics (MD) simulations (Steinbrecher et al. 2012). In contrast to typical pore-forming antimicrobial peptides, pronounced dye leakage was only observed at high TisB concentrations (Steinbrecher et al. 2012). A Hill coefficient of 1.93, calculated from the dye leakage experiments, suggested that TisB acts as a dimer. MD simulations suggested the formation of stable antiparallel dimers in model lipid bilayers (Steinbrecher et al. 2012). Hypothetically, the intermolecular salt bridges between the positively and

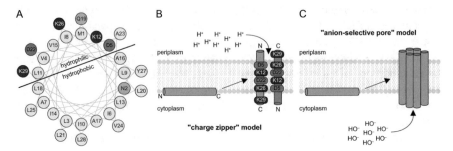

Fig. 5.3 Current models on TisB-dependent depolarization of the inner membrane. (**a**) Helical wheel projection of toxin TisB illustrating the positions of all 29 amino acids in the α-helix. Hydrophobic side chains (yellow); polar residues (light blue); positively charged residues (dark blue); negatively charged residues (red). Hydrophilic and hydrophobic sites of the α-helix are indicated. (**b**) "Charge zipper" model for the action of TisB. Upon alignment of TisB monomers with the inner membrane, formation of antiparallel dimers is supported by at least four intermolecular salt bridges between positively and negatively charged amino acid residues. Protons traverse the inner membrane along a wire of water molecules inside the TisB channels [based on (Steinbrecher et al. 2012)]. (**c**) "Anion-selective model" for the action of TisB. Upon initial alignment of TisB monomers, narrow pores are formed through which hydroxyl anions migrate across the membrane. Anions are selected by the +1 net charge of TisB [based on (Gurnev et al. 2012)]

negatively charged amino acid residues both stabilize dimer formation and explain collapse of the PMF (Fig. 5.3b). Driven by the electrochemical gradient, protons might pass the lipid bilayer along a wire of water molecules inside the TisB channel (Steinbrecher et al. 2012; Walther et al. 2013). Since in vivo experiments are still lacking, the "charge zipper" model remains to be demonstrated in its appropriate cellular environment.

An alternative model stems from in vitro experiments with black lipid membranes. Planar membranes of diphytanoyl-phosphatidylcholine were applied to conductance measurements after TisB pore formation (Gurnev et al. 2012). In this setup, TisB pores were selective for anions. Changing the net charge of TisB from +1 (wild-type TisB) to zero (TisB K26A) decreased the selectivity for anions, as expected. By probing polyethylene glycols (PEGs) with varying molecular weights as pore blockers, the authors concluded that TisB forms narrow pores within lipid bilayers, and that the net charge of +1 favors anion selectivity of the pores. In this model, hydroxyl anions migrate from the cytoplasm to the periplasm through TisB pores, leading to collapse of the PMF (Fig. 5.3c). The "charge zipper" and "anion-selective pore" models are very different in their predictions, and clearly, in vivo experiments are needed to confirm the mechanism by which TisB depolarizes bacterial membranes.

It is worthwhile to compare TisB to the type I toxin HokB, which is activated in an Obg-dependent manner, leading to depolarization and persistence in *E. coli* (Verstraeten et al. 2015). Conductance measurements of HokB pores in planar lipid bilayers suggested that a high membrane potential favors the formation of mature pores with an effective radius of ~0.59 nm in synthetic membranes and ~0.64 nm in natural membranes (Wilmaerts et al. 2018). Since the estimated pore size is ~0.15 nm for TisB (Gurnev et al. 2012), HokB pores are larger and capable of causing ATP leakage in vivo, which has been linked to persister formation (Wilmaerts et al. 2018). Interestingly, the high membrane potential in the in vitro model for TisB causes multiple TisB pores to be organized in honeycomb-like aggregates (Gurnev et al. 2012), rather than increasing the pore radius as observed for HokB (Wilmaerts et al. 2018). It seems that different type I toxins form pores of varying sizes, and this determines whether ions (narrow pores) or small molecules like ATP (bigger pores) traverse the membrane. The outcome, however, is similar: intracellular ATP levels are depleted to favor persister formation.

5.8 Outlook

Our current knowledge on the *tisB/istR-1* system with regard to persistence stems from work on the model bacterium *E. coli*, mainly non-pathogenic K-12 wild-type MG1655. The *tisB/istR* locus is, however, well conserved among pathogenic *E. coli* strains (e.g., shiga toxin-producing strain O157:H7; 99% identity), among diverse *Shigella* species (e.g., *Shigella dysenteriae* and *Shigella flexneri*; 99% identity), and in *Salmonella* Typhimurium (86% identity). Formation of persister cells is a valuable strategy of pathogenic bacteria to survive defense mechanisms of their hosts and withstand antibiotic therapy (Lewis 2007; Van den Bergh et al. 2017). It remains an intriguing question to which extent the *tisB/istR-1* system contributes to the long-term survival of pathogenic enterobacteria within their hosts. Deletion of *tisB* in *Salmonella* Typhimurium might reduce persister frequency in macrophages, as it was observed for type II TA systems (Helaine et al. 2014). Macrophages produce reactive oxygen species (ROS) during the so-called "respiratory burst" to kill internalized bacteria. Since ROS have the potential to damage DNA and, hence, activate the SOS response (Imlay and Linn 1987; Goerlich et al. 1989), it is tempting to speculate that *tisB* transcription is triggered in macrophages, ultimately resulting in TisB-dependent depolarization and persister formation. This remains to be tested in the future.

In order to repopulate their environments, and eventually cause relapsing infections in case of pathogens, bacteria have to leave the persistent state, a process called awakening. Across all TA systems linked to persisters, there is a surprising paucity of information on this event. Awakening must depend on mechanisms that inhibit the toxins and/or reverse the toxin-dependent, growth-arresting effects. In type II TA systems, "conditional cooperativity" allows for replenishing of the antitoxin pool and, hence, inhibition of toxin activity on the protein level (Chan et al. 2016; Page and Peti 2016). In the *tisB/istR-1* system (type I), replenishing the IstR-1 pool would curtail further toxin production but fail to inhibit the action of TisB proteins already in the inner membrane. To achieve recovery, cells might degrade TisB proteins or inactivate TisB pores. Possibly, cells could reverse TisB toxicity. In *Salmonella*

Typhimurium, the acetylation of tRNAs by toxin TacT is reversed by a peptidyl-tRNA hydrolase to facilitate awakening (Cheverton et al. 2016). Similarly, TisB-producing cells could repolarize their membranes to reverse toxicity. Alternatively, remodeling of the energy metabolism, to gain substantial amounts of ATP by substrate-level phosphorylation, might override the growth-inhibiting effect of TisB-dependent ATP depletion. As soon as cell division is restarted, TisB is diluted out and new TisB production repressed by IstR-1. Understanding the process of awakening is fundamental to the persister phenomenon, and might help to develop treatments for chronic infections caused by persister cells.

Acknowledgements We acknowledge support from The Swedish Research Council (to E.G.H. Wagner) and the DFG Priority Program SPP2002 *Small Proteins in Prokaryotes, an Unexplored World* (to B.A. Berghoff). We thank Erik Holmqvist and Alisa Rizvanovic (Uppsala University) for critical reading of the manuscript.

References

Aldred, K. J., Kerns, R. J., & Osheroff, N. (2014). Mechanism of quinolone action and resistance. *Biochemistry, 53*, 1565–1574. https://doi.org/10.1021/bi5000564.

Amitai, S., Yassin, Y., & Engelberg-Kulka, H. (2004). MazF-mediated cell death in *Escherichia coli*: A point of no return. *Journal of Bacteriology, 186*, 8295–8300. https://doi.org/10.1128/JB.186.24.8295-8300.2004.

Arnion, H., Korkut, D. N., Masachis Gelo, S., Chabas, S., Reignier, J., Iost, I., & Darfeuille, F. (2017). Mechanistic insights into type I toxin antitoxin systems in *Helicobacter pylori*: The importance of mRNA folding in controlling toxin expression. *Nucleic Acids Research, 45*, 4782–4795. https://doi.org/10.1093/nar/gkw1343.

Balaban, N. Q., Merrin, J., Chait, R., Kowalik, L., & Leibler, S. (2004). Bacterial persistence as a phenotypic switch. *Science, 305*, 1622–1625. https://doi.org/10.1126/science.1099390.

Barker, M. M., Gaal, T., & Gourse, R. L. (2001). Mechanism of regulation of transcription initiation by ppGpp. II. Models for positive control based on properties of RNAP mutants and competition for RNAP. *Journal of Molecular Biology, 305*, 689–702. https://doi.org/10.1006/JMBI.2000.4328.

Bayles, K. W. (2000). The bactericidal action of penicillin: New clues to an unsolved mystery. *Trends in Microbiology, 8*, 274–278.

Berghoff, B. A., & Wagner, E. G. H. (2017). RNA-based regulation in type I toxin–antitoxin systems and its implication for bacterial persistence. *Current Genetics, 63*, 1011–1016. https://doi.org/10.1007/s00294-017-0710-y.

Berghoff, B. A., Hoekzema, M., Aulbach, L., & Wagner, E. G. H. (2017a). Two regulatory RNA elements affect TisB-dependent depolarization and persister formation. *Molecular Microbiology, 103*, 1020–1033. https://doi.org/10.1111/mmi.13607.

Berghoff, B. A., Karlsson, T., Källman, T., Wagner, E. G. H., & Grabherr, M. G. (2017b). RNA-sequence data normalization through in silico prediction of reference genes: The bacterial response to DNA damage as case study. *BioData Mining, 10*, 30. https://doi.org/10.1186/s13040-017-0150-8.

Brauner, A., Fridman, O., Gefen, O., & Balaban, N. Q. (2016). Distinguishing between resistance, tolerance and persistence to antibiotic treatment. *Nature Reviews Microbiology, 14*, 320–330.

Chan, W. T., Espinosa, M., & Yeo, C. C. (2016). Keeping the wolves at bay: Antitoxins of prokaryotic type II toxin-antitoxin systems. *Frontiers in Molecular Biosciences, 3*, 9. https://doi.org/10.3389/fmolb.2016.00009.

Cheverton, A. M., Gollan, B., Przydacz, M., Wong, C. T., Mylona, A., Hare, S. A., & Helaine, S. (2016). A *Salmonella* toxin promotes persister formation through acetylation of tRNA. *Molecular Cell, 63*, 86–96. https://doi.org/10.1016/j.molcel.2016.05.002.

Conlon, B. P., Rowe, S. E., Gandt, A. B., Nuxoll, A. S., Donegan, N. P., Zalis, E. A., Clair, G., Adkins, J. N., Cheung, A. L., & Lewis, K. (2016). Persister formation in *Staphylococcus aureus* is associated with ATP depletion. *Nature Microbiology, 1*, 16051. https://doi.org/10.1038/nmicrobiol.2016.51.

Courcelle, J., Khodursky, A., Peter, B., Brown, P. O., & Hanawalt, P. C. (2001). Comparative gene expression profiles following UV exposure in wild-type and SOS-deficient *Escherichia coli*. *Genetics, 158*, 41–64.

Darfeuille, F., Unoson, C., Vogel, J., & Wagner, E. G. H. (2007). An antisense RNA inhibits translation by competing with standby ribosomes. *Molecular Cell, 26*, 381–392. https://doi.org/10.1016/j.molcel.2007.04.003.

de Smit, M. H., & van Duin, J. (1993). Translational initiation at the coat-protein gene of phage MS2: Native upstream RNA relieves inhibition by local secondary structure. *Molecular Microbiology, 9*, 1079–1088.

de Smit, M. H., & van Duin, J. (1994). Translational initiation on structured messengers. Another role for the Shine-Dalgarno interaction. *Journal of Molecular Biology, 235*, 173–184.

de Smit, M. H., & van Duin, J. (2003). Translational standby sites: How ribosomes may deal with the rapid folding kinetics of mRNA. *Journal of Molecular Biology, 331*, 737–743.

Dörr, T., Lewis, K., & Vulic, M. (2009). SOS response induces persistence to fluoroquinolones in *Escherichia coli*. *PLoS Genetics, 5*, e1000760. https://doi.org/10.1371/journal.pgen.1000760.

Dörr, T., Vulic, M., & Lewis, K. (2010). Ciprofloxacin causes persister formation by inducing the TisB toxin in *Escherichia coli*. *PLoS Biology, 8*, e1000317. https://doi.org/10.1371/journal.pbio.1000317.

Fernandez De Henestrosa, A. R., Ogi, T., Aoyagi, S., Chafin, D., Hayes, J. J., Ohmori, H., & Woodgate, R. (2000). Identification of additional genes belonging to the LexA regulon in *Escherichia coli*. *Molecular Microbiology, 35*, 1560–1572. https://doi.org/10.1046/j.1365-2958.2000.01826.x.

Fozo, E. M., Kawano, M., Fontaine, F., Kaya, Y., Mendieta, K. S., Jones, K. L., Ocampo, A., Rudd, K. E., & Storz, G. (2008). Repression of small toxic protein synthesis by the Sib and OhsC small RNAs. *Molecular Microbiology, 70*, 1076–1093. https://doi.org/10.1111/j.1365-2958.2008.06394.x.

Franch, T., Petersen, M., Wagner, E. G., Jacobsen, J. P., & Gerdes, K. (1999). Antisense RNA regulation in prokaryotes: Rapid RNA/RNA interaction facilitated by a general U-turn loop structure. *Journal of Molecular Biology, 294*, 1115–1125. https://doi.org/10.1006/jmbi.1999.3306.

Garcia-Pino, A., De Gieter, S., Talavera, A., De Greve, H., Efremov, R. G., & Loris, R. (2016). An intrinsically disordered entropic switch determines allostery in Phd-Doc regulation. *Nature Chemical Biology, 12*, 490–496. https://doi.org/10.1038/nchembio.2078.

Gerdes, K., & Wagner, E. G. H. (2007). RNA antitoxins. *Current Opinion in Microbiology, 10*, 117–124. https://doi.org/10.1016/j.mib.2007.03.003.

Gerdes, K., Bech, F. W., Jørgensen, S. T., Løbner-Olesen, A., Rasmussen, P. B., Atlung, T., Boe, L., Karlstrom, O., Molin, S., & von Meyenburg, K. (1986a). Mechanism of postsegregational killing by the hok gene product of the *parB* system of plasmid R1 and its homology with the *relF* gene product of the *E. coli relB* operon. *The EMBO Journal, 5*, 2023–2029.

Gerdes, K., Rasmussen, P. B., & Molin, S. (1986b). Unique type of plasmid maintenance function: Postsegregational killing of plasmid-free cells. *Proceedings of the National Academy of Sciences of the United States of America, 83*, 3116–3120.

Gerdes, K., Nielsen, A., Thorsted, P., & Wagner, E. G. (1992). Mechanism of killer gene activation. Antisense RNA-dependent RNase III cleavage ensures rapid turn-over of the stable *hok*, *srnB* and *pndA* effector messenger RNAs. *Journal of Molecular Biology, 226*, 637–649.

Germain, E., Castro-Roa, D., Zenkin, N., & Gerdes, K. (2013). Molecular mechanism of bacterial persistence by HipA. *Molecular Cell, 52*, 248–254. https://doi.org/10.1016/j.molcel.2013.08.045.

Goerlich, O., Quillardet, P., & Hofnung, M. (1989). Induction of the SOS response by hydrogen peroxide in various *Escherichia coli* mutants with altered protection against oxidative DNA damage. *Journal of Bacteriology, 171*, 6141–6147.

Golding, I., Paulsson, J., Zawilski, S. M., & Cox, E. C. (2005). Real-time kinetics of gene activity in individual bacteria. *Cell, 123*, 1025–1036. https://doi.org/10.1016/j.cell.2005.09.031.

Goormaghtigh, F., Fraikin, N., Putrinš, M., Hallaert, T., Hauryliuk, V., Garcia-Pino, A., Sjödin, A., Kasvandik, S., Udekwu, K., Tenson, T., Kaldalu, N., & Van Melderen, L. (2018). Reassessing the role of type II toxin-antitoxin systems in formation of *Escherichia coli* type ii persister cells. *MBio, 9*, e00640–e00618. https://doi.org/10.1128/mBio.00640-18.

Gotfredsen, M., & Gerdes, K. (1998). The *Escherichia coli relBE* genes belong to a new toxin-antitoxin gene family. *Molecular Microbiology, 29*, 1065–1076.

Gurnev, P. A., Ortenberg, R., Dörr, T., Lewis, K., & Bezrukov, S. M. (2012). Persister-promoting bacterial toxin TisB produces anion-selective pores in planar lipid bilayers. *FEBS Letters, 586*, 2529–2534. https://doi.org/10.1016/j.febslet.2012.06.021.

Harms, A., Fino, C., Sørensen, M. A., Semsey, S., & Gerdes, K. (2017). Prophages and growth dynamics confound experimental results with antibiotic-tolerant persister cells. *MBio, 8*, e01964–e01917. https://doi.org/10.1128/mBio.01964-17.

Harms, A., Brodersen, D. E., Mitarai, N., & Gerdes, K. (2018). Toxins, targets, and triggers: An overview of toxin-antitoxin biology. *Molecular Cell, 70*, 768–784. https://doi.org/10.1016/j.molcel.2018.01.003.

Harrison, J. J., Wade, W. D., Akierman, S., Vacchi-Suzzi, C., Stremick, C. A., Turner, R. J., & Ceri, H. (2009). The chromosomal toxin gene *yafQ* is a determinant of multidrug tolerance for *Escherichia coli* growing in a biofilm. *Antimicrobial Agents and Chemotherapy, 53*, 2253–2258. https://doi.org/10.1128/AAC.00043-09.

Hayes, F., & Van Melderen, L. (2011). Toxins-antitoxins: Diversity, evolution and function. *Critical Reviews in Biochemistry and Molecular Biology, 46*, 386–408. https://doi.org/10.3109/10409238.2011.600437.

Helaine, S., Cheverton, A. M., Watson, K. G., Faure, L. M., Matthews, S. A., & Holden, D. W. (2014). Internalization of *Salmonella* by macrophages induces formation of nonreplicating persisters. *Science, 343*, 204–208. https://doi.org/10.1126/science.1244705.

Imlay, J. A., & Linn, S. (1987). Mutagenesis and stress responses induced in *Escherichia coli* by hydrogen peroxide. *Journal of Bacteriology, 169*, 2967–2976.

Jahn, N., & Brantl, S. (2016). Heat-shock-induced refolding entails rapid degradation of *bsrG* toxin mRNA by RNases Y and J1. *Microbiology, 162*, 590–599. https://doi.org/10.1099/mic.0.000247.

Kawano, M., Aravind, L., & Storz, G. (2007). An antisense RNA controls synthesis of an SOS-induced toxin evolved from an antitoxin. *Molecular Microbiology, 64*, 738–754. https://doi.org/10.1111/j.1365-2958.2007.05688.x.

Keren, I., Shah, D., Spoering, A., Kaldalu, N., & Lewis, K. (2004). Specialized persister cells and the mechanism of multidrug tolerance in *Escherichia coli*. *Journal of Bacteriology, 186*, 8172–8180. https://doi.org/10.1128/JB.186.24.8172-8180.2004.

Kim, J.-S., & Wood, T. K. (2016). Persistent persister misperceptions. *Frontiers in Microbiology, 7*, 2134. https://doi.org/10.3389/fmicb.2016.02134.

Kreuzer, K. N. (2013). DNA damage responses in prokaryotes: Regulating gene expression, modulating growth patterns, and manipulating replication forks. *Cold Spring Harbor Perspectives in Biology, 5*, a012674. https://doi.org/10.1101/cshperspect.a012674.

Kristiansen, K. I., Weel-Sneve, R., Booth, J. A., & Bjørås, M. (2016). Mutually exclusive RNA secondary structures regulate translation initiation of DinQ in *Escherichia coli*. *RNA, 22*, 1739–1749. https://doi.org/10.1261/rna.058461.116.

Kwan, B. W., Valenta, J. A., Benedik, M. J., & Wood, T. K. (2013). Arrested protein synthesis increases persister-like cell formation. *Antimicrobial Agents and Chemotherapy, 57*, 1468–1473. https://doi.org/10.1128/AAC.02135-12.

Lewis, K. (2007). Persister cells, dormancy and infectious disease. *Nature Reviews. Microbiology, 5*, 48–56. https://doi.org/10.1038/nrmicro1557.

Lewis, L., Harlow, G. R., Gregg-Jolly, L. A., & Mount, D. W. (1994). Identification of high affinity binding sites for LexA which define new DNA damage-inducible genes in *Escherichia coli*. *Journal of Molecular Biology, 241*, 507–523. https://doi.org/10.1006/jmbi.1994.1528.

Little, J. W. (1991). Mechanism of specific LexA cleavage: Autodigestion and the role of RecA coprotease. *Biochimie, 73*, 411–422. https://doi.org/10.1016/0300-9084(91)90108-D.

Miller, C., Thomsen, L. E., Gaggero, C., Mosseri, R., Ingmer, H., & Cohen, S. N. (2004). SOS response induction by beta-lactams and bacterial defense against antibiotic lethality. *Science, 305*, 1629–1631. https://doi.org/10.1126/science.1101630.

Moyed, H. S., & Bertrand, K. P. (1983). *hipA*, a newly recognized gene of *Escherichia coli* K-12 that affects frequency of persistence after inhibition of murein synthesis. *Journal of Bacteriology, 155*, 768–775.

Neubauer, C., Gao, Y.-G., Andersen, K. R., Dunham, C. M., Kelley, A. C., Hentschel, J., Gerdes, K., Ramakrishnan, V., & Brodersen, D. E. (2009). The structural basis for mRNA recognition and cleavage by the ribosome-dependent endonuclease RelE. *Cell, 139*, 1084–1095. https://doi.org/10.1016/j.cell.2009.11.015.

Orman, M. A., & Brynildsen, M. P. (2013). Dormancy is not necessary or sufficient for bacterial persistence. *Antimicrobial Agents and Chemotherapy, 57*, 3230–3239. https://doi.org/10.1128/AAC.00243-13.

Overgaard, M., Borch, J., Jørgensen, M. G., & Gerdes, K. (2008). Messenger RNA interferase RelE controls *relBE* transcription by conditional cooperativity. *Molecular Microbiology, 69*, 841–857. https://doi.org/10.1111/j.1365-2958.2008.06313.x.

Page, R., & Peti, W. (2016). Toxin-antitoxin systems in bacterial growth arrest and persistence. *Nature Chemical Biology, 12*, 208–214. https://doi.org/10.1038/nchembio.2044.

Paul, B. J., Barker, M. M., Ross, W., Schneider, D. A., Webb, C., Foster, J. W., & Gourse, R. L. (2004). DksA: A critical component of the transcription initiation machinery that potentiates the regulation of rRNA promoters by ppGpp and the initiating NTP. *Cell, 118*(3), 311–322. https://doi.org/10.1016/j.cell.2004.07.009.

Pennington, J. M., & Rosenberg, S. M. (2007). Spontaneous DNA breakage in single living *Escherichia coli* cells. *Nature Genetics, 39*, 797–802. https://doi.org/10.1038/ng2051.

Pu, Y., Zhao, Z., Li, Y., Zou, J., Ma, Q., Zhao, Y., Ke, Y., Zhu, Y., Chen, H., Baker, M. A. B., Ge, H., Sun, Y., Xie, X. S., & Bai, F. (2016). Enhanced efflux activity facilitates drug tolerance in dormant bacterial cells. *Molecular Cell, 62*, 284–294. https://doi.org/10.1016/j.molcel.2016.03.035.

Radzikowski, J. L., Vedelaar, S., Siegel, D., Ortega, Á. D., Schmidt, A., & Heinemann, M. (2016). Bacterial persistence is an active σS stress response to metabolic flux limitation. *Molecular Systems Biology, 12*, 882. https://doi.org/10.15252/msb.20166998.

Romilly, C., Deindl, S., & Wagner, E. G. H. (2019). The ribosomal protein S1-dependent standby site in tisB mRNA consists of a single-stranded region and a 5' structure element. *Proceedings of the National Academy of Sciences of the United States of America, 116*, 15901–15906. https://doi.org/10.1073/pnas.1904309116

Ronneau, S., & Helaine, S. (2019) Clarifying the Link between Toxin-Antitoxin Modules and Bacterial Persistence. *Journal of Molecular Biology, 431*, 3462–3471. https://doi.org/10.1016/j.jmb.2019.03.019

Rycroft, J. A., Gollan, B., Grabe, G. J., Hall, A., Cheverton, A. M., Larrouy-Maumus, G., Hare, S. A., & Helaine, S. (2018). Activity of acetyltransferase toxins involved in *Salmonella* persister formation during macrophage infection. *Nature Communications, 9*, 1993. https://doi.org/10.1038/s41467-018-04472-6.

Schneider, D. A., Gaal, T., & Gourse, R. L. (2002). NTP-sensing by rRNA promoters in *Escherichia coli* is direct. *Proceedings of the National Academy of Sciences of the United States of America, 99*, 8602–8607. https://doi.org/10.1073/pnas.132285199.

Shah, D., Zhang, Z., Khodursky, A., Kaldalu, N., Kurg, K., & Lewis, K. (2006). Persisters: A distinct physiological state of *E. coli*. *BMC Microbiology, 6*, 53. https://doi.org/10.1186/1471-2180-6-53.

Shan, Y., Brown Gandt, A., Rowe, S. E., Deisinger, J. P., Conlon, B. P., & Lewis, K. (2017). ATP-dependent persister formation in *Escherichia coli*. *MBio, 8*, e02267–e02216. https://doi.org/10.1128/mBio.02267-16.

Sharma, C. M., Hoffmann, S., Darfeuille, F., Reignier, J., Findeiß, S., Sittka, A., Chabas, S., Reiche, K., Hackermüller, J., Reinhardt, R., Stadler, P. F., & Vogel, J. (2010). The primary transcriptome of the major human pathogen *Helicobacter pylori*. *Nature, 464*, 250–255. https://doi.org/10.1038/nature08756.

Song, S., & Wood, T. K. (2018). Post-segregational killing and phage inhibition are not mediated by cell death through toxin/antitoxin systems. *Frontiers in Microbiology, 9*, 814. https://doi.org/10.3389/fmicb.2018.00814.

Stapels, D. A. C., Hill, P. W. S., Westermann, A. J., Fisher, R. A., Thurston, T. L., Saliba, A.-E., Blommestein, I., Vogel, J., & Helaine, S. (2018). *Salmonella* persisters undermine host immune defenses during antibiotic treatment. *Science, 362*, 1156–1160. https://doi.org/10.1126/science.aat7148.

Steinbrecher, T., Prock, S., Reichert, J., Wadhwani, P., Zimpfer, B., Bürck, J., Berditsch, M., Elstner, M., & Ulrich, A. S. (2012). Peptide-lipid interactions of the stress-response peptide TisB that induces bacterial persistence. *Biophysical Journal, 103*, 1460–1469. https://doi.org/10.1016/j.bpj.2012.07.060.

Sterk, M., Romilly, C., & Wagner, E. G. H. (2018). Unstructured 5′-tails act through ribosome standby to override inhibitory structure at ribosome binding sites. *Nucleic Acids Research, 46*, 4188–4199. https://doi.org/10.1093/nar/gky073.

Thisted, T., & Gerdes, K. (1992). Mechanism of post-segregational killing by the *hok/sok* system of plasmid R1. Sok antisense RNA regulates *hok* gene expression indirectly through the overlapping *mok* gene. *Journal of Molecular Biology, 223*, 41–54. https://doi.org/10.1016/0022-2836(92)90714-U.

Thisted, T., Sørensen, N. S., & Gerdes, K. (1995). Mechanism of post-segregational killing: Secondary structure analysis of the entire Hok mRNA from plasmid R1 suggests a fold-back structure that prevents translation and antisense RNA binding. *Journal of Molecular Biology, 247*, 859–873. https://doi.org/10.1006/JMBI.1995.0186.

Tuomanen, E., Cozens, R., Tosch, W., Zak, O., & Tomasz, A. (1986). The rate of killing of *Escherichia coli* by beta-lactam antibiotics is strictly proportional to the rate of bacterial growth. *Journal of General Microbiology, 132*, 1297–1304. https://doi.org/10.1099/00221287-132-5-1297.

Unoson, C., & Wagner, E. G. H. (2008). A small SOS-induced toxin is targeted against the inner membrane in *Escherichia coli*. *Molecular Microbiology, 70*, 258–270. https://doi.org/10.1111/j.1365-2958.2008.06416.x.

Van den Bergh, B., Fauvart, M., & Michiels, J. (2017). Formation, physiology, ecology, evolution and clinical importance of bacterial persisters. *FEMS Microbiology Reviews, 41*, 219–251. https://doi.org/10.1093/femsre/fux001.

Van Melderen, L., & Wood, T. K. (2017). Commentary: What is the link between stringent response, endoribonuclease encoding type ii toxin-antitoxin systems and persistence? *Frontiers in Microbiology, 8*, 191. https://doi.org/10.3389/fmicb.2017.00191.

Veening, J.-W., Smits, W. K., & Kuipers, O. P. (2008). Bistability, epigenetics, and bet-hedging in bacteria. *Annual Review of Microbiology, 62*, 193–210. https://doi.org/10.1146/annurev.micro.62.081307.163002.

Verstraeten, N., Knapen, W. J., Kint, C. I., Liebens, V., Van den Bergh, B., Dewachter, L., Michiels, J. E., Fu, Q., David, C. C., Fierro, A. C., Marchal, K., Beirlant, J., Versées, W., Hofkens, J., Jansen, M., Fauvart, M., & Michiels, J. (2015). Obg and membrane depolarization are part of a microbial bet-hedging strategy that leads to antibiotic tolerance. *Molecular Cell, 59*, 9–21. https://doi.org/10.1016/j.molcel.2015.05.011.

Vogel, J., Argaman, L., Wagner, E. G. H., & Altuvia, S. (2004). The small RNA IstR inhibits synthesis of an SOS-induced toxic peptide. *Current Biology, 14*, 2271–2276. https://doi.org/10.1016/j.cub.2004.12.003.

Wagner, E. G. H., & Unoson, C. (2012). The toxin-antitoxin system *tisB-istR1*: Expression, regulation, and biological role in persister phenotypes. *RNA Biology, 9*, 1513–1519. https://doi.org/10.4161/rna.22578.

Walther, T. H., Gottselig, C., Grage, S. L., Wolf, M., Vargiu, A. V., Klein, M. J., Vollmer, S., Prock, S., Hartmann, M., Afonin, S., Stockwald, E., Heinzmann, H., Nolandt, O. V., Wenzel, W., Ruggerone, P., & Ulrich, A. S. (2013). Folding and self-assembly of the TatA translocation pore based on a charge zipper mechanism. *Cell, 152*, 316–326. https://doi.org/10.1016/j.cell.2012.12.017.

Weel-Sneve, R., Kristiansen, K. I., Odsbu, I., Dalhus, B., Booth, J., Rognes, T., Skarstad, K., & Bjørås, M. (2013). Single transmembrane peptide DinQ modulates membrane-dependent activities. *PLoS Genetics, 9*, e1003260. https://doi.org/10.1371/journal.pgen.1003260.

Wen, J., Won, D., & Fozo, E. M. (2014). The ZorO-OrzO type i toxin-Antitoxin locus: Repression by the OrzO antitoxin. *Nucleic Acids Research, 42*, 1930–1946. https://doi.org/10.1093/nar/gkt1018.

Wen, J., Harp, J. R., & Fozo, E. M. (2016). The 5' UTR of the type I toxin ZorO can both inhibit and enhance translation. *Nucleic Acids Research*, 1–15. https://doi.org/10.1093/nar/gkw1172.

Wilmaerts, D., Bayoumi, M., Dewachter, L., Knapen, W., Mika, J. T., Hofkens, J., Dedecker, P., Maglia, G., Verstraeten, N., & Michiels, J. (2018). The persistence-inducing toxin HokB forms dynamic pores that cause ATP leakage. *MBio, 9*, e00744–e00718. https://doi.org/10.1128/mBio.

Yamaguchi, Y., Park, J.-H., & Inouye, M. (2009). MqsR, a crucial regulator for quorum sensing and biofilm formation, is a GCU-specific mRNA interferase in Escherichia coli. *The Journal of Biological Chemistry, 284*, 28746–28753. https://doi.org/10.1074/jbc.M109.032904.

Zhang, Y., Zhang, J., Hoeflich, K. P., Ikura, M., Qing, G., & Inouye, M. (2003). MazF cleaves cellular mRNAs specifically at ACA to block protein synthesis in *Escherichia coli*. *Molecular Cell, 12*, 913–923. https://doi.org/10.1016/S1097-2765(03)00402-7.

Chapter 6
Nutrient Depletion and Bacterial Persistence

Wendy W. K. Mok and Mark P. Brynildsen

Abstract Most antibiotics do not work well on starving bacteria. In environments that are missing one or more essential nutrient, bacteria shut down the growth-related processes that most antibiotics target and ready themselves for stressful times. Such nutrient-depleted conditions can occur within a host, and they are prevalent within biofilms. For antibiotics that retain some bactericidal activity against starved populations, treatments of those cultures often leave many persisters, which can go on to spawn new populations. Persisters are bacterial cells with non-inherited abilities to survive antibiotic treatments that kill the majority of their genetically identical kin. The capacity of persisters to tolerate such treatments originates from phenotypic differences between them and the bacteria that die, and understanding those survival mechanisms promises to improve treatments for chronic and recurring infections. Here we review knowledge of bacterial starvation physiology and provide an overview of nutritional challenges bacteria face in the host and in biofilms. We then describe those antibiotic classes with the capacity to kill nutrient-deprived bacteria and summarize understanding of persistence in those populations. Finally, we discuss approaches that could be used to develop treatments that eradicate starved bacterial populations and the persisters within them.

6.1 Introduction

Bacterial persistence is intimately linked to metabolism, and the nutrient environment present before, during, and after antibiotic treatment is instrumental to this extreme form of tolerance (Amato et al. 2013, 2014; Radzikowski et al. 2016, 2017).

W. W. K. Mok (✉)
Department of Chemical and Biological Engineering, Princeton University, Princeton, NJ, USA

Department of Molecular Biology and Biophysics, UConn Health, Farmington, CT, USA
e-mail: mok@uchc.edu

M. P. Brynildsen (✉)
Department of Chemical and Biological Engineering, Princeton University, Princeton, NJ, USA
e-mail: mbrynild@princeton.edu

In response to nutrient depletion, bacteria execute a myriad of metabolic, transcriptional, translational, and morphological changes, which cease growth and augment their ability to cope with various stresses, including those brought on by antibiotic treatment (Siegele and Kolter 1992; Nystrom 2004). Upon entering the host, nutrient limitation is a common stress pathogens experience, as host anatomy, its response to infection, and endogenous microbiomes can restrict nutrient availability at infection sites (Appelberg 2006; Belkaid and Segre 2014; Alteri and Mobley 2012; Brooks and Keevil 1997; Pereira and Berry 2017). Pathogens can further assemble into multicellular aggregates known as biofilms, which can develop nutrient gradients and pockets of starvation (De Beer et al. 1994; Folsom et al. 2010; Stewart 2003; Stewart and Franklin 2008; Stewart et al. 2016). Given that the majority of antibiotics available today were selected for their ability to target biosynthetic processes that bacteria rely on to produce biomass (Walsh 2003; Walsh and Wencewicz 2014), most drugs in our inventory are ineffective at eradicating starved pathogens (Hu and Coates 2012), which makes infections involving nutrient-depleted bacterial populations difficult to treat.

In the laboratory setting, the recalcitrance of nutrient-depleted cultures to existing antibiotics is demonstrated by an increase, often by orders of magnitude, in bacterial survival (Eng et al. 1991; Fung et al. 2010). For antibiotics that retain some activity against starved bacteria, persisters complicate treatments because of their high abundances. This higher proportion of persisters in starved cultures compared to their exponentially growing counterparts has been observed with diverse bacterial species treated with distinct classes of antibiotics, which target different cellular processes (Keren et al. 2004; Sharma et al. 2015; Van Den Bergh et al. 2016; Verstraeten et al. 2015; Volzing and Brynildsen 2015). In the clinical realm, colonization of *Mycobacterium tuberculosis* in stressful and nutrient-deprived host sites, such as granulomas and activated macrophages, has been proposed to contribute to persistent infections (Evangelopoulos et al. 2015; Gengenbacher and Kaufmann 2012). Analogously, nutrient limitation and reduction in cellular metabolism have also been linked to chronic and relapsing infections in patients with other pathogens, including *Escherichia coli*, *Staphylococcus aureus*, and *Pseudomonas aeruginosa* (Meylan et al. 2018). These examples highlight the serious threat that nutrient-deprived pathogens pose to the success of antibiotic treatments.

In this chapter, we focus on starved bacterial populations and the persisters that are contained within them. We begin by summarizing the physiological responses of bacteria to starvation and discussing how host niches and biofilms can deprive bacteria of nutrients. We then provide an overview of existing antimicrobial compounds that retain activity against nutrient-deprived bacteria and discuss mechanisms that enable persisters in those populations to survive treatment. We conclude by highlighting research aimed at eradicating starved bacterial populations, which can improve the chances of achieving durable cures for chronic infections.

6.2 Nutrient-Depleted Physiology of Bacteria

The major elemental constituents of biomass are carbon, hydrogen, oxygen, and nitrogen, and if the composition of *E. coli* were expressed as a carbon-normalized chemical formula it would approximately be $CH_{1.8}O_{0.5}N_{0.25}$ (Stephanopoulos et al. 1998). Additional elements, such as phosphorous, sulfur, iron, and magnesium to name a few, are also present in biomass, though at lower abundances (Feist et al. 2007). Bacterial growth requires the elements of biomass in forms that can be catabolized to generate energy and the metabolic building blocks that anabolism transforms into new cells. The absence of such essential nutrients prevent growth and lead to a multitude of physiological changes that can influence the capacity of bacteria to cope with toxic stresses, such as antibiotics (Eng et al. 1991; Jenkins et al. 1988; Fung et al. 2010). Such changes include those that are shared between different starved states, and thus reflect modifications that occur due to growth arrest, whereas others depend on the identity of the depleted nutrient, which illustrates that starvation is context dependent (Ballesteros et al. 2001; Brauer et al. 2006; Chubukov and Sauer 2014; Groat et al. 1986; Peterson et al. 2005). Here we will summarize several of the major changes associated with metabolism, transcription, and translation under starvation, and discuss how bacteria change their morphology and subsist on the products of self-digestion. We note that shared and distinct mechanisms to cope with nutrient depletion are used by different bacteria (Bergkessel et al. 2016; Chubukov and Sauer 2014; O'Neal et al. 1994; Watson et al. 1998), and to provide a cohesive portrait of these physiological states, we will focus this section on *E. coli*.

6.2.1 Metabolic Adjustments to Nutrient Depletion

Under carbon starvation, which is usually achieved experimentally with glucose deprivation, *E. coli* synthesizes the well-known regulatory metabolites cyclic AMP (cAMP) and guanosine $3',5'$-bispyrophosphate (ppGpp) (Metzger et al. 1989; Notley-Mcrobb et al. 1997; Xiao et al. 1991). Increases in phosphoenolpyruvate (PEP) and decreases in fructose 1,6-bisphosphate (FBP), which both can be over an order of magnitude, have also been observed (Brauer et al. 2006; Chubukov and Sauer 2014). PEP and FBP are glycolytic intermediates with important regulatory functions (Keseler et al. 2017; Kochanowski et al. 2013; Litsios et al. 2018), and large changes to cAMP, PEP, and FBP reflect a massive reprogramming of central carbon metabolism. Accumulation of ppGpp also has far-reaching impacts, which generally correspond to a transition away from growth (Potrykus and Cashel 2008). Nitrogen starvation, which similarly leads to ppGpp accumulation (Irr 1972), was not observed to impact cAMP and FBP levels appreciably, but had an opposite effect on PEP compared to carbon starvation (Brauer et al. 2006). Glutamine and α-ketoglutarate, which are metabolites involved in ammonia assimilation, are decreased and increased, respectively, in nitrogen-starved cells, whereas their levels are only slightly altered under carbon starvation (Brauer et al. 2006, Chubukov and Sauer 2014). Glutamine and glutamate, which is a metabolic node between glutamine and α-ketoglutarate, are the main intracellular nitrogen carriers for the biosynthesis of nitrogenous cellular building blocks, such as nucleic and amino acids (Keseler et al. 2017). This knowledge suggests that while anabolic activities are severely limited in nitrogen-starved cells, catabolism can continue to function. Indeed, when O_2 consumption, CO_2 evolution, and heat production were measured, each declined less rapidly in nitrogen-starved cultures compared to carbon-starved cultures (Ballesteros et al. 2001). Interestingly, phosphorous-starved populations were observed to be much more metabolically active, consuming O_2 and producing heat and CO_2 at rates that were about an order of magnitude higher than carbon-starved cultures and three- to fourfold higher than nitrogen-starved populations (Ballesteros et al. 2001). Chubukov and Sauer found that sulfur- and magnesium-starved *E. coli* consumed glucose at a faster rate than phosphorous- and nitrogen-starved cultures (Chubukov and Sauer 2014). Specifically, magnesium-starved populations consumed glucose at ~50% the rate of cultures growing exponentially on glucose, whereas nitrogen-starved populations consumed glucose approximately an order of magnitude slower. The authors explained that this large difference in growth-inhibited metabolic activity was likely to originate from allosteric inhibition of glucose transport by α-ketoglutarate (Doucette et al. 2011), which builds up in nitrogen-starved cultures, and the incomplete utilization of glucose under magnesium-starvation conditions, which was detected as excretion of vast amounts of pyruvate and rationalized to result from the use of magnesium as a cofactor of pyruvate dehydrogenase (Chubukov and Sauer 2014). In addition, energy storage molecules, such as polyphosphate, that accumulate under certain nutrient-depleted conditions have been found to influence the survival of *E. coli* during stationary phase (Ault-Riche et al. 1998; Rao and Kornberg 1996). Overall, metabolic changes that occur upon starvation are widespread and dependent on the limiting nutrient. The intracellular abundances of many metabolites change and those perturbations can have local effects, such as on fluxes through reactions that they participate in, as well as more global impacts by modulating the activity of regulators or macromolecular machinery.

6.2.2   Transcriptional Regulation During Starvation

Transcriptional control is important to *E. coli* starvation physiology, and this is reflected by exacerbated loss of culturability in mutants with inactivated transcriptional regulators (Lange and Hengge-Aronis 1991; Nystrom et al. 1996; Farewell et al. 1996). RpoS, the stationary phase RNA polymerase sigma factor (σ_S), is the master transcriptional regulator under starvation conditions with hundreds of genes under its control (Keseler et al. 2017). In response to starvation, RpoS interacts with RNA polymerase to ready *E. coli* for lean and stressful times (Nystrom 2004;

Peterson et al. 2005; Jenkins et al. 1988). RpoS itself is subject to regulation at multiple levels, including at the transcription, transcript, translation, and protein levels (Keseler et al. 2017; Lange and Hengge-Aronis 1994), and that control depends on the type of starvation (Peterson et al. 2005). Under exponential growth, RpoS is synthesized but actively degraded by the ClpXP protease with the assistance of adaptor protein RssB (Pratt and Silhavy 1996; Schweder et al. 1996). Under starvation conditions for different nutrients, RpoS levels will increase to different extents and through different mechanisms (Peterson et al. 2005). These differences are explained in part by anti-adaptor proteins that have been found to interact directly with RssB to prevent RpoS proteolysis (Bougdour et al. 2008, 2006; Bougdour and Gottesman 2007). IraM interferes with RssB upon magnesium starvation to stabilize RpoS, whereas IraP acts similarly in the absence of phosphorous (Bougdour et al. 2008, 2006). In fact, the induction of *iraP* in response to phosphorous starvation was found to depend on ppGpp, which similar to during carbon and nitrogen starvation increases in response to phosphorous starvation (Bougdour and Gottesman 2007; Spira et al. 1995). ppGpp directly binds to RNA polymerase to exert its influence on transcription, and for some genes its activity synergizes with that of DksA, which is a regulatory protein that binds directly to RNA polymerase (Potrykus and Cashel 2008). Two binding sites for ppGpp have been identified on RNAP; the first is at the interface between the ω and β' subunit, whereas the second is at an interface between β' and DksA (Ross et al. 2016, 2013). Both are associated with ppGpp regulation, whereas only site 2 is responsible for the synergy between ppGpp and DksA. The result is a transcriptional overhaul that funnels resources away from macromolecular synthesis and toward stress responses and the generation of cellular building blocks (Durfee et al. 2008; Traxler et al. 2008). Another regulator that directly modulates RNA polymerase in stationary phase is the 6S RNA, which directly binds to the RNA polymerase catalytic site when it is complexed with σ_{70}, the exponential growth σ factor, and interferes with its ability to bind DNA (Wassarman and Saecker 2006). cAMP is an effector of the DNA-binding regulator CRP, which influences the expression of well over 100 genes, whereas NtrBC and PhoBR are two-component systems that sense and modulate gene expression in response to nitrogen and phosphorous depletion (Gorke and Stulke 2008; Keseler et al. 2017; Reitzer 2003; Peterson et al. 2005; Makino et al. 1989). In addition, ArcA, which is the DNA-binding regulator of the ArcAB two-component system, has a significant impact on *E. coli* starvation physiology (Nystrom et al. 1996). ArcAB is classically associated with controlling the expression of enzymes involved in respiratory metabolism (Salmon et al. 2005); however, the survival of Δ*arcA* is highly compromised in stationary phase (Nystrom et al. 1996). Specifically, Δ*arcA* continues to synthesize Krebs cycle enzymes, produce more heat, and consume more O_2 in stationary phase than wild-type *E. coli*, which suggests that ArcA is important for repressing respiration in the absence of essential nutrients (Nystrom et al. 1996). Further, the fatty acid degradation regulator FadR is important for survival under carbon-starved conditions, and this is thought to be associated with the catabolism of membrane phospholipids as a carbon and energy source (Farewell et al. 1996; Nystrom 2004). Collectively, transcriptional regulation is important for executing a program of physiological modifications to prepare *E. coli* for adversity in environments with limited resources.

6.2.3   Translation in the Absence of Growth

De novo synthesis of proteins in carbon-starved cultures has been found to be important for survival (Reeve et al. 1984a). Groat and colleagues found that a common set of proteins was produced in response to carbon, nitrogen, and phosphorous starvation, whereas other proteins were nutrient specific (Groat et al. 1986). Translation slows at the onset of nutrient deprivation by 50–90% and has then been observed to remain at a constant level for approximately 2 days (Ballesteros et al. 2001; Gefen et al. 2014; Reeve et al. 1984a). Upon entry into stationary phase, ribosome modulation factor (RMF) and hibernation promoting factor (HPF) work together to inactivate 70S ribosomes by dimerization (Ueta et al. 2008; Wada et al. 1995, 1990). Protein oxidation in nutrient-depleted cultures is higher than their exponential counterparts, and the extent of oxidation is dependent on the missing nutrient (Ballesteros et al. 2001). On 2D protein gels, Ballesteros and coworkers observed "protein stuttering," which is representative of different protein isoforms formed from the incorporation of improper amino acids (Ballesteros et al. 2001). Ribosome frame-shifting and stop codon read-through occur more frequently in stationary phase *E. coli* (Barak et al. 1996; Wenthzel et al. 1998), which led Ballesteros and colleagues to hypothesize that protein oxidation increases in non-growing *E. coli* due to the higher abundance of aberrant proteins (Ballesteros et al. 2001). Consistent with this hypothesis were results from strains with error-prone and hyper-accurate ribosomes that exhibited increased and decreased levels of protein oxidation, respectively (Ballesteros et al. 2001). Interestingly, an investigation of translation under carbon-, nitrogen-, and phosphorous-limited conditions revealed separate coping strategies (Li et al. 2018). Specifically, translation in nitrogen-limited *E. coli* tended to stall at codons that encoded for glutamine, carbon-limited cultures had many ribosomes that were not actively translating, and phosphorous-limited cells had ribosomes with higher relative activity but fewer of them, which probably reflects the high phosphorous requirements of ribosomal RNA (Li et al. 2018). Overall, translation continues in nutrient-deprived *E. coli*, although at a reduced rate and in an error-prone manner, and the identity of the missing nutrient will dictate the way in which translation adjusts and to some extent the proteins expressed.

6.2.4   Harvesting from Thyself

Degradation of cellular components is also a feature of nutrient-starved bacteria. In addition to inactivating its ribosomes, *E. coli* degrades them, which leads to a progressive deterioration of ribosomal RNA (Mandelstam 1963; Matin et al. 1989; Orman and Brynildsen 2015). Proteins are also subjected to degradation to provide carbon, nitrogen, and energy to starving cells, as well as remove damaged or misfolded-proteins and restructure the proteome (Bergkessel et al. 2016; Gottesman and Maurizi 2001). In the absence of growth, proteins cannot be diluted by cellular volume expansion, and thus degradation and recycling are an economic means of protein removal in resource-limited conditions. In accordance with this notion, deletion of components of the ClpP proteases (*clpP*, *clpX*, *clpA*) had little impact on the proteome of exponential phase *E. coli*, whereas the majority of the observed differences were in stationary-phase populations (Weichart et al. 2003). In addition, Δ*clpP* and Δ*clpX* exhibited compromised survival in stationary phase compared to wild-type cells (Weichart et al. 2003). Upon degradation of a protein, ClpP proteases release peptides that are 5–20 amino acids in length, which then need to be digested by peptidases in order to reenter metabolism or be used to synthesize new proteins (Sauer et al. 2004). Reeve and coworkers assayed peptidase-deficient mutants of *E. coli* and observed that they degraded and synthesized protein at reduced rates under carbon starvation compared to their wild-type counterpart. These mutants also lost culturability far faster (Reeve et al. 1984b). Recently, Link and colleagues found that amino acids in carbon-starved *E. coli* cultures exhibited separate trends, with some accumulating and others depleting or staying at constant levels (Link et al. 2015). Interestingly, the amino acids that accumulated had a higher metabolic cost for synthesis than those that were constant or lost abundance, and those more valuable amino acids were rapidly incorporated into proteins once carbon became available again (Link et al. 2015). This suggested that *E. coli* is programmed to preserve some amino acids and catabolize the others based on the extent of resources that would be needed to resynthesize them (Link et al. 2015). In addition, phospho-lipids are degraded in cultures depleted of carbon in a process to harvest carbon and energy, which results in the dwarfing of non-growing bacteria (Farewell et al. 1996; Nystrom 2004). Altogether, degradation of various macromolecules provides *E. coli* with the material, energy, and removal capabilities required to subsist under starvation.

6.2.5   Morphological Features of Starvation

Nutrient-depleted *E. coli* assume a different shape than exponentially growing cells. Specifically, they are smaller and more spherical (Orman and Brynildsen 2015; Peterson et al. 2005), and the regulator BolA is involved in that process (Santos et al. 2002). In addition, reductive division, which are cell division events within starving populations, contribute to cell shrinkage (Akerlund et al. 1995; Nystrom 2004). Interestingly, *E. coli* in stationary-phase cultures often have more than one copy of the chromosome (Akerlund et al. 1995). Akerlund and colleagues observed that cultures grown in rich media that had been in stationary phase for 20 h generally contained 2, 4, or 8 chromosomes, with 4 being the most prevalent (Akerlund et al.

1995). As nutrient-depleted conditions continued for another 24 h, the chromosome distribution of the population shifted due to reductive division, with gains in the subpopulations of cells with 1 and 2 chromosomes (Akerlund et al. 1995). Also, the nucleoid becomes compact and crystalline within stationary phase due to the action of Dps, which has been shown to protect DNA from a variety of stresses (Nair and Finkel 2004; Wolf et al. 1999). These adjustments, along with those described in the previous sections, reflect changes to maximize survival of starving *E. coli*.

6.3   Nutrient Availability in Host Sites

Host environments are not all reservoirs rich in nutrients, as the gut is, but rather different sites can provide distinct nutritional challenges to invading bacteria (Fig. 6.1). Such compositional differences are dictated by host variables, such as

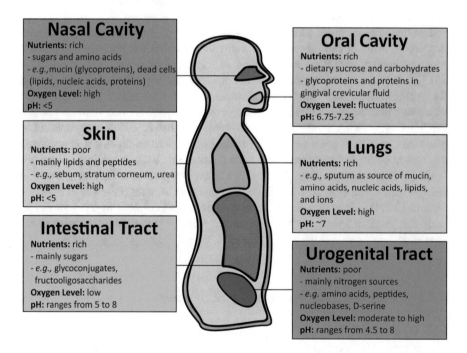

Fig. 6.1 Nutrient availability and conditions in six different host environments. The skin, our largest organ and barrier, is a challenging environment for microbes, as it is nutrient-limited and acidic (Belkaid and Segre 2014). Likewise, urine and the urogenital tract provide a variable and relatively nutrient-limited environment, where microbes are fed on a mainly nitrogen-based diet (Alteri and Mobley 2012; Brooks and Keevil 1997). By comparison, in the oral cavity (Passalacqua et al. 2016; Olsen 2005) and intestinal tract (Pereira and Berry 2017), microbes are offered a carbon-rich niche due to our carbohydrate-rich diets. In the respiratory tract, such as the nasal cavity and the lungs (Marks et al. 2012; Armstrong and Miller 2010), host mucin and enzymes provide microbes with sources of carbon and nitrogen

the vasculature that controls the transport of fluids and gases, but also by the microbiomes in residence at specific sites. Further, pathogens can secrete toxins, effectors, and siderophores to modulate host cell metabolism or sequester nutrients, thereby altering the nutritional composition at the infection site (Escoll et al. 2017; Freyberg and Harvill 2017; Holden et al. 2016). As mentioned in the preceding section, nutritional restrictions can render bacteria less likely to be killed by antibiotic treatments (Eng et al. 1991; Fung et al. 2010), and thus here we discuss several examples of how bacteria can be exposed to nutrient shortages within a host.

6.3.1 Compositional Differences in Host Microenvironments

Depending on their colonization sites in the host, bacteria are exposed to variable nutrient availability and limitations, which can impact their gene expression and sensitivity to antimicrobials. For example, in the nutrient-replete intestinal tract, bacteria can primarily catabolize sugars and glucoconjugates (Pereira and Berry 2017). Should they exit the glucose-rich gut and enter the urinary tract, as extraintestinal pathogenic *E. coli* (e.g., strain CFT073) would, nutrients become less abundant and more variable. In the urinary tract, the main nutrient sources become urea, amino acids, peptides, nucleobases, lactate, and citrate (Brooks and Keevil 1997). Further, D-serine, which acts as a neurotransmitter in the mammalian brain and is found in serum owing to dietary uptake and expression of serine racemase in peripheral tissue, is present at levels in urine that are potentially toxic to some strains of *E. coli* (Huang et al. 1998; Sasabe et al. 2014); however, uropathogenic *E. coli* (UPEC) are able to catabolize D-serine, which confers an advantage in colonizing and infecting the urinary tract (Brown et al. 2008). In individuals with cystic fibrosis, the production of large volumes of viscous mucus in the lungs provides an amino acid-rich but oxygen-limited environment, which prevents the clearance of pathogens such as *Pseudomonas aeruginosa* (Palmer et al. 2005, 2007).

Besides being dictated by host anatomy, nutrient availability can be modulated by the host in response to infections. Phagocytic cells can restrict glucose, amino acids, and essential trace metals in order to starve and limit the growth of invading microorganisms (Sprenger et al. 2017; Appelberg 2006). Alternatively, they can elevate levels of toxic metals, such as zinc and copper, which can lead to the generation of DNA-damaging radicals (Sprenger et al. 2017). In response to pathogen invasion, production of interferon-γ (INF-γ) can stimulate resting macrophages (Held et al. 1999). This immunomodulatory compound can also stimulate the production and secretion of tryptophan-degrading indoleamine-2,3-dioxygenase, thus, resulting in tryptophan starvation and growth suppression in intracellular pathogens (Yoshida et al. 1981; Takikawa et al. 1986; Mackenzie et al. 1998). These examples demonstrate that bacteria can encounter diverse and dynamic nutrient niches upon entering the host.

6.3.2 Impacts of the Microbiome on Nutrient Availability

Microbiomes in host microenvironments can also dictate nutrient availability at different body sites. Specifically, the metabolic activity of local microbial constituents can produce byproducts to support or suppress the growth and colonization of other microbial species (Pereira and Berry 2017). For instance, Bacteroides and Clostridiales species residing in the intestinal microbiota can digest complex polysaccharides from host diet or intestinal mucin, releasing simple sugars that can be utilized by Proteobacteria that lack enzymes to break down those complex substrates (Kamada et al. 2013). Commensal *E. coli* strains HS and Nissle 1917 compete for nutrients including sugars, organic acids, and amino acids with enterohemorragic *E. coli* EDL933, which can prevent colonization by that pathogen (Alteri and Mobley 2012). Similarly, gut commensals can decrease the availability of primary bile acids, increase concentrations of secondary bile acids, and compete for available nutrients, such as monosaccharides, which can limit *Clostridioides* (formerly *Clostridium*) *difficile* spore germination and growth (Schäffler and Breitrück 2018; Wilson and Perini 1988). It was observed that when the endogenous microbiota is suppressed following antibiotic treatments, a window of opportunity opens for *C. difficile* to use the pool of unconsumed sialic acid and proliferate (Ng et al. 2013). These examples demonstrate that the host microbiota can play important roles in maintaining the nutrient pool at certain host sites and provide checks and balances to suppress the growth of pathogens (Dethlefsen and Relman 2011; Blaser and Falkow 2009).

6.3.3 Pathogen Invasion Alters Nutrient Availability

Similar to endogenous commensal species, invading pathogens can alter their metabolic environments (Beisel 1975; Dong et al. 2012; Escoll and Buchrieser 2018). In patients with kidney infections caused by UPEC, rapid bacterial colonization can lead to clotting and obstructed blood flow (Melican et al. 2008, 2011). This ischemia can cause local oxygen tension to decrease to 0 mmHg and alter nutrient delivery (Melican et al. 2008, 2011). Phagocytized *M. tuberculosis* can internalize host-derived holotransferrin to acquire iron necessary for intracellular growth (Boradia et al. 2014). *Legionella pneumophila*, an intracellular pathogen that is the causative agent of Legionnaires' disease, can induce the expression of a host amino acid transporter to manipulate the amino acid pool to support its intracellular growth (Wieland et al. 2005). *L. pneumophila* can also secrete enzymes to breakdown host components for nutrients, including phospholipase that target host membranes (Fonseca and Swanson 2014). Furthermore, *L. pneumophila* can secrete effectors via their type IV secretion system, which enable the fusion of *L. pneumophila*-containing vacuoles with the host endoplasmic reticulum in lieu of lysosomes (Isberg et al. 2009). This decorates the membranes of *Legionella*-containing vacuoles with several host transporters for amino acids, carbohydrates, and fatty acids, which allow the bacteria to hijack the host and establish a favorable nutrient niche for growth and replication (Isberg et al. 2009). These host–pathogen interactions, together with the activities of the host and its associated microbiome, can constantly alter the nutrient microenvironment at the site of infection before, during, and after antibiotic treatment, which can have a considerable impact on antibiotic treatment outcomes.

6.4 Biofilms and Their Nutrient Heterogeneity

It is well known that bacteria can assemble into multicellular structures, known as biofilms, where distinct nutrient niches can be established (Stewart and Franklin 2008). Biofilms offer bacteria a protected environment to grow and survive under hostile and fluctuating conditions, shielding cells from stresses that include desiccation, ionizing radiation, predation, antimicrobial therapy, and host immunity (Hall-Stoodley et al. 2004; Stoodley et al. 2002). Compared with their planktonic counterparts, bacteria in biofilms can be 100-fold or more tolerant to antibiotics, and a major reason why that occurs is associated with the availability of nutrients in densely packed films (Spoering and Lewis 2001; Walters et al. 2003). As such, biofilms impose further challenges for the treatment of chronic, relapsing infections (Buhmann et al. 2016). To better understand the recalcitrance of biofilm infections to antibiotic treatment, we provide an overview of infections involving biofilms, the compositions of their extracellular matrices, and their intrinsic nutrient gradients in this section.

6.4.1 Biofilms in Acute and Chronic Infections

Bacterial biofilms can establish at air–liquid interfaces, on biotic surfaces, and on abiotic surfaces (Hall-Stoodley et al. 2004). Their ability to form and persist within diverse environments facilitates the transmission of pathogens from these films (Hall-Stoodley et al. 2004; Potera 1999). *L. pneumophila* is an aquatic pathogen that can adhere to and form biofilms on environmental sediments and anthropogenic water systems, such as plastic pipes used for plumbing (Abdel-Nour et al. 2013). They can naturally form multispecies biofilms together with other microorganisms, including different species of protozoa, which *L. pneumophila* use for intracellular replication (Abdel-Nour et al. 2013). As *L. pneumophila* has coevolved with multiple species of protozoa in these mixed-species biofilms, they can occupy a broad host range, including human macrophages (Abdel-Nour et al. 2013). Upon inhalation of aerosolized biofilms, *L. pneumophila* can cause severe, and sometimes fatal, respiratory illnesses (Abdel-Nour et al. 2013). Similar to *L. pneumophila*, *P. aeruginosa* is an environmental waterborne pathogen that can adhere to diverse surfaces. In addition to being able to colonize and form monospecies or polymicrobial biofilms at different host sites, including the airways of cystic fibrosis patients or on wounds (Mulcahy et al. 2014), *P. aeruginosa* biofilms can form on plumbing fixtures and showerheads, medical equipment, and implanted medical devices (Perkins et al. 2009). Biofilm formation on implanted medical devices accounts for over 25% of healthcare-related infections (Buhmann et al. 2016). Besides *P. aeruginosa*, biofilms of other pathogens belonging to the notorious ESKAPE (*Enterococcus faecalis, Staphylococcus aureus, Klebsiella pneumoniae, Acinetobacter baumannii, P. aeruginosa*, and *Enterobacter* spp.) group of bacteria that are often multidrug resistant and culprits of nosocomial infections are frequently found in device-associated infections (Percival et al. 2015). Collectively, these pathogens have been linked to catheter-associated urinary tract infections, central-line-associated septicemia, ventilator-associated pneumonia, and prosthesis-related infections (Percival et al. 2015; De Sanctis et al. 2014). Unfortunately, since pathogens in biofilm infections can be recalcitrant to antibiotic treatment and host defenses, total replacement of the implanted device is often necessary to eradicate severe infections (Percival et al. 2015; Mulcahy et al. 2014).

6.4.2 Composition of Biofilm Extracellular Matrices

Bacteria in biofilms are encased in a thick, self-produced, and protective matrix, which makes up to 90% of the biofilm dry mass (Flemming and Wingender 2010). The matrix can act as a barrier, impeding the penetration of some antimicrobials and host defense factors (Flemming and Wingender 2010; Stewart 1996). The matrix also physically interconnects cells, immobilizes the biofilm to surfaces, and provides mechanical stability to the structure. The matrix is typically composed of a complex mixture of extracellular polymeric substance (EPS) that includes polysaccharides, proteins, lipids, and nucleic acids (Flemming and Wingender 2010). Extracellular structures, including flagella, fimbrae, and pili, can also be found (Schooling and Beveridge 2006). The exact composition of the matrix is variable and depends on a number of factors, including hydrodynamic conditions, nutrient availability, and the microbial residents of the film (Flemming and Wingender 2010). For instance, streptococci species in oral biofilms produce sucrose-derived glucans and fructans, whereas cellulose is an important polymer in biofilms produced by *E. coli, K. pneumoniae, Enterobacter* spp., *Citrobacter* spp., and *Salmonella enterica* serovar Typhimurium (Koo et al. 2010; Zogaj et al. 2001; Flemming and Wingender 2010). Besides acting as a scaffold and barrier, the matrix keeps a consortium of extracellular digestive enzymes in close proximity of producing cells, allowing them to more efficiently capture metabolites from biopolymers and their lysed siblings. The availability of EPS and dead cell remnants produces a nutritive environment for cells occupying the exterior of the biofilm, but, as discussed below, the scenario is quite different for cells encased deep within the structure.

6.4.3   Nutrient Gradients in Biofilms

A prominent feature of biofilms is the presence of nutrient gradients (De Beer et al. 1994; Folsom et al. 2010; Stewart 2003; Stewart and Franklin 2008; Stewart et al. 2016). Cells at the periphery experience the highest substrate concentrations, whereas cells far from the exterior experience nutrient depletion (Stewart and Franklin 2008). Oxygen is commonly a substrate with steep gradients in biofilms because it is sparingly soluble in aqueous solutions and rapidly consumed through aerobic respiration (De Beer et al. 1994; Folsom et al. 2010; Stewart and Franklin 2008; Stewart et al. 2016; Xu et al. 1998; James et al. 2016). This produces spatial heterogeneity with respect to growth, where cells at the periphery are respiring and growing rapidly, whereas bacteria in the interior are fermenting, respiring anaerobically, or for obligate aerobes, not growing. Such growth heterogeneity has been visualized with the use of inducible fluorophores where the thickness of the translationally active layer corresponded to the oxygenated positions in the film (Folsom et al. 2010; Stewart et al. 2016; Xu et al. 1998). Nutrients produced and released by cells can also have spatial gradients in biofilms (Liu et al. 2015; Stewart and Franklin 2008). For instance, Liu and colleagues used a microfluidic device to grow a *Bacillus subtilis* biofilm, and they observed at specific biofilm sizes that the growth would oscillate (Liu et al. 2015). They found that only cells at the periphery were growing and that their growth depended on the release of ammonia from bacteria within the biofilm, which would then diffuse to the periphery (Liu et al. 2015). Interestingly, this metabolite exchange rendered the biofilm more resilient to insult, because the supply chain (interior bacteria) remained alive and thus able to provide reinforcements when the leading edges of the biofilm were decimated by an antimicrobial, whereas a genetically modified strain that did not require the interior bacteria for growth did not fare as well against the same antibacterial attack (Liu et al. 2015). Further, due to nutrient gradients in biofilms, complex communities can arise, where their spatial position is governed by metabolite availability (Mark Welch et al. 2016). Mark Welch and coworkers examined the community structure of oral biofilms, and found that in general facultative or obligate aerobes were at the periphery, obligate anaerobes were within the depths of the film, and species that catabolized specific substrates, such as lactate, were co-localized with species that excreted those compounds (Mark Welch et al. 2016). Biofilms are complex microbial communities and due to their structures and metabolic activities of their residents, nutrient gradients form and pockets of starvation can exist.

6.5   Antibiotics that Can Kill Starving Bacteria

Traditionally, antibiotics were developed for their ability to inhibit rapidly growing bacteria cultured in nutrient-rich media (Hu et al. 2010; Hu and Coates 2012). As many of these existing antibiotics target mechanisms of cell growth, they are effective against exponentially growing populations, but they often fail against slow- or non-growing bacteria (Hu et al. 2010; Hu and Coates 2012; Eng et al. 1991; Fung et al. 2010). For instance, β-lactams that target cell wall synthesis readily kill growing bacteria, but they generally are ineffective against non-growing bacteria (Cozens et al. 1986; Balaban et al. 2004; Eng et al. 1991; Tuomanen et al. 1986). Aminoglycosides act on the 30S ribosomal subunit to impair translational proof-reading, but they depend on proton motive force for uptake, which renders them largely ineffective against starving bacteria unless they are present at very high concentrations (Allison et al. 2011; Davis 1987; Shan et al. 2015; Taber et al. 1987; Van Den Bergh et al. 2016). Given the prevalence of non-growing bacteria at infection sites (Eng et al. 1991; Hu and Coates 2012), it is important to have antibiotics that retain bactericidal activity against growth-inhibited populations. In this section, we summarize those main antibiotic classes that can kill starved bacteria, as well as their mechanisms of action.

6.5.1 Fluoroquinolones Target Enzymes that Modify DNA Topologies

Fluoroquinolones are broad-spectrum antibiotics that target topoisomerase IV and gyrase, which are type II topoisomerases that help to maintain the supercoiling state of DNA during replication and transcription (Drlica and Zhao 1997). To modify DNA topology, these enzymes covalently bind DNA to form DNA–enzyme complexes before breaking one segment of the DNA, passing another segment through the break, and sealing the broken ends (Redgrave et al. 2014). When fluoroquinolones act on these enzymes, they bind helix 4 of gyrase or topoisomerase IV, thereby trapping the type II topoisomerases on the cleaved DNA and preventing religation (Drlica et al. 2008). These cleaved complexes can then produce DNA damage and cell death can occur (Drlica et al. 2008). Under nutrient deprivation, DNA is no longer being synthesized; however, RNA transcription continues to occur (Ballesteros et al. 2001; Gefen et al. 2014; Reeve et al. 1984a), and lethal doses of fluoroquinolones have been shown to kill 90–98% of starved populations (Volzing and Brynildsen 2015; Mok and Brynildsen 2018; Keren et al. 2004; Theodore et al. 2013).

6.5.2 Membrane-Targeting Antimicrobials Breach Bacterial Permeability Barriers

Membrane-targeting compounds and peptides, including many derived from natural products and host immunity, can kill bacteria independent of cell division and active metabolism (Bahar and Ren 2013; Reffuveille et al. 2014). Since the membranes of starving cells are still exposed to the environment, membrane-targeting antimicrobials can still access their primary target. These compounds either contain a cationic domain or assemble into structures with a net positive charge, which enables them to preferentially target negatively charged (e.g., phosphatidylglycerol, cardiolipin) or zwitterionic (e.g., phosphatidylethanolamine) phospholipid head groups that are abundant in microbial membranes but rare in mammalian membranes (Hurdle et al. 2011; Stark et al. 2002). Upon altering membrane architecture and properties, membrane-targeting antibacterials decrease transmembrane potentials, increase membrane permeability, and, in some cases, mislocalize membrane proteins (Hurdle et al. 2011). For example, daptomycin is a cyclic lipopeptide isolated from soil bacterium *Streptomyces roseosporus* that oligomerizes into micelles with positively charged surfaces in a calcium (Ca^{2+})-dependent manner and inserts into bacterial phospholipid bilayers (Mascio et al. 2007; Silverman et al. 2003; Pogliano et al. 2012). Although previous reports suggested that daptomycin kills by pore formation and ion leakage or improper recruitment of cell envelope machinery to areas of distorted membrane curvature (Silverman et al. 2003, Pogliano et al. 2012), recent work contends that daptomycin binds to and clusters fluid lipid microdomains in the cell membrane, which impacts the localization of peripheral membrane proteins involved in cell envelope biosynthesis (Müller et al. 2016). Recently, it was demonstrated that daptomycin exhibited activity against stationary phase *Borrelia burgdorferi*, which is the causative agent of Lyme disease (Sharma et al. 2015).

6.5.3   Targeting Proteases to Kill Starving Pathogens

Bacterial proteases regulate key processes, including cell division, stress tolerance, morphology maintenance, and virulence (Culp and Wright 2017), which make them interesting targets for novel antibiotics. As described in previous sections, nutrient-depleted bacteria rely on proteases to remove damaged or misfolded proteins and provide essential building blocks for continued translation (Prouty and Goldberg 1972; Damerau and St John 1993; Groat et al. 1986; Reeve et al. 1984b). This is exemplified by the importance of ClpP proteases to starvation survival of *E. coli* (Weichart et al. 2003). Recently, antibacterials that target proteases were found to kill stationary-phase bacteria. Lassomycin is a basic cyclic peptide isolated from soil bacterium *Lentzea kentukyensis* that can bind to the highly acidic region of *M. tuberculosis* ClpC1 (Gavrish et al. 2014). In doing so, it stimulates and uncouples the ATPase activity of ClpP1P2 from its protease activity (Gavrish et al. 2014). As the protease function is essential to the viability of mycobacteria, lassomycin readily kills *M. tuberculosis,* including stationary-phase cells. Acyldepsipeptide ADEP4 is another example of a ClpP-targeting antimicrobial (Conlon et al. 2013). Unlike lassomycin, ADEP4 directly binds ClpP and keeps its catalytic chamber open. As a result, ClpP non-specifically degrades proteins, essentially forcing the cell to indiscriminately self-digest. ADEP4 effectively kills stationary-phase *S. aureus,* whereas rifampicin, vancomycin, linezolid, and even ciprofloxacin could not (Conlon et al. 2013).

6.5.4   Pyrazinamide Kills Non-growing Tuberculosis

Pyrazinamide has been used against tuberculosis for over 60 years and has been a part of first-line regimens since the 1980s (Zhang et al. 2013b). Pyrazinamide is paradoxical in that it has little activity against growing bacilli and is primarily active against slow- or non-growing cells (Zhang et al. 2013a). It is effective in killing nutrient-starved cells (Peterson et al. 2015) and those cultured under hypoxic conditions (Dillon et al. 2017). However, its exact mechanism of action and cellular targets remain ill defined. Pyrazinamide has been shown to diffuse into *M. tuberculosis*, where it is activated to pyrazinoic acid (POA) by mycobacterium pyrazinamidase/ nicotinamidase PncA (Zhang et al. 2013b). Host-mediated bioactivation of the drug has also been reported (Via et al. 2015). POA can effectively penetrate lung tissues and granulomas (Via et al. 2015), where the pathogen is subjected to a plethora of stresses, which include oxygen, iron, and carbon limitations (Ehlers and Schaible 2012). POA can exit the bacilli, and in an acidic extracellular milieu (e.g., at a site of inflammation), it becomes protonated to HPOA and passively diffuses back into the mycobacteria (Zhang et al. 2013b). As efflux of HPOA requires energy, it accumulates in cells with reduced energy charge, where it can acidify the cytoplasm and inhibit various cellular targets (Zhang et al. 2013b). POA has been proposed to perturb a range of cellular processes, including stalled ribosome rescue via *trans*-translation (Shi et al. 2011), fatty acid biosynthesis (Zimhony et al. 2000), and pantothenate biosynthesis (Zhang et al. 2013a; Dillon et al. 2017). At present, it remains to be determined whether cell death following pyrazinamide treatment results from the collapse of one or multiple cellular processes (Hu et al. 2006). In various studies, pyrazinamide has been shown to shorten the treatment of drug-sensitive, drug-resistant, active, and latent tuberculosis (Zhang et al. 2003; Wade and Zhang 2006; Via et al. 2015).

6.6   Persisters in Nutrient-Depleted Populations

Antibiotics are less effective against starved bacterial populations (Fung et al. 2010; Hu and Coates 2012), and for those compounds that have retained their bactericidal activity in such situations, persisters will complicate efforts to achieve sterilization. Persisters are phenotypic variants with a higher capacity to tolerate antibiotic treatments than their genetically identical kin, and their levels can be as high as 1–10% of the population in nutrient-depleted conditions (Henry and Brynildsen 2016; Luidalepp et al. 2011; Mok and Brynildsen 2018; Shah et al. 2006; Volzing and Brynildsen 2015). That level is orders of magnitude higher than the incidence of spontaneously resistant mutants, and thus persisters are a more likely cause of antibiotic failure in populations that were originally susceptible to the antibiotic. Thus far, we have summarized the physiology of *E. coli* in different nutrient-depleted environments, described the nutrient limitations at different locations in the host, explained how gradients in biofilms can produce regions of depleted substrates, and delineated how some antibiotics retain activity against starved bacteria. In this section, we provide an overview of persisters in starved cultures and highlight several non-intuitive aspects of their physiology. As we did in Sect. 6.2, we will focus this section on *E. coli* because starvation physiology and thus tolerance toward antibiotics under nutrient depletion can differ between organisms.

6.6.1   Heterogeneous Tolerance in Starving Populations

Persistence describes a phenomenological outcome of assays where bacteria are treated with antibiotics and survival is measured as a function of time. When data from those assays is plotted as the logarithm of culturability (or survival) versus time, it is common to observe more than one death rate (Fig. 6.2) (Brauner et al. 2016; Lewis 2010). The initial killing is typically faster and most of the population dies off in that phase, whereas within the second phase slower cell death occurs. When survivors from that second phase are re-cultured and the same experiment is performed, indistinguishable killing dynamics are observed, which suggests that the reduced susceptibility of bacteria within the second phase was phenotypic and not genetic in origin (Keren et al. 2004; Barrett et al. 2019). Two different death rates within biphasic survival plots reflect populations where tolerance is heterogeneous (one characteristic death rate would reflect homogeneous tolerance). Persistence has been measured in a variety of experimental formats and as one would expect, the assay conditions have a strong impact on results (Hansen et al. 2008; Luidalepp et al. 2011). Here we will focus on results from assays where antibiotics were added

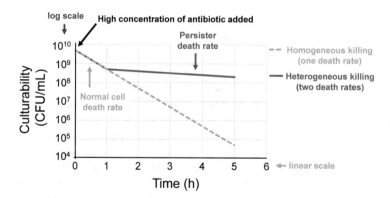

Fig. 6.2 Schematic description of persistence. Culturability is plotted on a log scale as a function of time, which is on a linear scale, after a high concentration of an antibiotic has been added to a bacterial culture. If a single slope is observed, a single death rate characterizes the population. If a line with two slopes is observed, two death rates characterize the population. In general, the first slope is steeper and the majority of the bacterial population is killed during that period. The second slope tends to be less steep, and it reflects the increased tolerance of persisters to the antibiotic

directly to starving bacterial populations (Allison et al. 2011; Hansen et al. 2008; Henry and Brynildsen 2016; Mok and Brynildsen 2018; Shah et al. 2006; Van Den Bergh et al. 2016; Verstraeten et al. 2015; Volzing and Brynildsen 2015), rather than those from assays where starving bacterial cultures were mixed with nutritive media containing antibiotics (Keren et al. 2004; Luidalepp et al. 2011; Orman and Brynildsen 2015; Spoering et al. 2006). We make this distinction because the former reflects the survival of starving bacteria treated with antibiotics, whereas the latter reflects the survival of formerly starved bacteria exposed to nutrients concurrently with antibiotics.

The most common antibiotic class used to measure persistence in starving bacterial populations are the fluoroquinolones (Hansen et al. 2008; Henry and Brynildsen 2016; Mok and Brynildsen 2018; Shah et al. 2006; Verstraeten et al. 2015; Volzing and Brynildsen 2015; Allison et al. 2011), although aminoglycosides at high concentrations (100–400 µg/mL) have also been used (Van Den Bergh et al. 2016). For fluoroquinolone persisters, biphasic survival curves have been observed, cultures grown from persisters exhibit similar killing dynamics under the same treatment conditions, and whole genome sequencing of persisters and controls did not reveal genetic differences (Henry and Brynildsen 2016; Mok and Brynildsen 2018; Volzing and Brynildsen 2015; Barrett et al. 2019). How those persisters survive while the majority of starving bacteria die remains poorly understood. Growth heterogeneity does not explain the difference, because all of the bacteria, regardless of whether they die or survive, are deprived of one or more essential nutrient. We note that starvation of 10 or more days can produce what is known as the "growth advantage in stationary phase" (GASP) phenotype, where bacteria are dying and growing in equal proportion (Finkel 2006); however, the time scales we discuss here are shorter than those where GASP manifests, and thus the bacteria are effectively uniform in their lack of growth. The capacity to synthesize new protein can be variable in some nutrient-deprived populations, and it was observed that the likelihood that the most translationally active bacteria would be fluoroquinolone persisters was approximately threefold less than other members of the population (Henry and Brynildsen 2016). Interestingly, Guido and colleagues predicted from a mathematical model and confirmed experimentally that the cessation of growth and cell division can impact the stochasticity of gene expression (Guido et al. 2007, 2006). Notably, experiments suggested that RMF and ppGpp serve to increase gene expression noise in stationary-phase populations (Guido et al. 2007).

Additional heterogeneous characteristics of nutrient-depleted bacteria include the "protein stuttering" that reflects different protein isoforms resulting from increased translational errors that occur in starved populations (Ballesteros et al. 2001), and variable chromosome abundances in stationary-phase bacteria (Akerlund et al. 1995). Both of these features could potentially impact cellular components that are present in low abundance. Differences in chromosome abundances directly change the level of DNA, which is present in very few copies, and if any low abundant protein suffers a translational error, the impact of that error could be significant depending on its functional role in the cell. Currently, it remains unclear what single cell distinctions separate persisters from cells that will die in starved populations treated with antibiotics; however, knowledge of the physiological diversity in nutrient-depleted cultures will likely provide clues to identify those persister survival mechanisms.

6.6.2 Genetic Indications of How Starving Bacteria Become Fluoroquinolone Persisters

Genetic approaches have been used to identify loci that impact the level of fluoro-quinolone persistence in nutrient-deprived cultures. Li and Zhang found that Δ*phoU* had significantly reduced survival in stationary phase when treated with norfloxacin, and microarray analysis of a *phoU* mutant suggested that it was in a hypermetabolic state (Li and Zhang 2007). PhoU is a regulator of phosphate metabolism and deletion mutants accumulate polyphosphate (Morohoshi et al. 2002), which as mentioned above, is thought to be used for energy storage by starving *E. coli* (Morohoshi et al. 2002). Hansen and colleagues screened the Keio collection (Baba et al. 2006) of *E. coli* deletion mutants for persistence to ofloxacin in stationary-phase cultures and found that deletions of *dksA*, *dnaK*, *ygfA*, and *yigB* had lower levels compared with wild-type cells (Hansen et al. 2008). DksA participates in the stringent response and influences DNA repair (Meddows et al. 2005; Potrykus and Cashel 2008; Ross et al. 2016), DnaK is a chaperone that assists in protein folding (Slepenkov and Witt 2002), YgfA is involved in folate biosynthesis (Jeanguenin et al. 2010), and YigB is involved in flavin biosynthesis (Haase et al. 2013). Fung and coworkers observed that cultures depleted for nutrients by growth to stationary phase or inoculation into non-nutritive buffer both required RecA for persistence to ofloxacin (Fung et al. 2010). Theodore and colleagues found that deletions of *dinG*, *uvrD*, and *ruvA* lowered ciprofloxacin persister levels in stationary-phase cultures (Theodore et al. 2013). DinG and UvrD are DNA helicases involved in DNA repair, RuvA is part of a complex that corrects Holliday junctions, and all of them are part of the SOS response (Keseler et al. 2017). ObgE, which is a GTPase involved in ribosome assembly, DNA replication, chromosome segregation, and DNA repair, was also found to influence stationary-phase persistence to fluoroquinolones, and that effect was dependent on ppGpp (Verstraeten et al. 2015). Although genetic studies have identified mediators with diverse functions, a recurring theme has been the importance of DNA repair to fluoroquinolone persistence in non-growing populations, and we also found that to be the case with Δ*recA*, Δ*recB*, Δ*ruvA*, and Δ*recN* mutants exhibiting lower ofloxacin persistence levels in stationary-phase cultures (Volzing and Brynildsen 2015).

6.6.3 Fluoroquinolone Persisters Survive Despite DNA Damage

A paradigm in persister research had been that their survival was due to limited primary target corruption compared to other bacteria in the culture (Balaban 2011;

Balaban et al. 2013; Gefen and Balaban 2009; Lewis 2007, 2010). Volzing and Brynildsen treated stationary-phase populations of *E. coli* that contained four different DNA damage reporters with ofloxacin, and observed subpopulations of cells that responded to the antibiotic and those that did not (Volzing and Brynildsen 2015). Sorting of the populations based on fluorescence from those reporters did not indicate any survival differences between the responding and non-responding subpopulations (Volzing and Brynildsen 2015). These data showed that response to the fluoroquinolone during treatment had no bearing on whether bacteria would survive to be persisters. Additional analyses suggested that persisters experienced comparable DNA damage from the treatment as cells that died, and that DNA repair machinery was only required for persistence after the fluoroquinolone treatment had ended (Volzing and Brynildsen 2015). Collectively, these data established that in nutrient-depleted conditions, fluoroquinolone persisters do not arise because of a lack of fluoroquinolone-induced damage, but rather that they survive in spite of that damage. In addition, it suggested that the events following treatments, also called the post-antibiotic recovery period, might hold clues to understanding fluoroquinolone persistence in starving bacterial cultures.

6.6.4 Events After Treatments Conclude Are Critical to Survival

Using a model system of persistence where the MazF endoribonuclease toxin was expressed to inhibit translation (Mok et al. 2015), Mok and Brynildsen found that the survival of MazF inhibited cultures after ofloxacin treatment far exceeded that of cultures where translation was inhibited by chloramphenicol (Mok and Brynildsen 2018). Further analyses of those populations suggested that the timing between DNA repair and growth resumption during the recovery period was an important variable that influenced the survival of growth-inhibited populations treated with fluoroquinolones (Mok and Brynildsen 2018). Interestingly, starving populations treated with ofloxacin or ciprofloxacin could approach almost complete survival if starvation continued for several hours after the fluoroquinolone had been removed, whereas immediate exposure to nutrients following fluoroquinolone treatment killed 90% or more of the population (Mok and Brynildsen 2018). The ability of starvation during recovery to enhance survival depended on the availability of RecA during that period, and if RecA was not expressed until after nutrients were introduced, survival returned to levels observed for populations exposed to nutrients immediately after treatment (Mok and Brynildsen 2018). Starvation following treatment was thought to allow cells sufficient time to repair damaged DNA before growth-related processes, such as DNA replication, resumed, and experiments with starving biofilms gave similar results. Collectively, these data indicated that events following fluoroquinolone treatment were important for persistence in starved *E. coli* populations.

6.7 Strategies to Kill Persisters in Nutrient-Depleted Populations

Non-growing bacteria are hard to treat with conventional antibiotics and for those that retain some activity, the levels of persisters are extremely high (Volzing and Brynildsen 2015; Mok and Brynildsen 2018; Keren et al. 2004; Theodore et al. 2013). Treatments that can kill persisters in such populations promise to improve outcomes and reduce the incidences of chronic and recurring infections (Gold and Nathan 2017). To identify such treatments, understanding how persister physiology enables survival as well as high-throughput screening methodologies can be empowering. In this section, we discuss how knowledge of persister physiology can provide a roadmap to more efficacious treatments, and highlight several studies where clever screening procedures identified exciting molecules with anti-persister activity in starving bacterial cultures.

6.7.1 Physiology-Guided Approaches

As mentioned above, aminoglycosides can lose activity in starved cultures based on insufficient proton motive force for import (Davis 1987). Hypothesizing that persisters in stationary-phase populations were protected from aminoglycosides due to a lack of import, a panel of metabolites were tested for their capacity to sensitize *E. coli* persisters to aminoglycosides (Allison et al. 2011). Glucose, fructose, mannitol, and pyruvate potentiated the activity of aminoglycosides in persisters, and it was shown to be associated with increased uptake due to PMF generation (Allison et al. 2011). An analogous phenomenon was observed in *P. aeruginosa* persisters, though the potentiating metabolites were somewhat different (Meylan et al. 2017), which likely reflects metabolic differences between *P. aeruginosa* and *E. coli* (Gorke and Stulke 2008; Wolff et al. 1991). Using a different approach that was similarly motivated, Schmidt and colleagues developed a hybrid antibiotic called Pentobra, which is part aminoglycoside (tobramycin) and part membrane-permeabilizing peptide (Schmidt et al. 2014). The impressive killing of *S. aureus* in non-nutritive buffer was observed for Pentobra compared to tobramycin by itself (Schmidt et al. 2014). In a similar vein, Cui and colleagues used the membrane disruptive antibiotic colistin to increase uptake of aminoglycosides and killing of persisters in starved cultures (Cui et al. 2016). These studies were motivated by the knowledge that nutrient-deprived bacteria tolerate aminoglycoside due to low uptake, and each one found a way to kill persisters in starved cultures by addressing that limitation.

Fluoroquinolone persisters in nutrient-deprived cultures do not suffer from a lack of drug import (Gutierrez et al. 2017), but rather survive despite antibiotic-induced DNA damage by using the SOS response and DNA repair machinery (Mok and Brynildsen 2018; Volzing and Brynildsen 2015; Barrett et al. 2019). Thus, targeting DNA repair could improve fluoroquinolone treatments of starved bacterial populations. In fact, chemical- and peptide-based inhibitors of RecA have been identified (Wigle et al. 2009; Nautiyal et al. 2014; Yakimov et al. 2017), and bacteriophage have been engineered to deliver dominant negative mutants of LexA, which suppress the SOS response (Lu and Collins 2009). However, the caveat is that inhibition would have to be present from when fluoroquinolone treatments ended until nutrients became available to those bacteria again since continued starvation for several hours after treatment significantly boosted survival in a DNA repair-dependent manner (Mok and Brynildsen 2018). In addition, nutrient supplementation of starving cultures has been explored as a potentiation strategy for fluoroquinolones, and unlike aminoglycosides that only required a carbon source, a carbon and terminal electron acceptor were required for fluoroquinolone killing to improve (Gutierrez et al. 2017).

6.7.2   Screening Approaches

Drug discovery efforts that begin with screens have also shown promise for the identification of agents with the capacity to eradicate nutrient-deprived bacteria. Recognizing the capacity of fluoroquinolones to kill non-growing bacteria, Hu and colleagues used chemical similarity to that antibiotic class to perform an in silico screening of almost one million compounds (Hu et al. 2010). After experimental assessment of killing of stationary phase *S. aureus* and derivatization of promising leads, HT-61 was found to eradicate non-growing *S. aureus* at concentrations where conventional treatments were largely ineffective (Hu et al. 2010). As respiration is essential to growing and non-growing *M. tuberculosis*, Sukheja and colleagues screened for respiratory inhibitors (Sukheja et al. 2017). They identified a compound that targeted demethylmenaquinone methyltransferase, which is involved in the final step of menaquinone biosynthesis, and it was found to be more potent against nutrient-depleted *M. tuberculosis* than the five other antituberculosis drugs tested (Sukheja et al. 2017). Using a *Caenorhabditis elegans* infection model, Kim and coworkers screened approximately 80,000 compounds for their ability to protect the nematodes from methicillin-resistant *S. aureus* (Kim et al. 2018). Several vitamin A analogues were found to reduce the culturability of stationary phase *S. aureus* by over 10,000-fold, and their mechanisms of action were centered on membrane perturbations (Kim et al. 2018). Interestingly, the vitamin A analogues also potentiated the activity of aminoglycosides against starved *S. aureus* populations (Kim et al. 2018).

6.8   Conclusion

In response to starvation, bacteria cease growing and adjust their physiology to cope with the absence of one or more essential nutrient. These phenotypic adjustments render starved populations extremely tolerant to antibiotics, which can complicate treatments of infections. Diversity appears to be hard-wired into the regulation of bacterial starvation with one outcome constituting high abundances of persisters. To better resolve infections that relapse due to persisters, understanding how subpopulations of nutrient-depleted bacteria tolerate antibiotic treatments better than the general population will be empowering. We highlighted several promising treatments that kill persisters in starving populations, and we anticipate that as knowledge of starvation and persistence improve, even more efficacious treatments will be realized.

Acknowledgements This work was supported by the National Institute of Allergy and Infectious Diseases of the National Institutes of Health (M.P.B: R21AI117009, R01AI130293), the Charles H. Revson Foundation (W.W.K.M.: Fellowship in Biomedical Science), and Princeton University (M.P.B.: startup funds). This content is solely the responsibility of the authors and does not necessarily represent the views of the funding agencies. The authors declare no conflicts of interest.

References

Abdel-Nour, M., Duncan, C., Low, D. E., & Guyard, C. (2013). Biofilms: The stronghold of *Legionella pneumophila*. *International Journal of Molecular Sciences, 14*, 21660–21675.

Akerlund, T., Nordstrom, K., & Bernander, R. (1995). Analysis of cell size and DNA content in exponentially growing and stationary-phase batch cultures of *Escherichia coli*. *Journal of Bacteriology, 177*, 6791–6797.

Allison, K. R., Brynildsen, M. P., & Collins, J. J. (2011). Metabolite-enabled eradication of bacterial persisters by aminoglycosides. *Nature, 473*, 216–220.

Alteri, C. J., & Mobley, H. L. (2012). *Escherichia coli* physiology and metabolism dictates adaptation to diverse host microenvironments. *Current Opinion in Microbiology, 15*, 3–9.

Amato, S. M., Orman, M. A., & Brynildsen, M. P. (2013). Metabolic control of persister formation in *Escherichia coli*. *Molecular Cell, 50*, 475–487.

Amato, S. M., Fazen, C. H., Henry, T. C., Mok, W. W., Orman, M. A., Sandvik, E. L., Volzing, K. G., & Brynildsen, M. P. (2014). The role of metabolism in bacterial persistence. *Frontiers in Microbiology, 5*, 70.

Appelberg, R. (2006). Macrophage nutriprive antimicrobial mechanisms. *Journal of Leukocyte Biology, 79*, 1117–1128.

Armstrong, E. S., & Miller, G. H. (2010). Combating evolution with intelligent design: The neoglycoside ACHN-490. *Current Opinion in Microbiology, 13*, 565–573.

Ault-Riche, D., Fraley, C. D., Tzeng, C. M., & Kornberg, A. (1998). Novel assay reveals multiple pathways regulating stress-induced accumulations of inorganic polyphosphate in *Escherichia coli*. *Journal of Bacteriology, 180*, 1841–1847.

Baba, T., Ara, T., Hasegawa, M., Takai, Y., Okumura, Y., Baba, M., Datsenko, K. A., Tomita, M., Wanner, B. L., & Mori, H. (2006). Construction of *Escherichia coli* K-12 in-frame, single-gene knockout mutants: The Keio collection. *Molecular Systems Biology, 2*, 2006.0008.

Bahar, A. A., & Ren, D. (2013). Antimicrobial peptides. *Pharmaceuticals (Basel), 6*, 1543–1575.

Balaban, N. Q. (2011). Persistence: Mechanisms for triggering and enhancing phenotypic variability. *Current Opinion in Genetics & Development, 21*, 768–775.

Balaban, N. Q., Merrin, J., Chait, R., Kowalik, L., & Leibler, S. (2004). Bacterial persistence as a phenotypic switch. *Science, 305*, 1622–1625.

Balaban, N. Q., Gerdes, K., Lewis, K., & Mckinney, J. D. (2013). A problem of persistence: Still more questions than answers? *Nature Reviews. Microbiology, 11*, 587–591.

Ballesteros, M., Fredriksson, A., Henriksson, J., & Nystrom, T. (2001). Bacterial senescence: Protein oxidation in non-proliferating cells is dictated by the accuracy of the ribosomes. *The EMBO Journal, 20*, 5280–5289.

Barak, Z., Gallant, J., Lindsley, D., Kwieciszewki, B., & Heidel, D. (1996). Enhanced ribosome frameshifting in stationary phase cells. *Journal of Molecular Biology, 263*, 140–148.

Barrett, T. C., Mok, W. W. K., Murawski, A. M., & Brynildsen, M. P. (2019). Enhanced antibiotic resistance development from fluoroquinolone persisters after a single exposure to antibiotic. *Nature Communications, 10*(1), 1177.

Beisel, W. R. (1975). Metabolic response to infection. *Annual Review of Medicine, 26*, 9–20.

Belkaid, Y., & Segre, J. A. (2014). Dialogue between skin microbiota and immunity. *Science, 346*, 954–959.

Bergkessel, M., Basta, D. W., & Newman, D. K. (2016). The physiology of growth arrest: Uniting molecular and environmental microbiology. *Nature Reviews. Microbiology, 14*, 549–562.

Blaser, M. J., & Falkow, S. (2009). What are the consequences of the disappearing human microbiota? *Nature Reviews. Microbiology, 7*, 887–894.

Boradia, V. M., Malhotra, H., Thakkar, J. S., Tillu, V. A., Vuppala, B., Patil, P., Sheokand, N., Sharma, P., Chauhan, A. S., Raje, M., & Raje, C. I. (2014). *Mycobacterium tuberculosis* acquires iron by cell-surface sequestration and internalization of human holo-transferrin. *Nature Communications, 5*, 4730.

Bougdour, A., & Gottesman, S. (2007). ppGpp regulation of RpoS degradation via anti-adaptor protein IraP. *Proceedings of the National Academy of Sciences of the United States of America, 104*, 12896–12901.

Bougdour, A., Wickner, S., & Gottesman, S. (2006). Modulating RssB activity: IraP, a novel regulator of sigma(S) stability in *Escherichia coli. Genes and Development, 20*, 884–897.

Bougdour, A., Cunning, C., Baptiste, P. J., Elliott, T., & Gottesman, S. (2008). Multiple pathways for regulation of sigma (RpoS) stability in *Escherichia coli* via the action of multiple anti-adaptors. *Molecular Microbiology, 68*, 298–313.

Brauer, M. J., Yuan, J., Bennett, B. D., Lu, W., Kimball, E., Botstein, D., & Rabinowitz, J. D. (2006). Conservation of the metabolomic response to starvation across two divergent microbes. *Proceedings of the National Academy of Sciences of the United States of America, 103*, 19302–19307.

Brauner, A., Fridman, O., Gefen, O., & Balaban, N. Q. (2016). Distinguishing between resistance, tolerance and persistence to antibiotic treatment. *Nature Reviews. Microbiology, 14*, 320–330.

Brooks, T., & Keevil, C. W. (1997). A simple artificial urine for the growth of urinary pathogens. *Letters in Applied Microbiology, 24*, 203–206.

Brown, S. A., Palmer, K. L., & Whiteley, M. (2008). Revisiting the host as a growth medium. *Nature Reviews. Microbiology, 6*, 657–666.

Buhmann, M. T., Stiefel, P., Maniura-Weber, K., & Ren, Q. (2016). In vitro biofilm models for device-related infections. *Trends in Biotechnology, 34*, 945–948.

Chubukov, V., & Sauer, U. (2014). Environmental dependence of stationary-phase metabolism in *Bacillus subtilis* and *Escherichia coli. Applied and Environmental Microbiology, 80*, 2901–2909.

Conlon, B. P., Nakayasu, E. S., Fleck, L. E., Lafleur, M. D., Isabella, V. M., Coleman, K., Leonard, S. N., Smith, R. D., Adkins, J. N., & Lewis, K. (2013). Activated ClpP kills persisters and eradicates a chronic biofilm infection. *Nature, 503*, 365–370.

Cozens, R. M., Tuomanen, E., Tosch, W., Zak, O., Suter, J., & Tomasz, A. (1986). Evaluation of the bactericidal activity of beta-lactam antibiotics on slowly growing bacteria cultured in the chemostat. *Antimicrobial Agents and Chemotherapy, 29*, 797–802.

Cui, P., Niu, H., Shi, W., Zhang, S., Zhang, H., Margolick, J., Zhang, W., & Zhang, Y. (2016). Disruption of membrane by colistin kills uropathogenic *Escherichia coli* persisters and enhances killing of other antibiotics. *Antimicrobial Agents and Chemotherapy, 60*, 6867–6871.

Culp, E., & Wright, G. D. (2017). Bacterial proteases, untapped antimicrobial drug targets. *Journal of Antibiotics (Tokyo), 70*, 366–377.

Damerau, K., & St John, A. C. (1993). Role of Clp protease subunits in degradation of carbon starvation proteins in *Escherichia coli*. *Journal of Bacteriology, 175*, 53–63.

Davis, B. D. (1987). Mechanism of bactericidal action of aminoglycosides. *Microbiological Reviews, 51*, 341–350.

De Beer, D., Stoodley, P., Roe, F., & Lewandowski, Z. (1994). Effects of biofilm structures on oxygen distribution and mass transport. *Biotechnology and Bioengineering, 43*, 1131–1138.

De Sanctis, J., Teixeira, L., Van Duin, D., Odio, C., Hall, G., Tomford, J. W., Perez, F., Rudin, S. D., Bonomo, R. A., Barsoum, W. K., Joyce, M., Krebs, V., & Schmitt, S. (2014). Complex prosthetic joint infections due to carbapenemase-producing *Klebsiella pneumoniae*: A unique challenge in the era of untreatable infections. *International Journal of Infectious Diseases, 25*, 73–78.

Dethlefsen, L., & Relman, D. A. (2011). Incomplete recovery and individualized responses of the human distal gut microbiota to repeated antibiotic perturbation. *Proceedings of the National Academy of Sciences of the United States of America, 108*(Suppl 1), 4554–4561.

Dillon, N. A., Peterson, N. D., Feaga, H. A., Keiler, K. C., & Baughn, A. D. (2017). Anti-tubercular activity of pyrazinamide is independent of trans-translation and RpsA. *Scientific Reports, 7*, 6135.

Dong, F., Wang, B., Zhang, L., Tang, H., Li, J., & Wang, Y. (2012). Metabolic response to *Klebsiella pneumoniae* infection in an experimental rat model. *PLoS One, 7*, E51060.

Doucette, C. D., Schwab, D. J., Wingreen, N. S., & Rabinowitz, J. D. (2011). Alpha-ketoglutarate coordinates carbon and nitrogen utilization via enzyme I inhibition. *Nature Chemical Biology, 7*, 894–901.

Drlica, K., & Zhao, X. (1997). DNA gyrase, topoisomerase IV, and the 4-quinolones. *Microbiology and Molecular Biology Review, 61*, 377–392.

Drlica, K., Malik, M., Kerns, R. J., & Zhao, X. (2008). Quinolone-mediated bacterial death. *Antimicrobial Agents and Chemotherapy, 52*, 385–392.

Durfee, T., Hansen, A. M., Zhi, H., Blattner, F. R., & Jin, D. J. (2008). Transcription profiling of the stringent response in *Escherichia coli*. *Journal of Bacteriology, 190*, 1084–1096.

Ehlers, S., & Schaible, U. E. (2012). The granuloma in tuberculosis: Dynamics of a host-pathogen collusion. *Frontiers in Immunology, 3*, 411.

Eng, R. H., Padberg, F. T., Smith, S. M., Tan, E. N., & Cherubin, C. E. (1991). Bactericidal effects of antibiotics on slowly growing and nongrowing bacteria. *Antimicrobial Agents and Chemotherapy, 35*, 1824–1828.

Escoll, P., & Buchrieser, C. (2018). Metabolic reprogramming of host cells upon bacterial infection: Why shift to a warburg-like metabolism? *The FEBS Journal, 285*, 2146–2160.

Escoll, P., Song, O. R., Viana, F., Steiner, B., Lagache, T., Olivo-Marin, J. C., Impens, F., Brodin, P., Hilbi, H., & Buchrieser, C. (2017). *Legionella pneumophila* modulates mitochondrial dynamics to trigger metabolic repurposing of infected macrophages. *Cell Host and Microbe, 22*, 302–316.E7.

Evangelopoulos, D., Da Fonseca, J. D., & Waddell, S. J. (2015). Understanding anti-tuberculosis drug efficacy: Rethinking bacterial populations and how we model them. *International Journal of Infectious Diseases, 32*, 76–80.

Farewell, A., Diez, A. A., Dirusso, C. C., & Nystrom, T. (1996). Role of the *Escherichia coli* FadR regulator in stasis survival and growth phase-dependent expression of the UspA, fad, and fab genes. *Journal of Bacteriology, 178*, 6443–6450.

Feist, A. M., Henry, C. S., Reed, J. L., Krummenacker, M., Joyce, A. R., Karp, P. D., Broadbelt, L. J., Hatzimanikatis, V., & Palsson, B. O. (2007). A genome-scale metabolic reconstruction for *Escherichia coli* K-12 MG1655 that accounts for 1260 ORFs and thermodynamic information. *Molecular Systems Biology, 3*, 121.

Finkel, S. E. (2006). Long-term survival during stationary phase: Evolution and the GASP phenotype. *Nature Reviews. Microbiology, 4*, 113–120.

Flemming, H. C., & Wingender, J. (2010). The biofilm matrix. *Nature Reviews. Microbiology, 8*, 623–633.

Folsom, J. P., Richards, L., Pitts, B., Roe, F., Ehrlich, G. D., Parker, A., Mazurie, A., & Stewart, P. S. (2010). Physiology of *Pseudomonas aeruginosa* in biofilms as revealed by transcriptome analysis. *BMC Microbiology, 10*, 294.

Fonseca, M. V., & Swanson, M. S. (2014). Nutrient salvaging and metabolism by the intracellular pathogen *Legionella pneumophila*. *Frontiers in Cellular and Infection Microbiology, 4*, 12.

Freyberg, Z., & Harvill, E. T. (2017). Pathogen manipulation of host metabolism: A common strategy for immune evasion. *PLoS Pathogens, 13*, e1006669.

Fung, D. K., Chan, E. W., Chin, M. L., & Chan, R. C. (2010). Delineation of a bacterial starvation stress response network which can mediate antibiotic tolerance development. *Antimicrobial Agents and Chemotherapy, 54*, 1082–1093.

Gavrish, E., Sit, C. S., Cao, S., Kandror, O., Spoering, A., Peoples, A., Ling, L., Fetterman, A., Hughes, D., Bissell, A., Torrey, H., Akopian, T., Mueller, A., Epstein, S., Goldberg, A., Clardy, J., & Lewis, K. (2014). Lassomycin, a ribosomally synthesized cyclic peptide, kills *Mycobacterium tuberculosis* by targeting the ATP-dependent protease Clpc1p1p2. *Chemistry and Biology, 21*, 509–518.

Gefen, O., & Balaban, N. Q. (2009). The importance of being persistent: Heterogeneity of bacterial populations under antibiotic stress. *FEMS Microbiology Reviews, 33*, 704–717.

Gefen, O., Fridman, O., Ronin, I., & Balaban, N. Q. (2014). Direct observation of single stationary-phase bacteria reveals a surprisingly long period of constant protein production activity. *Proceedings of the National Academy of Sciences of the United States of America, 111*, 556–561.

Gengenbacher, M., & Kaufmann, S. H. (2012). *Mycobacterium tuberculosis*: Success through dormancy. *FEMS Microbiology Reviews, 36*, 514–532.

Gold, B., & Nathan, C. (2017). Targeting phenotypically tolerant *Mycobacterium tuberculosis*. *Microbiology Spectrum, 5*. https://doi.org/10.1128/microbiolspec

Gorke, B., & Stulke, J. (2008). Carbon catabolite repression in bacteria: Many ways to make the most out of nutrients. *Nature Reviews. Microbiology, 6*, 613–624.

Gottesman, S., & Maurizi, M. R. (2001). Cell biology. Surviving starvation. *Science, 293*, 614–615.

Groat, R. G., Schultz, J. E., Zychlinsky, E., Bockman, A., & Matin, A. (1986). Starvation proteins in *Escherichia coli*: Kinetics of synthesis and role in starvation survival. *Journal of Bacteriology, 168*, 486–493.

Guido, N. J., Wang, X., Adalsteinsson, D., Mcmillen, D., Hasty, J., Cantor, C. R., Elston, T. C., & Collins, J. J. (2006). A bottom-up approach to gene regulation. *Nature, 439*, 856–860.

Guido, N. J., Lee, P., Wang, X., Elston, T. C., & Collins, J. J. (2007). A pathway and genetic factors contributing to elevated gene expression noise in stationary phase. *Biophysical Journal, 93*, L55–L57.

Gutierrez, A., Jain, S., Bhargava, P., Hamblin, M., Lobritz, M. A., & Collins, J. J. (2017). Understanding and sensitizing density-dependent persistence to quinolone antibiotics. *Molecular Cell, 68*, 1147–1154.e3.

Haase, I., Sarge, S., Illarionov, B., Laudert, D., Hohmann, H. P., Bacher, A., & Fischer, M. (2013). Enzymes from the haloacid dehalogenase (HAD) superfamily catalyse the elusive dephosphorylation step of riboflavin biosynthesis. *Chembiochem, 14*, 2272–2275.

Hall-Stoodley, L., Costerton, J. W., & Stoodley, P. (2004). Bacterial biofilms: From the natural environment to infectious diseases. *Nature Reviews. Microbiology, 2*, 95–108.

Hansen, S., Lewis, K., & Vulic, M. (2008). Role of global regulators and nucleotide metabolism in antibiotic tolerance in *Escherichia coli*. *Antimicrobial Agents and Chemotherapy, 52*, 2718–2726.

Held, T. K., Weihua, X., Yuan, L., Kalvakolanu, D. V., & Cross, A. S. (1999). Gamma interferon augments macrophage activation by lipopolysaccharide by two distinct mechanisms, at the signal transduction level and via an autocrine mechanism involving tumor necrosis factor alpha and interleukin-1. *Infection and Immunity, 67*, 206–212.

Henry, T. C., & Brynildsen, M. P. (2016). Development of persister-FACSeq: A method to massively parallelize quantification of persister physiology and its heterogeneity. *Scientific Reports, 6*, 25100.

Holden, V. I., Breen, P., Houle, S., Dozois, C. M., & Bachman, M. A. (2016). *Klebsiella pneumoniae* siderophores induce inflammation, bacterial dissemination, and HIF-1α stabilization during pneumonia. *MBio, 7*, e01397-16.

Hu, Y., & Coates, A. (2012). Nonmultiplying bacteria are profoundly tolerant to antibiotics. *Handbook of experimental pharmacology*, 99–119.

Hu, Y., Coates, A. R., & Mitchison, D. A. (2006). Sterilising action of pyrazinamide in models of dormant and rifampicin-tolerant *Mycobacterium tuberculosis*. *The International Journal of Tuberculosis and Lung Disease, 10*, 317–322.

Hu, Y., Shamaei-Tousi, A., Liu, Y., & Coates, A. (2010). A new approach for the discovery of antibiotics by targeting non-multiplying bacteria: A novel topical antibiotic for staphylococcal infections. *PLoS One, 5*, e11818.

Huang, Y., Nishikawa, T., Satoh, K., Iwata, T., Fukushima, T., Santa, T., Homma, H., & Imai, K. (1998). Urinary excretion of D-serine in human: Comparison of different ages and species. *Biological and Pharmaceutical Bulletin, 21*, 156–162.

Hurdle, J. G., O'neill, A. J., Chopra, I., & Lee, R. E. (2011). Targeting bacterial membrane function: An underexploited mechanism for treating persistent infections. *Nature Reviews. Microbiology, 9*, 62–75.

Irr, J. D. (1972). Control of nucleotide metabolism and ribosomal ribonucleic acid synthesis during nitrogen starvation of *Escherichia coli*. *Journal of Bacteriology, 110*, 554–561.

Isberg, R. R., O'connor, T. J., & Heidtman, M. (2009). The *Legionella pneumophila* replication vacuole: Making a cosy niche inside host cells. *Nature Reviews. Microbiology, 7*, 13–24.

James, G. A., Ge Zhao, A., Usui, M., Underwood, R. A., Nguyen, H., Beyenal, H., Delancey Pulcini, E., Agostinho Hunt, A., Bernstein, H. C., Fleckman, P., Olerud, J., Williamson, K. S., Franklin, M. J., & Stewart, P. S. (2016). Microsensor and transcriptomic signatures of oxygen depletion in biofilms associated with chronic wounds. *Wound Repair and Regeneration, 24*, 373–383.

Jeanguenin, L., Lara-Nunez, A., Pribat, A., Mageroy, M. H., Gregory, J. F., 3rd, Rice, K. C., De Crecy-Lagard, V., & Hanson, A. D. (2010). Moonlighting glutamate formiminotransferases can functionally replace 5-formyltetrahydrofolate cycloligase. *The Journal of Biological Chemistry, 285*, 41557–41566.

Jenkins, D. E., Schultz, J. E., & Matin, A. (1988). Starvation-induced cross protection against heat or H_2O_2 challenge in *Escherichia coli*. *Journal of Bacteriology, 170*, 3910–3914.

Kamada, N., Chen, G. Y., Inohara, N., & Núñez, G. (2013). Control of pathogens and pathobionts by the gut microbiota. *Nature Immunology, 14*, 685–690.

Keren, I., Kaldalu, N., Spoering, A., Wang, Y., & Lewis, K. (2004). Persister cells and tolerance to antimicrobials. *FEMS Microbiology Letters, 230*, 13–18.

Keseler, I. M., Mackie, A., Santos-Zavaleta, A., Billington, R., Bonavides-Martinez, C., Caspi, R., Fulcher, C., Gama-Castro, S., Kothari, A., Krummenacker, M., Latendresse, M., Muniz-Rascado, L., Ong, Q., Paley, S., Peralta-Gil, M., Subhraveti, P., Velazquez-Ramirez, D. A., Weaver, D., Collado-Vides, J., Paulsen, I., & Karp, P. D. (2017). The ecocyc database: Reflecting new knowledge about *Escherichia coli* K-12. *Nucleic Acids Research, 45*, D543–D550.

Kim, W., Zhu, W., Hendricks, G. L., Van Tyne, D., Steele, A. D., Keohane, C. E., Fricke, N., Conery, A. L., Shen, S., Pan, W., Lee, K., Rajamuthiah, R., Fuchs, B. B., Vlahovska, P. M., Wuest, W. M., Gilmore, M. S., Gao, H., Ausubel, F. M., & Mylonakis, E. (2018). A new class of synthetic retinoid antibiotics effective against bacterial persisters. *Nature, 556*, 103–107.

Kochanowski, K., Volkmer, B., Gerosa, L., Haverkorn Van Rijsewijk, B. R., Schmidt, A., & Heinemann, M. (2013). Functioning of a metabolic flux sensor in *Escherichia coli*. *Proceedings of the National Academy of Sciences of the United States of America, 110*, 1130–1135.

Koo, H., Xiao, J., Klein, M. I., & Jeon, J. G. (2010). Exopolysaccharides produced by *Streptococcus mutans* glucosyltransferases modulate the establishment of microcolonies within multispecies biofilms. *Journal of Bacteriology, 192*, 3024–3032.

Lange, R., & Hengge-Aronis, R. (1991). Identification of a central regulator of stationary-phase gene expression in *Escherichia coli*. *Molecular Microbiology, 5*, 49–59.

Lange, R., & Hengge-Aronis, R. (1994). The cellular concentration of the sigma S subunit of RNA polymerase in *Escherichia coli* is controlled at the levels of transcription, translation, and protein stability. *Genes and Development, 8*, 1600–1612.

Lewis, K. (2007). Persister cells, dormancy and infectious disease. *Nature Reviews. Microbiology, 5*, 48–56.

Lewis, K. (2010). Persister cells. *Annual Review of Microbiology, 64*, 357–372.

Li, Y., & Zhang, Y. (2007). Phou is a persistence switch involved in persister formation and tolerance to multiple antibiotics and stresses in *Escherichia coli*. *Antimicrobial Agents and Chemotherapy, 51*, 2092–2099.

Li, S. H., Li, Z., Park, J. O., King, C. G., Rabinowitz, J. D., Wingreen, N. S., & Gitai, Z. (2018). *Escherichia coli* translation strategies differ across carbon, nitrogen and phosphorus limitation conditions. *Nature Microbiology, 3*, 939–947.

Link, H., Fuhrer, T., Gerosa, L., Zamboni, N., & Sauer, U. (2015). Real-time metabolome profiling of the metabolic switch between starvation and growth. *Nature Methods, 12*, 1091–1097.

Litsios, A., Ortega, A. D., Wit, E. C., & Heinemann, M. (2018). Metabolic-flux dependent regulation of microbial physiology. *Current Opinion in Microbiology, 42*, 71–78.

Liu, J., Prindle, A., Humphries, J., Gabalda-Sagarra, M., Asally, M., Lee, D. Y., Ly, S., Garcia-Ojalvo, J., & Suel, G. M. (2015). Metabolic co-dependence gives rise to collective oscillations within biofilms. *Nature, 523*, 550–554.

Lu, T. K., & Collins, J. J. (2009). Engineered bacteriophage targeting gene networks as adjuvants for antibiotic therapy. *Proceedings of the National Academy of Sciences of the United States of America, 106*, 4629–4634.

Luidalepp, H., Joers, A., Kaldalu, N., & Tenson, T. (2011). Age of inoculum strongly influences persister frequency and can mask effects of mutations implicated in altered persistence. *Journal of Bacteriology, 193*, 3598–3605.

Mackenzie, C. R., Hadding, U., & Däubener, W. (1998). Interferon-gamma-induced activation of indoleamine 2,3-dioxygenase in cord blood monocyte-derived macrophages inhibits the growth of group B streptococci. *The Journal of Infectious Diseases, 178*, 875–878.

Makino, K., Shinagawa, H., Amemura, M., Kawamoto, T., Yamada, M., & Nakata, A. (1989). Signal transduction in the phosphate regulon of *Escherichia coli* involves phosphotransfer between PhoR and PhoB proteins. *Journal of Molecular Biology, 210*, 551–559.

Mandelstam, J. (1963). Protein turnover and its function in economy of cell. *Annals of the New York Academy of Sciences, 102*, 621–636.

Mark Welch, J. L., Rossetti, B. J., Rieken, C. W., Dewhirst, F. E., & Borisy, G. G. (2016). Biogeography of a human oral microbiome at the micron scale. *Proceedings of the National Academy of Sciences of the United States of America, 113*, E791–E800.

Marks, L. R., Reddinger, R. M., & Hakansson, A. P. (2012). High levels of genetic recombination during nasopharyngeal carriage and biofilm formation in *Streptococcus pneumoniae*. *MBio, 3*, e00200-12.

Mascio, C. T., Alder, J. D., & Silverman, J. A. (2007). Bactericidal action of daptomycin against stationary-phase and nondividing *Staphylococcus aureus* cells. *Antimicrobial Agents and Chemotherapy, 51*, 4255–4260.

Matin, A., Auger, E. A., Blum, P. H., & Schultz, J. E. (1989). Genetic basis of starvation survival in nondifferentiating bacteria. *Annual Review of Microbiology, 43*, 293–316.

Meddows, T. R., Savory, A. P., Grove, J. I., Moore, T., & Lloyd, R. G. (2005). RecN protein and transcription factor DksA combine to promote faithful recombinational repair of DNA double-strand breaks. *Molecular Microbiology, 57*, 97–110.

Melican, K., Boekel, J., Månsson, L. E., Sandoval, R. M., Tanner, G. A., Källskog, O., Palm, F., Molitoris, B. A., & Richter-Dahlfors, A. (2008). Bacterial infection-mediated mucosal signalling induces local renal ischaemia as a defence against sepsis. *Cellular Microbiology, 10*, 1987–1998.

Melican, K., Sandoval, R. M., Kader, A., Josefsson, L., Tanner, G. A., Molitoris, B. A., & Richter-Dahlfors, A. (2011). Uropathogenic *Escherichia coli* P and type 1 fimbriae act in synergy in a living host to facilitate renal colonization leading to nephron obstruction. *PLoS Pathogens, 7*, e1001298.

Metzger, S., Schreiber, G., Aizenman, E., Cashel, M., & Glaser, G. (1989). Characterization of the *relA1* mutation and a comparison of *relA1* with new *relA* null alleles in *Escherichia coli*. *The Journal of Biological Chemistry, 264*, 21146–21152.

Meylan, S., Porter, C. B. M., Yang, J. H., Belenky, P., Gutierrez, A., Lobritz, M. A., Park, J., Kim, S. H., Moskowitz, S. M., & Collins, J. J. (2017). Carbon sources tune antibiotic susceptibility in *Pseudomonas aeruginosa* via tricarboxylic acid cycle control. *Cell Chemical Biology, 24*, 195–206.

Meylan, S., Andrews, I. W., & Collins, J. J. (2018). Targeting antibiotic tolerance, pathogen by pathogen. *Cell, 172*, 1228–1238.

Mok, W. W. K., & Brynildsen, M. P. (2018). Timing of DNA damage responses impacts persistence to fluoroquinolones. *Proceedings of the National Academy of Sciences of the United States of America, 115*, e6301–e6309.

Mok, W. W., Park, J. O., Rabinowitz, J. D., & Brynildsen, M. P. (2015). RNA futile cycling in model persisters derived from MazF accumulation. *MBio, 6*, E01588–E01515.

Morohoshi, T., Maruo, T., Shirai, Y., Kato, J., Ikeda, T., Takiguchi, N., Ohtake, H., & Kuroda, A. (2002). Accumulation of inorganic polyphosphate in *phoU* mutants of *Escherichia coli* and *Synechocystis* sp. strain Pcc6803. *Applied and Environmental Microbiology, 68*, 4107–4110.

Mulcahy, L. R., Isabella, V. M., & Lewis, K. (2014). *Pseudomonas aeruginosa* biofilms in disease. *Microbial Ecology, 68*, 1–12.

Müller, A., Wenzel, M., Strahl, H., Grein, F., Saaki, T. N. V., Kohl, B., Siersma, T., Bandow, J. E., Sahl, H. G., Schneider, T., & Hamoen, L. W. (2016). Daptomycin inhibits cell envelope synthesis by interfering with fluid membrane microdomains. *Proceedings of the National Academy of Sciences of the United States of America, 113*, E7077–E7086.

Nair, S., & Finkel, S. E. (2004). Dps protects cells against multiple stresses during stationary phase. *Journal of Bacteriology, 186*, 4192–4198.

Nautiyal, A., Patil, K. N., & Muniyappa, K. (2014). Suramin is a potent and selective inhibitor of *Mycobacterium tuberculosis* RecA protein and the SOS response: RecA as a potential target for antibacterial drug discovery. *The Journal of Antimicrobial Chemotherapy, 69*, 1834–1843.

Ng, K. M., Ferreyra, J. A., Higginbottom, S. K., Lynch, J. B., Kashyap, P. C., Gopinath, S., Naidu, N., Choudhury, B., Weimer, B. C., Monack, D. M., & Sonnenburg, J. L. (2013). Microbiota-liberated host sugars facilitate post-antibiotic expansion of enteric pathogens. *Nature, 502*, 96–99.

Notley-Mcrobb, L., Death, A., & Ferenci, T. (1997). The relationship between external glucose concentration and cAMP levels inside *Escherichia coli*: Implications for models of phosphotransferase-mediated regulation of adenylate cyclase. *Microbiology, 143*(Pt 6), 1909–1918.

Nystrom, T. (2004). Stationary-phase physiology. *Annual Review of Microbiology, 58*, 161–181.

Nystrom, T., Larsson, C., & Gustafsson, L. (1996). Bacterial defense against aging: Role of the *Escherichia coli* ArcA regulator in gene expression, readjusted energy flux and survival during stasis. *The EMBO Journal, 15*, 3219–3228.

O'Neal, C. R., Gabriel, W. M., Turk, A. K., Libby, S. J., Fang, F. C., & Spector, M. P. (1994). Rpos is necessary for both the positive and negative regulation of starvation survival genes during phosphate, carbon, and nitrogen starvation in *Salmonella typhimurium*. *Journal of Bacteriology, 176*, 4610–4616.

Olsen, I. (2005). New principles in ecological regulation—Features from the oral cavity. *Microbial Ecology in Health and Disease, 18*, 26–31.

Orman, M. A., & Brynildsen, M. P. (2015). Inhibition of stationary phase respiration impairs persister formation in *E. coli*. *Nature Communications, 6*, 7983.

Palmer, K. L., Mashburn, L. M., Singh, P. K., & Whiteley, M. (2005). Cystic fibrosis sputum supports growth and cues key aspects of *Pseudomonas aeruginosa* physiology. *Journal of Bacteriology, 187*, 5267–5277.

Palmer, K. L., Aye, L. M., & Whiteley, M. (2007). Nutritional cues control *Pseudomonas aeruginosa* multicellular behavior in cystic fibrosis sputum. *Journal of Bacteriology, 189*, 8079–8087.

Passalacqua, K. D., Charbonneau, M. E., & O'riordan, M. X. (2016). Bacterial metabolism shapes the host-pathogen interface. *Microbiology Spectrum, 4*. https://doi.org/10.1128/microbiolspec. VMBF-0027-2015

Percival, S. L., Suleman, L., Vuotto, C., & Donelli, G. (2015). Healthcare-associated infections, medical devices and biofilms: Risk, tolerance and control. *Journal of Medical Microbiology, 64*, 323–334.

Pereira, F. C., & Berry, D. (2017). Microbial nutrient niches in the gut. *Environmental Microbiology, 19*, 1366–1378.

Perkins, S. D., Mayfield, J., Fraser, V., & Angenent, L. T. (2009). Potentially pathogenic bacteria in shower water and air of a stem cell transplant unit. *Applied and Environmental Microbiology, 75*, 5363–5372.

Peterson, C. N., Mandel, M. J., & Silhavy, T. J. (2005). *Escherichia coli* starvation diets: Essential nutrients weigh in distinctly. *Journal of Bacteriology, 187*, 7549–7553.

Peterson, N. D., Rosen, B. C., Dillon, N. A., & Baughn, A. D. (2015). Uncoupling environmental pH and intrabacterial acidification from pyrazinamide susceptibility in *Mycobacterium tuberculosis*. *Antimicrobial Agents and Chemotherapy, 59*, 7320–7326.

Pogliano, J., Pogliano, N., & Silverman, J. A. (2012). Daptomycin-mediated reorganization of membrane architecture causes mislocalization of essential cell division proteins. *Journal of Bacteriology, 194*, 4494–4504.

Potera, C. (1999). Forging a link between biofilms and disease. *Science, 283*(1837), 1839.

Potrykus, K., & Cashel, M. (2008). (p)ppGpp: Still magical? *Annual Review of Microbiology, 62*, 35–51.

Pratt, L. A., & Silhavy, T. J. (1996). The response regulator SprE controls the stability of RpoS. *Proceedings of the National Academy of Sciences of the United States of America, 93*, 2488–2492.

Prouty, W. F., & Goldberg, A. L. (1972). Effects of protease inhibitors on protein breakdown in *Escherichia coli*. *The Journal of Biological Chemistry, 247*, 3341–3352.

Radzikowski, J. L., Vedelaar, S., Siegel, D., Ortega, Á., Schmidt, A., & Heinemann, M. (2016). Bacterial persistence is an active σs stress response to metabolic flux limitation. *Molecular Systems Biology, 12*, 882.

Radzikowski, J. L., Schramke, H., & Heinemann, M. (2017). Bacterial persistence from a system-level perspective. *Current Opinion in Biotechnology, 46*, 98–105.

Rao, N. N., & Kornberg, A. (1996). Inorganic polyphosphate supports resistance and survival of stationary-phase *Escherichia coli*. *Journal of Bacteriology, 178*, 1394–1400.

Redgrave, L. S., Sutton, S. B., Webber, M. A., & Piddock, L. J. (2014). Fluoroquinolone resistance: Mechanisms, impact on bacteria, and role in evolutionary success. *Trends in Microbiology, 22*, 438–445.

Reeve, C. A., Amy, P. S., & Matin, A. (1984a). Role of protein synthesis in the survival of carbon-starved *Escherichia coli* K-12. *Journal of Bacteriology, 160*, 1041–1046.

Reeve, C. A., Bockman, A. T., & Matin, A. (1984b). Role of protein degradation in the survival of carbon-starved *Escherichia coli* and *Salmonella typhimurium*. *Journal of Bacteriology, 157*, 758–763.

Reffuveille, F., De La Fuente-Nunez, C., Mansour, S., & Hancock, R. E. (2014). A broad-spectrum antibiofilm peptide enhances antibiotic action against bacterial biofilms. *Antimicrobial Agents and Chemotherapy, 58*, 5363–5371.

Reitzer, L. (2003). Nitrogen assimilation and global regulation in *Escherichia coli*. *Annual Review of Microbiology, 57*, 155–176.

Ross, W., Vrentas, C. E., Sanchez-Vazquez, P., Gaal, T., & Gourse, R. L. (2013). The magic spot: A ppGpp binding site on *E. coli* RNA polymerase responsible for regulation of transcription initiation. *Molecular Cell, 50*, 420–429.

Ross, W., Sanchez-Vazquez, P., Chen, A. Y., Lee, J. H., Burgos, H. L., & Gourse, R. L. (2016). PpGpp binding to a site at the RNAP-DksA interface accounts for its dramatic effects on transcription initiation during the stringent response. *Molecular Cell, 62*, 811–823.

Salmon, K. A., Hung, S. P., Steffen, N. R., Krupp, R., Baldi, P., Hatfield, G. W., & Gunsalus, R. P. (2005). Global gene expression profiling in *Escherichia coli* K12: Effects of oxygen availability and ArcA. *The Journal of Biological Chemistry, 280*, 15084–15096.

Santos, J. M., Lobo, M., Matos, A. P., De Pedro, M. A., & Arraiano, C. M. (2002). The gene *bolA* regulates *dacA* (PBP5), *dacC* (PBP6) and *ampC* (AmpC), promoting normal morphology in *Escherichia coli*. *Molecular Microbiology, 45*, 1729–1740.

Sasabe, J., Suzuki, M., Miyoshi, Y., Tojo, Y., Okamura, C., Ito, S., Konno, R., Mita, M., Hamase, K., & Aiso, S. (2014). Ischemic acute kidney injury perturbs homeostasis of serine enantiomers in the body fluid in mice: Early detection of renal dysfunction using the ratio of serine enantiomers. *PLoS One, 9*, e86504.

Sauer, R. T., Bolon, D. N., Burton, B. M., Burton, R. E., Flynn, J. M., Grant, R. A., Hersch, G. L., Joshi, S. A., Kenniston, J. A., Levchenko, I., Neher, S. B., Oakes, E. S., Siddiqui, S. M., Wah, D. A., & Baker, T. A. (2004). Sculpting the proteome with AAA(+) proteases and disassembly machines. *Cell, 119*, 9–18.

Schäffler, H., & Breitrück, A. (2018). From colonization to infection. *Frontiers in Microbiology, 9*, 646.

Schmidt, N. W., Deshayes, S., Hawker, S., Blacker, A., Kasko, A. M., & Wong, G. C. (2014). Engineering persister-specific antibiotics with synergistic antimicrobial functions. *ACS Nano, 8*, 8786–8793.

Schooling, S. R., & Beveridge, T. J. (2006). Membrane vesicles: An overlooked component of the matrices of biofilms. *Journal of Bacteriology, 188*, 5945–5957.

Schweder, T., Lee, K. H., Lomovskaya, O., & Matin, A. (1996). Regulation of *Escherichia coli* starvation sigma factor (sigma s) by ClpXP protease. *Journal of Bacteriology, 178*, 470–476.

Shah, D., Zhang, Z., Khodursky, A., Kaldalu, N., Kurg, K., & Lewis, K. (2006). Persisters: A distinct physiological state of *E. coli*. *BMC Microbiology, 6*, 53.

Shan, Y., Lazinski, D., Rowe, S., Camilli, A., & Lewis, K. (2015). Genetic basis of persister tolerance to aminoglycosides in *Escherichia coli*. *MBio, 6*, e00078-15.

Sharma, B., Brown, A. V., Matluck, N. E., Hu, L. T., & Lewis, K. (2015). *Borrelia burgdorferi*, the causative agent of Lyme disease, forms drug-tolerant persister cells. *Antimicrobial Agents and Chemotherapy, 59*, 4616–4624.

Shi, W., Zhang, X., Jiang, X., Yuan, H., Lee, J. S., Barry, C. E., Wang, H., Zhang, W., & Zhang, Y. (2011). Pyrazinamide inhibits trans-translation in *Mycobacterium tuberculosis*. *Science, 333*, 1630–1632.

Siegele, D. A., & Kolter, R. (1992). Life after log. *Journal of Bacteriology, 174*, 345–348.

Silverman, J. A., Perlmutter, N. G., & Shapiro, H. M. (2003). Correlation of daptomycin bactericidal activity and membrane depolarization in *Staphylococcus aureus*. *Antimicrobial Agents and Chemotherapy, 47*, 2538–2544.

Slepenkov, S. V., & Witt, S. N. (2002). The unfolding story of the *Escherichia coli* Hsp70 DnaK: Is Dnak a holdase or an unfoldase? *Molecular Microbiology, 45*, 1197–1206.

Spira, B., Silberstein, N., & Yagil, E. (1995). Guanosine 3′,5′-Bispyrophosphate (ppGpp) synthesis in cells of *Escherichia coli* starved for P$_i$. *Journal of Bacteriology, 177*, 4053–4058.

Spoering, A. L., & Lewis, K. (2001). Biofilms and planktonic cells of *Pseudomonas aeruginosa* have similar resistance to killing by antimicrobials. *Journal of Bacteriology, 183*, 6746–6751.

Spoering, A. L., Vulic, M., & Lewis, K. (2006). GlpD And PlsB participate in persister cell formation in *Escherichia coli*. *Journal of Bacteriology, 188*, 5136–5144.

Sprenger, M., Kasper, L., Hensel, M., & Hube, B. (2017). Metabolic adaptation of intracellular bacteria and fungi to macrophages. *International Journal of Medical Microbiology, 308*(1), 215–227.

Stark, M., Liu, L. P., & Deber, C. M. (2002). Cationic hydrophobic peptides with antimicrobial activity. *Antimicrobial Agents and Chemotherapy, 46*, 3585–3590.

Stephanopoulos, G. N., Aristidou, A. A., & Nielsen, J. (1998). *Metabolic engineering: Principles and methodologies* (pp. 119–120). San Diego: Academic.

Stewart, P. S. (1996). Theoretical aspects of antibiotic diffusion into microbial biofilms. *Antimicrobial Agents and Chemotherapy, 40*, 2517–2522.

Stewart, P. S. (2003). Diffusion in biofilms. *Journal of Bacteriology, 185*, 1485–1491.

Stewart, P. S., & Franklin, M. J. (2008). Physiological heterogeneity in biofilms. *Nature Reviews. Microbiology, 6*, 199–210.

Stewart, P. S., Zhang, T., Xu, R., Pitts, B., Walters, M. C., Roe, F., Kikhney, J., & Moter, A. (2016). Reaction-diffusion theory explains hypoxia and heterogeneous growth within microbial biofilms associated with chronic infections. *NPJ Biofilms Microbiomes, 2*, 16012.

Stoodley, P., Sauer, K., Davies, D. G., & Costerton, J. W. (2002). Biofilms as complex differentiated communities. *Annual Review of Microbiology, 56*, 187–209.

Sukheja, P., Kumar, P., Mittal, N., Li, S. G., Singleton, E., Russo, R., Perryman, A. L., Shrestha, R., Awasthi, D., Husain, S., Soteropoulos, P., Brukh, R., Connell, N., Freundlich, J. S., & Alland, D. (2017). A novel small-molecule inhibitor of the *Mycobacterium tuberculosis* demethylmenaquinone methyltransferase MenG is bactericidal to both growing and nutritionally deprived persister cells. *Mbio, 8*, e02022-16.

Taber, H. W., Mueller, J. P., Miller, P. F., & Arrow, A. S. (1987). Bacterial uptake of aminoglycoside antibiotics. *Microbiological Reviews, 51*, 439–457.

Takikawa, O., Yoshida, R., Kido, R., & Hayaishi, O. (1986). Tryptophan degradation in mice initiated by indoleamine 2,3-dioxygenase. *The Journal of Biological Chemistry, 261*, 3648–3653.

Theodore, A., Lewis, K., & Vulic, M. (2013). Tolerance of *Escherichia coli* to fluoroquinolone antibiotics depends on specific components of the SOS response pathway. *Genetics, 195*, 1265–1276.

Traxler, M. F., Summers, S. M., Nguyen, H. T., Zacharia, V. M., Hightower, G. A., Smith, J. T., & Conway, T. (2008). The global, ppGpp-mediated stringent response to amino acid starvation in *Escherichia coli. Molecular Microbiology, 68*, 1128–1148.

Tuomanen, E., Cozens, R., Tosch, W., Zak, O., & Tomasz, A. (1986). The rate of killing of *Escherichia coli* by beta-lactam antibiotics is strictly proportional to the rate of bacterial growth. *Journal of General Microbiology, 132*, 1297–1304.

Ueta, M., Ohniwa, R. L., Yoshida, H., Maki, Y., Wada, C., & Wada, A. (2008). Role of HPF (hibernation promoting factor) in translational activity in *Escherichia coli. Journal of Biochemistry, 143*, 425–433.

Van Den Bergh, B., Michiels, J. E., Wenseleers, T., Windels, E. M., Boer, P. V., Kestemont, D., De Meester, L., Verstrepen, K. J., Verstraeten, N., Fauvart, M., & Michiels, J. (2016). Frequency of antibiotic application drives rapid evolutionary adaptation of *Escherichia coli* persistence. *Nature Microbiology, 1*, 16020.

Verstraeten, N., Knapen, W. J., Kint, C. I., Liebens, V., Van Den Bergh, B., Dewachter, L., Michiels, J. E., Fu, Q., David, C. C., Fierro, A. C., Marchal, K., Beirlant, J., Versees, W., Hofkens, J., Jansen, M., Fauvart, M., & Michiels, J. (2015). Obg and membrane depolarization are part of a microbial bet-hedging strategy that leads to antibiotic tolerance. *Molecular Cell, 59*, 9–21.

Via, L. E., Savic, R., Weiner, D. M., Zimmerman, M. D., Prideaux, B., Irwin, S. M., Lyon, E., O'brien, P., Gopal, P., Eum, S., Lee, M., Lanoix, J. P., Dutta, N. K., Shim, T., Cho, J. S., Kim, W., Karakousis, P. C., Lenaerts, A., Nuermberger, E., Barry, C. E., & Dartois, V. (2015). Host-mediated bioactivation of pyrazinamide: Implications for efficacy, resistance, and therapeutic alternatives. *ACS Infectious Diseases, 1*, 203–214.

Volzing, K. G., & Brynildsen, M. P. (2015). Stationary-phase persisters to ofloxacin sustain DNA damage and require repair systems only during recovery. *MBio, 6*, e00731–e00715.

Wada, A., Yamazaki, Y., Fujita, N., & Ishihama, A. (1990). Structure and probable genetic location of a "ribosome modulation factor" associated with 100s ribosomes in stationary-phase *Escherichia coli* cells. *Proceedings of the National Academy of Sciences of the United States of America, 87*, 2657–2661.

Wada, A., Igarashi, K., Yoshimura, S., Aimoto, S., & Ishihama, A. (1995). Ribosome modulation factor: Stationary growth phase-specific inhibitor of ribosome functions from *Escherichia coli*. *Biochemical and Biophysical Research Communications, 214*, 410–417.

Wade, M. M., & Zhang, Y. (2006). Effects of weak acids, UV and proton motive force inhibitors on pyrazinamide activity against *Mycobacterium tuberculosis* in vitro. *The Journal of Antimicrobial Chemotherapy, 58*, 936–941.

Walsh, C. (2003). Where will new antibiotics come from? *Nature Reviews. Microbiology, 1*, 65–70.

Walsh, C. T., & Wencewicz, T. A. (2014). Prospects for new antibiotics: A molecule-centered perspective. *Journal of Antibiotics (Tokyo), 67*, 7–22.

Walters, M. C., 3rd, Roe, F., Bugnicourt, A., Franklin, M. J., & Stewart, P. S. (2003). Contributions of antibiotic penetration, oxygen limitation, and low metabolic activity to tolerance of *Pseudomonas aeruginosa* biofilms to ciprofloxacin and tobramycin. *Antimicrobial Agents and Chemotherapy, 47*, 317–323.

Wassarman, K. M., & Saecker, R. M. (2006). Synthesis-mediated release of a small RNA inhibitor of RNA polymerase. *Science, 314*, 1601–1603.

Watson, S. P., Clements, M. O., & Foster, S. J. (1998). Characterization of the starvation-survival response of *Staphylococcus aureus*. *Journal of Bacteriology, 180*, 1750–1758.

Weichart, D., Querfurth, N., Dreger, M., & Hengge-Aronis, R. (2003). Global role for ClpP-containing proteases in stationary-phase adaptation of *Escherichia coli*. *Journal of Bacteriology, 185*, 115–125.

Wenthzel, A. M., Stancek, M., & Isaksson, L. A. (1998). Growth phase dependent stop codon readthrough and shift of translation reading frame in *Escherichia coli*. *FEBS Letters, 421*, 237–242.

Wieland, H., Ullrich, S., Lang, F., & Neumeister, B. (2005). Intracellular multiplication of *Legionella pneumophila* depends on host cell amino acid transporter Slc1a5. *Molecular Microbiology, 55*, 1528–1537.

Wigle, T. J., Sexton, J. Z., Gromova, A. V., Hadimani, M. B., Hughes, M. A., Smith, G. R., Yeh, L. A., & Singleton, S. F. (2009). Inhibitors of RecA activity discovered by high-throughput screening: Cell-permeable small molecules attenuate the SOS response in *Escherichia coli*. *Journal of Biomolecular Screening, 14*, 1092–1101.

Wilson, K. H., & Perini, F. (1988). Role of competition for nutrients in suppression of *Clostridium difficile* by the colonic microflora. *Infection and Immunity, 56*, 2610–2614.

Wolf, S. G., Frenkiel, D., Arad, T., Finkel, S. E., Kolter, R., & Minsky, A. (1999). DNA protection by stress-induced biocrystallization. *Nature, 400*, 83–85.

Wolff, J. A., Macgregor, C. H., Eisenberg, R. C., & Phibbs, P. V., Jr. (1991). Isolation and characterization of catabolite repression control mutants of *Pseudomonas aeruginosa* PAO. *Journal of Bacteriology, 173*, 4700–4706.

Xiao, H., Kalman, M., Ikehara, K., Zemel, S., Glaser, G., & Cashel, M. (1991). Residual guanosine $3',5'$-bispyrophosphate synthetic activity of rela null mutants can be eliminated by spot null mutations. *The Journal of Biological Chemistry, 266*, 5980–5990.

Xu, K. D., Stewart, P. S., Xia, F., Huang, C. T., & Mcfeters, G. A. (1998). Spatial physiological heterogeneity in *Pseudomonas aeruginosa* biofilm is determined by oxygen availability. *Applied and Environmental Microbiology, 64*, 4035–4039.

Yakimov, A., Pobegalov, G., Bakhlanova, I., Khodorkovskii, M., Petukhov, M., & Baitin, D. (2017). Blocking the RecA activity and SOS-response in bacteria with a short α-helical peptide. *Nucleic Acids Research, 45*, 9788–9796.

Yoshida, R., Imanishi, J., Oku, T., Kishida, T., & Hayaishi, O. (1981). Induction of pulmonary indoleamine 2,3-dioxygenase by interferon. *Proceedings of the National Academy of Sciences of the United States of America, 78,* 129–132.

Zhang, Y., Wade, M. M., Scorpio, A., Zhang, H., & Sun, Z. (2003). Mode of action of pyrazinamide: Disruption of *Mycobacterium tuberculosis* membrane transport and energetics by pyrazinoic acid. *The Journal of Antimicrobial Chemotherapy, 52,* 790–795.

Zhang, S., Chen, J., Shi, W., Liu, W., Zhang, W., & Zhang, Y. (2013a). Mutations in *panD* encoding aspartate decarboxylase are associated with pyrazinamide resistance in *Mycobacterium tuberculosis*. *Emerging Microbes and Infections, 2,* e34.

Zhang, Y., Shi, W., Zhang, W., & Mitchison, D. (2013b). Mechanisms of pyrazinamide action and resistance. *Microbiology Spectrum, 2,* 1–12.

Zimhony, O., Cox, J. S., Welch, J. T., Vilchèze, C., & Jacobs, W. R. (2000). Pyrazinamide inhibits the eukaryotic-like fatty acid synthetase I (FASI) of *Mycobacterium tuberculosis*. *Nature Medicine, 6,* 1043–1047.

Zogaj, X., Nimtz, M., Rohde, M., Bokranz, W., & Römling, U. (2001). The multicellular morphotypes of *Salmonella typhimurium* and *Escherichia coli* produce cellulose as the second component of the extracellular matrix. *Molecular Microbiology, 39,* 1452–1463.

Chapter 7
Genetic Determinants of Persistence in *Escherichia coli*

Dorien Wilmaerts, Pauline Herpels, Jan Michiels, and Natalie Verstraeten

Abstract Persisters comprise a small fraction of cells within a bacterial population that transiently are tolerant to lethal doses of antibiotics. Following their discovery, persister cells went unheeded for nearly 40 years until Moyed and Bertrand revived the field of persister research in 1983. Ever since, an increasing body of literature has reported on genetic determinants of persistence. We here present a comprehensive overview of all currently known genes affecting persistence in *Escherichia coli*. We systematically group persister genes according to the biological processes they are involved in, more specifically a variety of stress responses and energy metabolism. We also briefly touch upon the role of toxin-antitoxin systems in persistence. In general, persister levels are positively correlated with expression levels of genes that yield protection against nutrient stress (e.g., *dksA*, *relA*), DNA damage (e.g., *recA*, *lexA*, *umuDC*), heat shock (e.g., *dnaJ*, *dnaK*), or oxidative stress (e.g., *soxS*, *oxyR*). This underlines the importance of these stress responses in the formation of persister cells. However, both elevated and decreased persister levels are found upon impeding the general stress response and energy metabolism, emphasizing the need for further research. Combined with additional persister genes that undoubtedly await discovery, the information presented in this work will support the development of new persister models that will in turn greatly contribute to our understanding of this intriguing phenomenon.

Dorien Wilmaerts and Pauline Herpels are the co-first authors.
Jan Michiels and Natalie Verstraeten are the co-last authors.

D. Wilmaerts · P. Herpels · J. Michiels (✉) · N. Verstraeten
VIB, Center for Microbiology, Leuven, Belgium

KU Leuven, Centre of Microbial and Plant Genetics, Leuven, Belgium
e-mail: jan.michiels@kuleuven.vib.be

© Springer Nature Switzerland AG 2019   133
K. Lewis (ed.), *Persister Cells and Infectious Disease*,
https://doi.org/10.1007/978-3-030-25241-0_7

7.1   Introduction

Literature on persistence has been steadily growing for the past two decades. As a consequence, it is becoming increasingly difficult to keep an overview of genetic determinants affecting persistence. We, therefore, performed an extensive search of the existing literature for persistence genes. On the basis of this search, we list in this chapter all persister genes currently known in *Escherichia coli*. Furthermore, as experimental conditions are well known to affect persistence tests, we also provide decisive elements in the used protocols that are known to alter persistence, including factors such as used antibiotics, growth medium, and growth phase. Persister genes are defined as genes that, when mutated, deleted, or overexpressed, change persistence in a specific condition. Furthermore, we discuss a selection of genes in light of the biological process they are involved in (stress responses, metabolism) and we highlight connections between these processes.

7.2   General Stress Response

The general stress response (GSR) is mastered by the sigma factor RpoS (σ^S) and regulates approximately 10% of all genes in *E. coli*. Although the RpoS regulon consists of many genes, they are not all specific for the GSR as many genes are also involved in other, more specific, stress responses (Weber et al. 2005). While many bacterial stress responses yield protection against a specific stressor, the GSR entails a more preventive strategy to survive exposure to a variety of stresses, for example, acid, osmotic and heat stress, which results in cross-protection (Rowe and Kirk 1999; Battesti et al. 2011; Behmardi et al. 2009).

RpoS is regulated at multiple levels as reviewed in (Battesti et al. 2011; Landini et al. 2014): transcription and translation of *rpoS*, degradation of RpoS and loading of the sigma factor on the polymerase are all controlled by many regulators, and different stresses may act at distinct levels (Battesti et al. 2011; Hengge-Aronis 2002). Cellular RpoS levels are low in exponential phase due to RssB-induced proteolysis (Muffler et al. 1996), but increase strongly during stationary phase (Battesti et al. 2011). Furthermore, the RpoS concentration in early exponential phase is much higher in minimal media as compared to LB medium (Dong and Schellhorn 2009).

Deletion of *rpoS* has been reported to increase the persister fraction in stationary phase after ciprofloxacin treatment and, after dilution, ampicillin and norfloxacin treatment (Wu et al. 2015; Hong et al. 2012). In contrast, a Δ*rpoS* strain exhibits a strongly reduced persister fraction following gentamicin treatment in (early) stationary phase (Wu et al. 2015; Liu et al. 2017) and treatments that induce *rpoS* transcription, including oxidative and acid stresses, cause the persister fraction to increase (Hong et al. 2012). Furthermore, when persistence is induced through nutrient shifts, expression of *rpoS* increases the persister fraction, while deletion of *rpoS* results in more growing cells and consequently fewer persisters (Radzikowski et al. 2016). Lastly, deletion of *rssB*, a negative regulator of RpoS, decreases the persister fraction, although this phenotype was only observed in 96-well plates and not in larger volumes (Hansen et al. 2008). Contrasting results presumably emerge from differences in used antibiotics and treatment conditions and emphasize the need for further research on the role of RpoS in persistence.

Several genes in the RpoS regulon have been linked with persistence (Table 7.1). For example, *osmY* (involved in the hyperosmotic response) is upregulated in non-growing cells that are enriched in persisters (Shah et al. 2006), and deletion of *osmY* (Weber et al. 2005; Yim et al. 1994), *gadB* and *gadX* (both involved in pH homeostasis) (Tramonti et al. 2002) increases the persister fraction tolerant to ampicillin (Hong et al. 2012). However, deletion of *osmY* might yield some resistance as a large-scale screen showed that a Δ*osmY* strain grows better than the wild type in the presence of subinhibitory concentrations of ampicillin (Nichols et al. 2011).

7.3 Stringent Response

Upon nutrient deprivation, bacteria adapt their gene expression profile from one that supports growth to one that supports survival. In *E. coli*, this switch is regulated by the RelA and SpoT proteins that control cellular levels of the alarmone (p)ppGpp, the hallmark of the stringent response (Boutte and Crosson 2013). (p)ppGpp directly interacts with RNA polymerase. Together with the transcription factor DksA, (p) ppGpp will bind to the RNA polymerase, thereby downregulating genes necessary for rapid growth (e.g., rRNA genes) and upregulating genes important for amino acid biosynthesis, stress survival, and nutrient uptake (Boutte and Crosson 2013). The stringent response and the GSR are linked as (p)ppGpp increases the efficacy of *rpoS* transcription (Brown et al. 2002; Girard et al. 2018; Gentry et al. 1993).

(p)ppGpp is present at low intracellular levels during exponential phase (Potrykus et al. 2011), but its concentration increases strongly upon nutrient limitation through RelA activation (Haseltine and Block 1973). Depletion of nutrients, resulting in amino acid starvation, leads to the accumulation of uncharged tRNAs that enter the ribosomal A site, which halts translation (Haseltine and Block 1973). This is the signal for RelA to dissociate from the ribosome (English et al. 2011) and produce (p) ppGpp (Haseltine and Block 1973). In contrast to RelA, SpoT synthesizes (p)ppGpp in response to different stresses, such as carbon starvation (Xiao et al. 1991), iron starvation (Vinella et al. 2005), diauxic shifts (Harshman and Yamazaki 1971), phosphorous limitation (Rao et al. 1998), hyperosmotic shock (Harshman and Yamazakif 1972) and fatty acid starvation (Battesti and Bouveret 2006). Furthermore, SpoT also functions as a (p)ppGpp hydrolase. This activity is repressed upon binding with free uncharged tRNAs (An et al. 1979) and/or upon binding with the conserved GTPase ObgE (Wout et al. 2004).

Table 7.1 Genetic determinants of persistence involved in the general stress response

Gene	Protein	Genetic background	Mutation	Persister fraction	Growth phase	Medium	Antibiotic	References
gadB	Glutamate decarboxylase	BW25113	Deletion	Increase	Stat	LB	Ap	Hong et al. (2012)
gadX	Transcriptional regulator	BW25113	Deletion	Increase	Stat	LB	Ap	Hong et al. (2012)
osmY	Osmotically inducible protein	BW25113	Deletion	Increase	Stat	LB	Ap	Hong et al. (2012)
		MG1655	Upregulated in non-growing cells		Exp	LB	/	Shah et al. (2006)
rpoS	RNA polymerase sigma factor	W3110	Deletion	Increase	Stat*	LB	Ap, Nor	Wu et al. (2015)
		W3110	Deletion	Decrease	Stat*	LB	Gm	Wu et al. (2015)
		W3110	Deletion	Decrease	Stat	LB	Gm	Liu et al. (2017)
		BW25113	Deletion	Increase	Stat	LB	Cip	Hong et al. (2012)
rssB	RpoS regulator	BW25113	Deletion	Decrease	Exp	MOPS + 0.1% Suc + 0.05% CAA	Of	Hansen et al. (2008)

Stat stationary, *Stat** stationary-phase cells treated after dilution, *Exp* exponential, *LB* lysogeny broth, *MOPS* (3-(*N*-morpholino) propanesulfonic acid), *Suc* succinate, *CAA* casamino acids, *Ap* ampicillin, *Cip* ciprofloxacin, *Gm* gentamicin, *Nor* norfloxacin, *Of* ofloxacin

Several studies have shown a positive correlation between the stringent response and persistence (Table 7.2). The first link between (p)ppGpp and persistence was demonstrated by Korch and colleagues, who showed that HipA7 (see below) induces persistence by increasing the level of (p)ppGpp synthesis (Korch et al. 2003). (p) ppGpp was also shown to be important for the induction of persistence upon ectopic expression of the wild-type HipA toxin (Bokinsky et al. 2013; Germain et al. 2013). Furthermore, deletion of *relAspoT* (Korch et al. 2003; Fung et al. 2010; Amato et al. 2013) or *relA* (Wu et al. 2015; Liu et al. 2017) decreases the persister fraction and both *relA* and *spoT* were found to be upregulated in persister cells (Pu et al. 2016). RelA and SpoT, in combination with the transcription factor DksA, mediate persister formation during carbon source transitions (Amato et al. 2013). Deletion of *dksA* also reduces persistence (Hansen et al. 2008; Amato et al. 2013) and the reduction in persister fraction caused by deletion of several genes (e.g., *dnaK* and *recA*) is dependent on RelA functioning (Liu et al. 2017). In addition, (p)ppGpp is linked with persistence as it is a prerequisite for ObgE overexpression to mediate persistence (Verstraeten et al. 2015).

Inducing amino acid starvation by deleting several biosynthesis genes was shown to strongly increase persistence. This effect is even more pronounced in biofilm setups (Bernier et al. 2013). Deletion of either biosynthesis genes of cysteine (*cysD*), arginine (*argE*, *argH*), proline (*proA*, *proC*), aromatic amino acids (*aroE*), lysine (*lysA*), phenylalanine (*pheA*), methionine (*metA*) and leucine, isoleucine and valine (*leuB*, *leuC*, *ilvA*, *ilvC*, *livJ*) leads to a significantly increased persister fractions (Bernier et al. 2013; Girgis et al. 2012). Notably, transposon mutants of genes that are functional in the early steps of the aromatic biosynthesis pathway [the *aro* genes (Bernier et al. 2013; Girgis et al. 2012; Shan et al. 2015)] and more toward the end [the *trp* genes (Bernier et al. 2013; Shan et al. 2015)] show decreased persister levels, thereby contradicting the hypothesis of increased persistence upon amino acid starvation.

Several downstream genes of the stringent response play a role in persistence. For example, (p)ppGpp positively regulates expression of CspD (Yamanaka and Inouye 1997), which inhibits chromosomal replication of nutrient-depleted cells (Yamanaka et al. 2001) and whose cellular levels are positively correlated with the persister fraction (Kim and Wood 2010). Interestingly, growth resumption after starvation depends on degradation of CspD by Lon (Langklotz and Narberhaus 2011), a protease associated with persistence (Pu et al. 2016; Harms et al. 2017; Germain et al. 2015). Next, the limitation of inorganic phosphate (Pi) results in SpoT-mediated accumulation of (p)ppGpp (Rao et al. 1998). This, in turn, causes an upregulation of *phoA*, coding for a Pi scavenger, and *pstS*, coding for a Pi-transporter, both members of the Pho regulon that is important for metabolism and transport of Pi (Santos-Beneit 2015; Spira et al. 1995). PhoU, a repressor of the phosphate metabolism, is deactivated upon Pi starvation. Deletion of *phoU* causes the Pho operon to be constitutively transcribed and decreases the persister fraction (Li and Zhang 2007; Luidalepp et al. 2011) and *phoU* is upregulated in persisters (Pu et al. 2016). Although it was originally stated that the formation of persisters by PhoU is independent of phosphate metabolism (Li and Zhang 2007), deletion of

Table 7.2 Genetic determinants of persistence involved in the stringent response

Gene	Protein	Genetic background	Mutation	Persister fraction	Growth phase	Medium	Antibiotic	References
argE	Acetylornithine deacetylase	TG1	Deletion	Increase	Biofilm	M63B1 + 0.4% Glc	Tic, Of	Bernier et al. (2013)
argH	Argininosuccinate lyase	TG1	Deletion	Increase	Biofilm	M63B1 + 0.4% Glc	Tic, Of	Bernier et al. (2013)
aroADF	3-Phosphoshikimate 1-carboxyvinyltransferase	MG1655	Transposon insertion	Decrease	Stat	MOPS + 0.2% Glc + 0.2% CAA	Gm	Shan et al. (2015)
aroE	Shikimate 5-dehydrogenase	TG1	Deletion	Increase	Biofilm	M63B1 + 0.4% Glc	Tic, Of	Bernier et al. (2013)
aroP	Aromatic amino acid transport protein	MG1655 (metG*)	Transposon insertion	Decrease	Plates	LB	Ap	Girgis et al. (2012)
aspC	l-Phenylalanine biosynthetic process	MG1655	Transposon insertion	Decrease	Stat	MOPS + 0.2% Glc + 0.2% CAA	Gm	Shan et al. (2015)
cspD	Cold-shock protein	BW25113	Overexpression	Decrease	Stat	LB	Ap	Kim and Wood (2010)
		HM22 (hipA7)	Upregulated in persister cells			LB	Ap	Keren et al. (2004a)
cysD	Sulfate adenylyltransferase	TG1	Deletion	Increase	Stat	M63B1 + 0.4% Glc	Tic	Bernier et al. (2013)
		TG1	Deletion	Increase	Biofilm	M63B1 + 0.4% Glc	Tic, Of	Bernier et al. (2013)
cysK	Cysteine synthase	MG1655	Transposon insertion	Decrease	Stat	MOPS + 0.2% Glc + 0.2% CAA	Gm	Shan et al. (2015)
dksA	RNA polymerase-binding transcription factor	MG1655	Deletion	Decrease	Exp	M9	Of	Amato et al. (2013)
		BW25113	Deletion	Decrease	Exp	MOPS + 0.1% Suc + 0.05% CAA	Ap	Hansen et al. (2008)
		BW25113	Deletion	Decrease	Stat*	LB	Carb	Pu et al. (2016)
		BW25113	Upregulated in persister cells		Exp	LB	Carb	Pu et al. (2016)

Gene	Function	Strain	Mutation	Change	Phase	Medium	Antibiotic	Reference
hisG	ATP phosphoribosyl-transferase	TG1	Deletion	Increase	Biofilm	M63B1 + 0.4% Glc	Tic, Of	Bernier et al. (2013)
ilvA	Threonine dehydratase	TG1	Deletion	Increase	Biofilm	M63B1 + 0.4% Glc	Tic, Of	Bernier et al. (2013)
ilvC	Ketol acid reductoisomerase	TG1	Deletion	Increase	Biofilm	M63B1 + 0.4% Glc	Tic, Of	Bernier et al. (2013)
leuB	3-Isopropylmalate dehydrogenase	TG1	Deletion	Increase	Biofilm	M63B1 + 0.4% Glc	Tic, Of	Bernier et al. (2013)
leuC	Isopropylmalate isomerase	TG1	Deletion	Increase	Biofilm	M63B1 + 0.4% Glc	Tic, Of	Bernier et al. (2013)
		TG1	Deletion	Increase	Stat	M63B1 + 0.4% Glc	Tic	Bernier et al. (2013)
livJ	Leucine/isoleucine/valine transporter	MG1655	Transposon insertion	Increase	Plates	LB	Ap	Girgis et al. (2012)
lrp	Leucine-responsive regulator	MG1655	Transposon insertion and deletion	Decrease	Stat	MOPS + 0.2% Glc + 0.2% CAA	Gm	Shan et al. (2015)
lysA	Diaminopimelate decarboxylase, PLP-binding	TG1	Deletion	Increase	Stat	M63B1 + 0.4% Glc	Tic	Bernier et al. (2013)
			Deletion	Increase	Biofilm	M63B1 + 0.4% Glc	Tic, Of	Bernier et al. (2013)
metA	Homoserine O-succinyltransferase	TG1	Deletion	Increase	Biofilm	M63B1 + 0.4% Glc	Tic, Of	Bernier et al. (2013)
mtr	Tryptophan-specific transport	EMG2	Deletion	Decrease	Stat	LB	Of	Vega et al. (2012)
obgE	GTPase	TOP10	Overexpression	Increase	Exp, Stat	LB	Ceft, Of, Tob	Verstraeten et al. (2015)
		BW25113	Overexpression	Increase	Stat	LB	Of	Verstraeten et al. (2015)
		TOP10	Downregulation	Decrease	Stat	LB	Of, Tob	Verstraeten et al. (2015)
		TOP10	Downregulation	Decrease	Exp	LB	Of, Ceft	Verstraeten et al. (2015)

(continued)

Table 7.2 (continued)

Gene	Protein	Genetic background	Mutation	Persister fraction	Growth phase	Medium	Antibiotic	References
pheA	Fused chorismate mutase P/prephenate dehydratase	TG1	Deletion	Increase	Biofilm	M63B1 + 0.4% Glc	Tic, Of	Bernier et al. (2013)
phoU	Phosphate-specific transport system accessory protein	W3110	Transposon insertion and deletion	Decrease	Exp, Stat	LB	Ap, Nor, Pza, Gm	Li and Zhang (2007)
		BW25113	Deletion	Decrease	Stat*	Lennox LB	Ap	Luidalepp et al. (2011)
		W3110	Deletion	Decrease	Stat	LB	Ap, Gm	Wu et al. (2015)
proA	γ-Glutamyl phosphate reductase	TG1	Deletion	Increase	Biofilm	M63B1 + 0.4% Glc	Tic, Of	Bernier et al. (2013)
proC	Pyrroline-5-carboxylate reductase	TG1	Deletion	Increase	Biofilm	M63B1 + 0.4% Glc	Tic, Of	Bernier et al. (2013)
relA	GTP pyrophosphokinase	MG1655	Deletion	Decrease	Exp	LB	Cip	Germain et al. (2015)
		MG1655	Deletion (ΔrelAΔspoT)	Decrease	Exp	LB	Cip	Germain et al. (2015)
		W3110	Deletion	Decrease	Stat*	LB	Ap	Wu et al. (2015)
		MG1655	Deletion (ΔrelAΔspoT)	Decrease	Exp	M9	Of	Amato et al. (2013)
		W3110	Deletion	Decrease	Stat	LB	Ap, Gm, Nor	Liu et al. (2017)
		BW25113	Upregulated in persister cells		Exp	LB	Carb	Pu et al. (2016)
		BW25113	Deletion (ΔrelAΔspoT)	Decrease	Stat	LB	Of	Verstraeten et al. (2015)
		BW25113	Deletion	Decrease	Stat	LB	Of	Verstraeten et al. (2015)

serA	D-3-Phosphoglycerate dehydrogenase	MG1655	Transposon insertion and deletion	Decrease	Stat	MOPS + 0.2% Glc + 0.2% CAA	Gm	Shan et al. (2015)
serB	Phosphoserine phosphatase	MG1655	Transposon insertion and deletion	Decrease	Stat	MOPS + 0.2% Glc + 0.2% CAA	Gm	Shan et al. (2015)
serC	Phosphoserine aminotransferase	MG1655	Transposon insertion and deletion	Decrease	Stat	MOPS + 0.2% Glc + 0.2% CAA	Gm	Shan et al. (2015)
tnaA	Tryptophanase	W3110	Deletion	Decrease	Stat	LB	Nor	Wu et al. (2015)
		EMG2	Deletion	Decrease	Stat	LB	Of	Giudice et al. (2014)
		W3110	Deletion	Decrease	Stat	LB	Ap, Gm	Liu et al. (2017)
		W3110 (Δ*relA*)	Deletion	Decrease	Stat	LB	Ap, Gm, Nor	Liu et al. (2017)
trpA	Tryptophan synthase	TG1	Deletion	Decrease	Biofilm	M63B1 + 0.4% Glc	Tic	Bernier et al. (2013)
		MG1655	Transposon insertion	Decrease	Stat	MOPS + 0.2% Glc + 0.2% CAA	Gm	Shan et al. (2015)
trpBCDE	Tryptophan synthase	MG1655	Transposon insertion	Decrease	Stat	MOPS + 0.2% Glc + 0.2% CAA	Gm	Shan et al. (2015)
tyrA	T-Protein	TG1	Deletion	Increase	Biofilm	M63B1 + 0.4% Glc	Tic, Of	Bernier et al. (2013)
		MG1655	Transposon insertion	Decrease	Stat	MOPS + 0.2% Glc + 0.2% CAA	Gm	Shan et al. (2015)

metG∗ *metG* missing 7 amino acids at the C-terminus, *Stat* stationary, *Stat*∗ stationary-phase cells treated after dilution, *Exp* exponential, *LB* lysogeny broth, *MHB* Mueller Hinton broth, *MOPS* 3-(*N*-morpholino)propanesulfonic acid, *Glc* glucose, *CAA* casamino acids, *Suc* sucrose, *Ap* ampicillin, *Carb* carbenicillin, *Ceft* ceftazidime, *Cip* ciprofloxacin, *Gm* gentamicin, *Nor* norfloxacin, *Of* ofloxacin, *Pza* pyrazinamide, *Tic* ticarcillin, *Tob* tobramycin

phoU results in an uncontrolled uptake of Pi, which is toxic for the cell and might, thus, be an alternative explanation for the sensitivity of Δ*phoU* strains toward antibiotics (Rice et al. 2009). Furthermore, *phoU* deletion mutants grow poorly and tend to accumulate compensatory mutations in the Pho regulon, which might conceal the effect of *phoU* deletion on the persister fraction (Steed and Wanner 1993).

7.4 SOS Response

The bacterial SOS response coordinates the response of the cell to DNA damage (Kreuzer 2013). In *E. coli*, the major regulators of this pathway are LexA, acting as a repressor, and RecA, acting as a de-repressor. LexA in its dimeric form binds to the promoter of multiple SOS genes, thereby inhibiting their expression (Brent and Ptashne 1980; Giese et al. 2008; Luo et al. 2001). Importantly, LexA regulates its own expression and that of *recA*, thereby creating a mechanism for both induction and repression of the SOS response (Brent and Ptashne 1980). Upon DNA damage, RecA binds to single-stranded DNA. This binding activates RecA to become a coprotease that enhances the self-cleavage of LexA. This weakens the DNA-binding properties of LexA, resulting in increased expression of the SOS regulon genes (Little 1991). Furthermore, RecA stabilizes the stalled replication fork (Courcelle and Hanawalt 2003). Importantly, not all LexA-regulated genes are induced by the same level of DNA damage (Kamenšek et al. 2010).

Several studies have revealed a link between genes from the SOS response and persistence (Table 7.3). In general, downregulating the SOS response by deleting *recA* or by expressing a non-cleavable LexA3 repressor causes a decrease in persistence (Wu et al. 2015; Luidalepp et al. 2011; Debbia et al. 2001; Dörr et al. 2009). Conversely, constitutively activating the SOS regulon (*lexA300*) induces the formation of persister cells (Dörr et al. 2009). In addition, *recA* is upregulated in persisters isolated by treating an exponential-phase culture with ampicillin (Keren et al. 2004a).

A study by the Lewis group showed that ciprofloxacin-mediated induction of persistence in exponential phase results from the emergence of double-stranded DNA breaks (DSB) that trigger the SOS response (Dörr et al. 2009). Noteworthy, a high level of SOS induction is not a prerequisite for transition to the persistent state in exponential phase as persisters display only weak induction, presumably resulting from only a few DSB (Dörr et al. 2009). Expression of the toxin gene *tisB*, part of the SOS regulon, was subsequently shown to result in the collapse of the membrane potential and a drop in ATP levels, thereby inducing persistence and preventing further DNA damage (Dörr et al. 2010). At both high and low ciprofloxacin concentrations, the SOS-inducible proteins DinG, UvrD, RuvA, and RuvB, play a role in bacterial persistence as deletion mutants display lower persister fractions following treatment with ciprofloxacin (Theodore et al. 2013) and the corresponding genes are upregulated in persister cells (Pu et al. 2016). *dinG* and *uvrD* encode DNA

Table 7.3 Genetic determinants of persistence involved in the SOS response

Gene	Protein	Genetic background	Mutation	Persister fraction	Growth phase	Medium	Antibiotic	References
dinG	ATP-dependent DNA helicase	MG1655	Deletion	Decrease	Exp	MHB	Cip	Theodore et al. (2013)
		MG1655	Deletion	Decrease	Stat	MHB	Cip	Theodore et al. (2013)
		BW25113	Upregulated in persister cells		Exp	LB	Carb	Pu et al. (2016)
hupA	DNA-binding protein	BW25113	Deletion	Decrease	Stat	LB	Carb	Pu et al. (2016)
		BW25113	Upregulated in persister cells		Exp	LB	Carb	Pu et al. (2016)
hupB	DNA-binding protein	BW25113	Deletion	Decrease	Stat	MOPS + 0.1% Suc + 0.05% CAA	Of	Hansen et al. (2008)
		MG1655	Deletion	Decrease	Stat	M9	Of	Amato et al. (2013)
		BW25113	Upregulated in persister cells		Exp	LB	Carb	Pu et al. (2016)
lexA	LexA repressor	AB1157	Downreg SOS (*lexA3*)	Decrease	Exp	MHB	Ap, Ceftr, Mer, Amk, Cip	Debbia et al. (2001)
		MG1655	Upregul SOS (*lexA300*)	Increase	Stat	MHB	Cip	Dörr et al. (2009)
		MG1655	Downreg SOS (*lexA3*)	Decrease	Stat	MHB	Cip	Dörr et al. (2009)
		BW25113	Downreg SOS (*lexA3*)	Decrease	Stat*	LB	Of	Wu et al. (2012)

(continued)

Table 7.3 (continued)

Gene	Protein	Genetic background	Mutation	Persister fraction	Growth phase	Medium	Antibiotic	References
recA	Recombinase A	W3110	Deletion	Decrease	Stat*	LB	Ap	Wu et al. (2015)
		BW25113	Deletion	Decrease	Stat*	Lennox LB	Ap	Luidalepp et al. (2011)
		MG1655	Deletion	Decrease	Stat	MHB	Cip	Dörr et al. (2009)
		HM22 (hipA7)	Upregulated in persister cells		Exp	LB	Ap	Keren et al. (2004a)
		MG1655	Deletion	Decrease	Stat	M9 + 10 mM Glc	Of	Völzing and Brynildsen (2015)
recB	RecBCD enzyme subunit	MG1655	Deletion	Decrease	Stat	M9 + 10 mM Glc	Of	Völzing and Brynildsen (2015)
		MG1655	Deletion	Decrease	Stat	MHB	Cip	Dörr et al. (2009)
recN	DNA-repair protein	MG1655	Deletion	Decrease	Stat	M9 + 10 mM Glc	Of	Völzing and Brynildsen (2015)
ruvA	Holliday junction ATP-dependent DNA helicase	MG1655	Deletion	Decrease	Stat	M9 + 10 mM Glc	Of	Völzing and Brynildsen (2015)
		BW25113	Deletion	Decrease	Stat*	LB	Car	Pu et al. (2016)
		MG1655	Deletion	Decrease	Exp	MHB	Cip	Theodore et al. (2013)
		MG1655	Deletion	Decrease	Stat	MHB	Cip	Theodore et al. (2013)
		BW25113	Upregulated in persister cells		Exp	LB	Carb	Pu et al. (2016)
ruvB	Holliday junction ATP-dependent DNA helicase	BW25113	Upregulated in persister cells		Exp	LB	Carb	Pu et al. (2016)
sulA	Cell division inhibitor	HM22 (hipA7)	Upregulated in persister cells		Exp	LB	Ap	Keren et al. (2004a)

umuC	Error-prone polymerase V	HM22 (*hipA7*)	Upregulated in persister cells		Exp	LB	Ap	Keren et al. (2004a)
umuD	Error-prone polymerase V	HM22 (*hipA7*)	Upregulated in persister cells		Exp	LB	Ap	Keren et al. (2004a)
uvrA	Excision nuclease subunit	HM22 (*hipA7*)	Upregulated in persister cells		Exp	LB	Ap	Keren et al. (2004a)
uvrB	Excision nuclease subunit	HM22 (*hipA7*)	Upregulated in persister cells		Exp	LB	Ap	Keren et al. (2004a)
uvrD	DNA helicase II	MG1655	Deletion	Decrease	Exp	MHB	Cip	Theodore et al. (2013)
		MG1655	Deletion	Decrease	Stat	MHB	Cip	Theodore et al. (2013)
		BW25113	Upregulated in persister cells		Exp	LB	Carb	Pu et al. (2016)

Stat stationary, *Stat** stationary-phase cells treated after dilution, *Exp* exponential, *LB* lysogeny broth, *MHB* Mueller Hinton broth, *MOPS* 3-(*N*-morpholino) propanesulfonic acid, *CAA* casamino acids, *Glc* glucose, *Suc* sucrose, *Amk* amikacin, *Ap* ampicillin, *Carb* carbenicillin, *Ceftr* ceftriaxone, *Cip* ciprofloxacin, *Mer* meropenem, *Of* ofloxacin

helicases, translocating 5'-3' (DinG) or 3'-5' (UvrD) (Runyon et al. 1990; Tuteja and Tuteja 2004). RuvAB forms a complex with RuvC and catalyzes migration and cleavage of Holliday junctions formed during recombinational repair of DNA damage (Parsons and West 1993). Noteworthy, deletion of *ruvA* also causes a decrease in persistence using ofloxacin (Völzing and Brynildsen 2015) or carbenicillin (Pu et al. 2016) as killing agents. Although the latter antibiotic does not lead to the formation of DSB, it has been shown that β-lactams also induce the SOS response (Miller et al. 2004).

In contrast to persisters in exponential phase that exhibit a low level of SOS induction compared with the rest of the population (Dörr et al. 2009), there is no difference in SOS induction in stationary phase (Völzing and Brynildsen 2015). In this case, persisters require DNA damage repair systems and the SOS response only during the post-treatment recovery period (Völzing and Brynildsen 2015). More specifically, persisters halt DNA synthesis until DNA damage repair is complete (Mok and Brynildsen 2018). Intriguingly, both *umuC* and *umuD* were found to be upregulated in isolated persisters (Keren et al. 2004a), and deletion of *umuD* decreases the persister fraction (Wu et al. 2015). These genes are expressed late in the SOS response (Kamenšek et al. 2010), and their gene products delay the initiation of DNA replication and cell growth after DNA damage. If the available repair mechanisms are insufficient, RecA activates $UmuD_2$, after which $UmuD_2$'C (Pol V, a low-fidelity polymerase) tolerates the DNA damage (Opperman et al. 1999; Simmons et al. 2008).

7.5   Heat Shock

Several heat shock proteins including the cytoplasmic ClpB (Wu et al. 2015), HslU (Girgis et al. 2012), HtpX (Keren et al. 2004a), IbpAB (Keren et al. 2004a), Lon (Pu et al. 2016; Harms et al. 2017; Germain et al. 2015), DnaK (Wu et al. 2015; Liu et al. 2017; Hansen et al. 2008; Pu et al. 2016; Goltermann et al. 2013) and DnaJ (Hansen et al. 2008; Luidalepp et al. 2011; Goltermann et al. 2013; Vázquez-Laslop et al. 2006), and the periplasmic DegP (Keren et al. 2004a), were found to be linked with persistence (Table 7.4). In general, the presence of heat shock proteins is positively correlated with persistence as *htpX, ibpAB, lon, dnaK, dnaJ,* and *degP* are upregulated in persister cells (Pu et al. 2016; Keren et al. 2004b) and deletion of *clpB* (Wu et al. 2015), *lon* (Pu et al. 2016; Harms et al. 2017; Germain et al. 2015), *dnaK* (Wu et al. 2015; Liu et al. 2017; Hansen et al. 2008; Pu et al. 2016; Goltermann et al. 2013), and *dnaJ* (Hansen et al. 2008; Luidalepp et al. 2011; Goltermann et al. 2013; Vázquez-Laslop et al. 2006) decreases persistence. The latter is not the case for *hslU,* although it is noteworthy that a transposon insertion mutant was assayed in this chapter instead of a clean knockout mutant (Girgis et al. 2012).

Heat shock proteins mainly function as proteases [HtpX (Sakoh et al. 2005), Lon (Gur 2013), DegP (Chang 2016)], chaperones [ClpB (Zolkiewski 1999), HslU (Seong et al. 2000), DnaK (Schröder et al. 1993), DnaJ (Schröder et al. 1993)], or

Table 7.4 Genetic determinants of persistence involved in heat shock and protein folding

Gene	Protein	Genetic background	Mutation	Persister fraction	Growth phase	Medium	Antibiotic	References
clpB	Chaperone	W3110	Deletion	Decrease	Stat*	LB	Ap	Wu et al. (2015)
degP	Periplasmic serine endoprotease	HM22 (*hipA7*)	Upregulated in persister cells		Exp	LB	Ap	Keren et al. (2004a)
dnaJ	Chaperone	BW25113	Deletion	Decrease	Stat	MOPS + 0.1% Suc + 0.05% CAA	Of	Hansen et al. (2008)
		BW25113	Deletion	Decrease	Exp	MOPS + 0.1% Suc + 0.05% CAA	Cip, Strep, Ap	Hansen et al. (2008)
		LMG194	Overexpression	Increase	Stat	M9, 2% CAA, 1% Glyc	Ap, Cip,	Vázquez-Laslop et al. (2006)
		BW25113	Deletion	Decrease	Stat*	Lennox LB	Ap	Luidalepp et al. (2011)
		MG1655	Overexpression	Increase	Exp*	LB	Gm	Goltermann et al. (2013)
		BW25113	Upregulated in persister cells		Exp	LB	Carb	Pu et al. (2016)
dnaK	Chaperone	W3110	Deletion	Decrease	Stat*	LB	Ap, Nor, Trim, Gm	Wu et al. (2015)
		W3110	Deletion	Decrease	Stat	LB	Ap, Gm, Nor	Liu et al. (2017)
		BW25113	Deletion	Decrease	Stat	MOPS + 0.1% Suc + 0.05% CAA	Of	Hansen et al. (2008)
		BW25113	Deletion	Decrease	Exp	MOPS + 0.1% Suc + 0.05% CAA	Of, Cip, Strep, Ap, BZK	Hansen et al. (2008)
		MG1655	Expression	Increase	Exp*	LB	Gm	Goltermann et al. (2013)
		BW25113	Deletion	Decrease	Stat*	LB	Carb	Pu et al. (2016)
		BW25113	Upregulated in persister cells		Exp	LB	Carb	Pu et al. (2016)

(continued)

Table 7.4 (continued)

Gene	Protein	Genetic background	Mutation	Persister fraction	Growth phase	Medium	Antibiotic	References
hslU	Protease	MG1655	Transposon insertion	Increase	Stat	LB	Ap	Girgis et al. (2012)
htpX	Protease	HM22 (hipA7)	Upregulated in persister cells		Exp	LB	Ap	Keren et al. (2004a)
ibpA	Small heat shock protein	HM22 (hipA7)	Upregulated in persister cells		Exp	LB	Ap	Keren et al. (2004a)
ibpB	Small heat shock protein	HM22 (hipA7)	Upregulated in persister cells		Exp	LB	Ap	Keren et al. (2004a)
lon	Protease	MG1655 (Δlon ΔsulA)	Deletion	Decrease	Exp	M9 + 0.4% CAA	Cip	Harms et al. (2017)
		MG1655	Deletion	Decrease	Exp	LB	Cip	Germain et al. (2015)
		BW25113	Deletion	Decrease	Stat*	LB	Carb	Pu et al. (2016)
		BW25113	Upregulated in persister cells		Exp	LB	Carb	Pu et al. (2016)

Stat stationary, *Stat** stationary-phase cells treated after dilution, *Exp* exponential, *LB* lysogeny broth, *MOPS* (3-(N-morpholino)propanesulfonic acid), *CAA* casamino acids, *Glyc* glycerol, *Suc* sucrose, *Ap* ampicillin, *BZK* benzalkonium chloride, *Carb* carbenecillin, *Cip* ciprofloxacin, *Gm* gentamicin, *Nor* norfloxacin, *Of* ofloxacin, *Strep* streptomycin, *Trim* trimethoprim

chaperone-helper proteins [IbpAB (Kuczyńska-Wiśnik et al. 2002)]. As the abovementioned genes were identified as persister genes using assays that did not include a heat shock, it is not unlikely that these genes are under the influence of stresses other than heat or have a function in the general metabolism. For example, at lower temperatures DegP might be important for the degradation of misfolded proteins after host-induced oxidative damage (Raivio 2005). Furthermore, while DnaK and DnaJ are well-known as heat shock chaperones under the influence of RpoH (Jenkins et al. 1991), they are also linked with error-prone repair (Grudniak et al. 2005). More specifically, DnaK is linked with tolerance to replication fork arrest, when the repair is RecA-independent, and DNA damage (Goldfless et al. 2006). Other studies have shown that DnaK and DnaJ are important for the stability of UmuC, part of the low-fidelity polymerase Pol V (Goldfless et al. 2006; Petit et al. 1994). Thus, a role for DnaK and DnaJ in the SOS response is not unlikely. Lastly, the Lon protease has been linked to the degradation of several antitoxins [YefM (Christensen et al. 2004), DinJ (Prysak et al. 2009), RelB (Christensen et al. 2001), MqsA (Christensen-Dalsgaard et al. 2010)], of which the cognate toxins (YoeB, YafQ, RelE, and MqsR, respectively) are implicated in persistence (see Table 7.6). The role of the Lon protease in persistence is under debate, as the deletion mutant does not have a phenotype in all conditions (Harms et al. 2017; Theodore et al. 2013; Shan et al. 2017; Ramisetty et al. 2017) and antitoxin degradation might be redundant and not performed by Lon alone (Ramisetty et al. 2017).

Interestingly, protein aggregation in stationary phase is positively linked with persister formation (Leszczynska et al. 2013; Pu et al. 2018), possibly due to the sequestering of essential proteins (Stewart et al. 2005). Of note, protein aggregates can be segregated asymmetrically during cell division and can, therefore, be a source of intrapopulation heterogeneity, which is a hallmark of bacterial persistence (Lindner et al. 2008). The presence of protein aggregates has been suggested to induce transcription or enhance translation of heat shock proteins (Gragerov et al. 1991). Only newly synthesized proteins aggregate after a heat shock (Gragerov et al. 1991) and therefore, the observed elevated concentrations of proteases and chaperones in persisters (Pu et al. 2016; Keren et al. 2004b) might prevent the aggregation of newly formed proteins or result in persister awakening by dissolving the formed aggregates (Pu et al. 2018).

7.6 Oxidative Stress

In general, oxidative stress is positively correlated with persistence (Table 7.5). Deletion of the oxidative stress regulator OxyR decreases the persister fraction (Wu et al. 2015) and SoxS, the transcriptional regulator of the superoxide response regulon, is upregulated in persister cells (Pu et al. 2016). Furthermore, oxidative stress induces expression of the AcrAB-TolC efflux pump, which reduces the concentration of fluoroquinolones in the cell and increases the number of tolerant persister cells (Wu et al. 2012). It is important to note that multidrug efflux pumps

Table 7.5 Genetic determinants of persistence involved in the oxidative stress

Gene	Protein	Genetic background	Mutation	Persister fraction	Growth phase	Medium	Antibiotic	References
acrA	Multidrug efflux pump subunit	BW25113	Upregulated in persister cells		Exp	LB	Carb	Pu et al. (2016)
acrB	Multidrug efflux pump subunit	BW25113	Deletion	Decrease	Exp	LB	Carb	Pu et al. (2016)
acrD	Aminoglycoside efflux pump	BW25113	Upregulated in persister cells		Exp	LB	Carb	Pu et al. (2016)
acrF	Multidrug export protein	BW25113	Upregulated in persister cells		Exp	LB	Carb	Pu et al. (2016)
emrA	Multidrug export protein	BW25113	Upregulated in persister cells		Exp	LB	Carb	Pu et al. (2016)
emrB	Multidrug export protein	BW25113	Upregulated in persister cells		Exp	LB	Carb	Pu et al. (2016)
macA	Macrolide export protein	BW25113	Upregulated in persister cells		Exp	LB	Carb	Pu et al. (2016)
macB	Macrolide export protein	BW25113	Upregulated in persister cells		Exp	LB	Carb	Pu et al. (2016)
mdtF	Multidrug efflux pump	BW25113	Deletion	Increase	Stat	LB	Ap	Hong et al. (2012)
oxyR	Hydrogen peroxide-inducible genes activator	W3110	Deletion	Decrease	Stat*	LB	Ap, Nor, Gm, Trim	Wu et al. (2015)
soxS	Regulatory protein	BW25113	Upregulated in persister cells		Exp	LB	Carb	Pu et al. (2016)
tolC	Multidrug efflux pump subunit	BW25113	Deletion	Decrease	Stat*	LB	Carb	Pu et al. (2016)

Stat stationary, *Stat** stationary-phase cells treated after dilution, *Exp* exponential, *LB* lysogeny broth, *Ap* ampicillin, *Carb* carbenicillin, *Gm* gentamicin, *Nor* norfloxacin, *Trim* trimethoprim

Table 7.6 Toxin-antitoxin modules implicated in *E. coli* persistence

Type	Gene	Protein	Genetic background	Mutation	Persister fraction	Growth phase	Medium	Antibiotic	References
Type I	hokA	Presumed pore former	BW25113	Deletion	Decrease	Exp	LB	Ap	Kim and Wood (2010)
			BW25113	Overexpression	Increase	Exp	LB	Ap	Kim and Wood (2010)
	hokB	Pore former	TOP10	Overexpression	Increase	Stat	LB	Of	Battesti et al. (2011)
			TOP10	Overexpression	Increase	Exp	LB	Ceft	Wilmaerts et al. (2018)
	tisB	Small toxic protein	MG1655	Deletion	Decrease	Exp	MHB	Cip	Dörr et al. (2010)
			MG1655	Overexpression	increase	Exp	MHB	Cip	Dörr et al. (2010)
Type II	dinJ	Antitoxin of YafQ	MG1655	Upregulated in non-growing cells		Exp	LB	/	Shah et al. (2006)
			HM22 (*hipA7*)	Upregulated in persister cells		Exp	LB	Ap	Keren et al. (2004a)
	hha	Hemolysin expression-modulating protein	BW25113	Overexpression	Increase	Exp	LB	Ap	Kim and Wood (2010)
			BW25113	Deletion	Decrease	Exp	LB	Ap	Kim and Wood (2010)
	hipA	Ser/Thr-protein kinase	HM22 (*hipA7*)	Mutation (*hipA7*)	Increase	Exp	LB	Ap, Phos, Cyclo	Moyed and Bertrand (1983)
			LMG194	Overexpression	Increase	Stat	M9, 2% CAA, 1% Glyc	Ap, Cip	Vázquez-Laslop et al. (2006)
			MG1655	Mutation (*hipA7*)	Increase	Exp	LB	Ap	Korch et al. (2003)
			W3110	Deletion	Decrease	Stat	LB	Ap	Wu et al. (2015)
			MG1655	Mutation (*hipA7*)	Increase	Stat*	Lennox LB	Gm	Luidalepp et al. (2011)

(continued)

Table 7.6 (continued)

Gene	Protein	Genetic background	Mutation	Persister fraction	Growth phase	Medium	Antibiotic	References
		MG1655	Overexpression	Increase	Exp	LB	Ap	Korch and Hill (2006)
		BW25113	Upregulated in persister cells		Exp	LB	Carb	Pu et al. (2016)
mazE	Antitoxin of MazF	HM22 (hipA7)	Upregulated in persister cells		Exp	LB	Ap	Keren et al. (2004a)
mazF	Endoribonuclease	MG1655	Upregulated in non-growing cells		Exp	LB	/	Shah et al. (2006)
		HM22 (hipA7)	Upregulated in persister cells		Exp	LB	Ap	Keren et al. (2004a)
		LMG194	Overexpression	Increase	Stat	M9, 2% CAA, 1% Glyc	Ap, Cip	Vázquez-Laslop et al. (2006)
		BW25113	Deletion	Decrease	Stat	LB	Cip	Tripathi et al. (2014)
mqsR	mRNA interferase	MG1655	Upregulated in non-growing cells		Exp	LB	/	Shah et al. (2006)
		MG1655	Overexpression	Increase	Exp	LB	Of, Cef, Mit	Shah et al. (2006)
		BW25113	Deletion	Decrease	Exp	LB	Ap	Kim and Wood (2010)
		BW25113	Overexpression	Increase	Stat	LB	Ap, Cip	Kim and Wood (2010)
		MG1655	Deletion	Decrease	Stat*	Lennox LB	Ap	Luidalepp et al. (2011)
pasT	Ribosome association toxin	CFT073	Deletion	Decrease	Exp	LB	Ap, Cip	Norton and Mulvery (2012)
relB	Antitoxin of RelE	HM22 (hipA7)	Upregulated in persister cells		Exp	LB	Ap	Keren et al. (2004a)

Type	Gene	Description	Strain	Manipulation	Increase	Stat	M9 + 0.2% CAA	Ap, Of, Km	Reference
	relE	mRNA interferase	MG1655	Overexpression	Increase	Stat	M9 + 0.2% CAA	Ap, Of, Km	Tashiro et al. (2012)
			MG1655	Upregulated in non-growing cells		Exp	LB	/	Shah et al. (2006)
			MC1000 (ΔrelBE)	Overexpression	Increase	Exp	LB	Cef, Of, Tob	Keren et al. (2004a)
			HM22 (hipA7)	Upregulated in persister cells		Exp	LB	Ap	Keren et al. (2004a)
	yafQ	mRNA interferase	BW25113	Deletion	Decrease	Stat	LB	Cefa, Tob	Harrison et al. (2009)
			BW25113	Overexpression	Increase	Stat	LB	Cefa, Tob	Harrison et al. (2009)
			MG1655	Upregulated in non-growing cells		Exp	LB	/	Shah et al. (2006)
			HM22 (hipA7)	Upregulated in persister cells		Exp	LB	Ap	Keren et al. (2004a)
			BW25113 (ΔyafQ)	Overexpression	Increase	Stat	LB	Ap, Cip	Hu et al. (2015)
	yefM	Antitoxin of YoeB	MG1655	Upregulated in non-growing cells		Exp	LB	/	Shah et al. (2006)
			HM22 (hipA7)	Upregulated in persister cells		Exp	LB	Ap	Keren et al. (2004a)
Type V	ghoT	Toxic membrane peptide	BW25113	Overexpression	Increase	Exp	LB	Ap	Wang et al. (2012)

Stat stationary, *Stat** stationary-phase cells treated after dilution, *Exp* exponential, *LB* lysogeny broth, *MHB* Mueller Hinton broth, *CAA* casamino acids, *Glyc* glycerol, *Ap* ampicillin, *Carb* carbenicillin, *Cef* cefotaxime, *Cefa* cefazolin, *Ceft* ceftazidim, *Cip* ciprofloxacin, *Gm* gentamicin, *Cyclo* cycloserine, *Km* kanamycin, *Mit* mitomycine C, *Of* ofloxacin, *Phos* phosphomycin, *Tob* tobramycine

are classical examples of resistance mechanisms. However, stochastic fluctuations in the expression level of efflux pumps might result in phenotypic heterogeneity at the population level. In accordance, persisters have an increased expression of multidrug efflux genes including *tolC, acrA, acrB, acrD, acrF, emrA, emrB, macA*, and *macB*, which likely results in reduced intracellular concentrations of antibiotics (Pu et al. 2016). In addition, deletion of TolC decreases the persister fraction (Pu et al. 2016). Also, the widely-spread signal molecule indole, which presumably induces oxidative stress (Garbe et al. 2000), enhances persister levels (Vega et al. 2012) by upregulating drug efflux genes *mdtEF* and *acrD* (Hirakawa et al. 2005). Furthermore, RpoS stimulates indole production, revealing a link between the general stress response and oxidative stress (Lacour and Landini 2004).

7.7 TA Modules

Toxin-antitoxin (TA) modules are genomic or plasmid-encoded elements. While plasmid-encoded modules are linked with post-segregational killing (Gerdes et al. 1986), genomic TA modules are abundant in free-living organisms and seem to be absent in obligate host-associated organisms facing a stable environment (Pandey and Gerdes 2005). This suggests that genomic TA modules play a role in survival in stressful conditions by reversibly shutting down metabolism in response to different stresses (Page and Peti 2016; Harms et al. 2018).

TA modules are classified into six groups, depending on the inhibitory action of the antitoxin on the toxin (Page and Peti 2016). Up to now, genomic type I, type II, and type V TA modules have been implicated in persistence (Page and Peti 2016). In type I systems, the antitoxin is an mRNA molecule that inhibits translation or triggers degradation of its cognate toxin mRNA. In Type II and Type V TA modules, the antitoxin is a protein that inhibits the protein toxin (type II) or degrades the toxin mRNA (type V) (Page and Peti 2016).

Persistence is induced when the toxin concentration reaches a certain threshold (Rotem et al. 2010). This can be achieved via upregulation of TA modules by stress or stochastic fluctuations, combined with the degradation of the intrinsically unstable antitoxins. Alternatively, the toxin can be specifically upregulated (e.g., TisB) (Keren et al. 2004a; Dörr et al. 2010). Stress responses were found not only to induce several TA modules (Verstraeten et al. 2015; Dörr et al. 2010; Shan et al. 2017) but also to activate toxins by degradation of the antitoxin (Muthuramalingam et al. 2016). However, few studies have succeeded in providing details on how toxin levels are controlled and experimental data are sometimes contradictory, especially in the case of type II TA modules. As a result, there is no general consensus on the regulation of cellular toxin levels to date (Ramisetty et al. 2017).

Ectopic expression of several toxins causes an increase in persister levels (Table 7.6), but deletion of a single TA module rarely affects persistence (Michiels et al. 2016), which is a recurring comment on the role of TA modules in persistence. However, there are several explanations for this discrepancy. First, deletion of a single TA module has been shown to decrease persistence only in very specific conditions (Kim and Wood 2010; Dörr et al. 2010; Norton and Mulvey 2012). Indeed, *Salmonella* Typhimurium mutants lacking a single TA module display decreased persistence after phagocytic uptake but not in planktonic cultures (Helaine et al. 2014) and deletion of *tisB* decreases persistence only in logarithmically growing cultures treated with ciprofloxacin (Dörr et al. 2010). It is therefore plausible that deletion of other single TA modules decreases persistence in conditions that have not yet been examined. Second, multiple TA modules are upregulated by one specific stress, as has been shown in *Mycobacterium tuberculosis* (Gupta et al. 2017) and *E. coli* (Shah et al. 2006, 2017; Muthuramalingam et al. 2016; Anders et al. 2013), resulting in a heterogeneous population of TA-induced cells. This might lead to a non-significant effect of a single-deletion mutant on the persister level of the population. Indeed, several reports demonstrate that the persister population is heterogeneous (Balaban et al. 2004; Amato and Brynildsen 2015). Third, there is transcriptional cross-activation between TA systems, presumably resulting from the accumulation of toxin-encoding mRNA fragments during toxin-induced selective mRNA cleavage (Kasari et al. 2013). This might partly conceal the effect of a single deletion. Alternatively, it might indicate that some TA systems need to work together in certain conditions in order to induce persistence (Kim and Wood 2010; Kasari et al. 2013; Wessner et al. 2015). Importantly, deletion of 10 TA modules does not decrease the persister fraction (Harms et al. 2017). In conclusion, the influence of TA modules on persistence might be masked by their complex regulation. Hence, more research is necessary to unravel the role of TA modules in persistence.

7.7.1 Type I TA Modules

In type I TA modules, the antitoxin is an mRNA molecule that base-pairs with the toxin mRNA, thereby inhibiting translation or inducing breakdown of the toxin mRNA (Harms et al. 2018). In general, type I toxins are small (<60 amino acids), and consist of a hydrophobic α-helix that spans the membrane (Brielle et al. 2016). To date, three type I toxins have been linked with persistence: TisB, HokB, and HokA (Verstraeten et al. 2015; Kim and Wood 2010; Dörr et al. 2009). TisB consists of 29 amino acids and has been shown to induce persistence in response to DNA damage (Dörr et al. 2009). TisB is a pore-forming peptide that collapses the membrane potential, thereby diminishing ATP levels (Dörr et al. 2010; Gurnev et al. 2012). The intracellular concentration of TisB positively affects survival after ciprofloxacin treatment (Dörr et al. 2010). HokB and HokA are members of the *hok/gef* family. HokB consists of 49 amino acids and is the effector of the ObgE-mediated persistence pathway (Verstraeten et al. 2015). It induces persistence via the formation of pores whose size depends on the membrane potential, suggesting that persistence is only induced in metabolically active cells (Wilmaerts et al. 2018). Furthermore, HokB pores induce the leakage of ATP, which is presumably linked with persistence (Wilmaerts et al. 2018). HokA consists of 50 amino acids and has been shown to increase the persister fraction upon overexpression and to lower the persister fraction upon deletion (Kim and Wood 2010).

7.7.2 Type II TA Modules

Isolated persisters display increased expression levels of several type II TA modules (Shah et al. 2006; Pu et al. 2016; Keren et al. 2004a). These modules encode protein toxins that typically target translation and protein antitoxins that inhibit their cognate toxin via direct binding (Harms et al. 2018). Stochastic fluctuations or environmental triggers resulting in the induction of a stress response result in degradation of the intrinsically unstable antitoxin, thereby activating the toxin (Lewis 2010).

The first TA module to be implicated in persistence was *hipAB* (Wu et al. 2015; Vázquez-Laslop et al. 2006; Korch and Hill 2006), of which a mutant (*hipA7*) was detected in high-persister strains that display 1000–10,000-fold increased persister fraction (Korch et al. 2003; Moyed and Bertrand 1983). Active HipA has kinase activity and phosphorylates glutamyl t-RNA synthetase (GltX), which results in the accumulation of uncharged tRNA^{Glu} (Germain et al. 2013; Kaspy et al. 2013). Eventually, this triggers the dissociation of RelA from the ribosome, which activates (p)ppGpp synthesis and eventually induces persistence (Bokinsky et al. 2013; Germain et al. 2013).

The type II toxins YafQ, RelE, MazF, and MqsR are endoribonucleases that block translation by cleaving mRNA (Prysak et al. 2009; Pedersen et al. 2003; Zhang et al. 2005; Yamaguchi et al. 2009). In general, there is a positive correlation between the expression of mRNA endoribonucleases and persistence. mRNA cleavage under moderate amino acid starvation is, however, toxin independent, suggesting that toxin-induced mRNA cleavage only occurs during strong amino acid starvation (Li et al. 2008). YafQ has been reported to induce persistence in biofilms, but not in planktonic cells (Harrison et al. 2009). However, another study has shown that ectopic expression of *yafQ* induces persistence in planktonic cells via reduction of indole (Hu et al. 2015), although this, in turn, contradicts other findings showing a positive correlation between indole production and persistence (Vega et al. 2012). Ectopic expression of *relE* increases the persister fraction mainly during nutritional stress (Christensen et al. 2001; Tashiro et al. 2012). Furthermore, the intracellular concentration of MazF is positively correlated with persistence (Vázquez-Laslop et al. 2006; Tripathi et al. 2014), but high concentrations of MazF, resulting from plasmid expression, in absence of its antitoxin MazE induce cell death (Aizenman et al. 1996; Sat et al. 2001). MqsR is induced in persister cells (Shah et al. 2006) and the intracellular concentration of MqsR positively correlates with persistence (Shah et al. 2006; Kim and Wood 2010).

Norton and Mulvey assessed the clinical relevance of type II TA systems by infecting mice with single-TA deletion mutants of extraintestinal *E. coli*. Deletion of toxin-encoding genes *hha*, *yoeB*, and *pasT* compromises infection by the bacteria of the bladder (Hha and YefM) and kidneys (PasT) (Norton and Mulvey 2012). PasT inhibits protein synthesis by binding with the 50S ribosomal subunit and preventing

Fig. 7.1 Expression of the toxin-encoding *relE* gene induces transcription of *mazF*, *yafQ*, and *mqsR*. *relE* is induced by expression of *hipA*, *mazF*, and *mqsR* (Kasari et al. 2013). Furthermore, *mqsR* is induced by YafQ and HipA, while expression of *mqsR* results in the activation of GhoT and induction of *hha* (Kim and Wood 2010; Kasari et al. 2013; Wang et al. 2013)

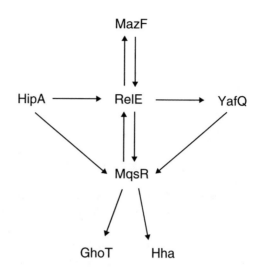

70S ribosome assembly (Zhang and Inouye 2011). In vitro, deletion of *pasT*, but not *hha* and *yoeB*, decrease persistence in the used genetic background (CFT073), indicating that toxins are functional in specific conditions (Norton and Mulvey 2012). However, isolated *E. coli* MG1655 persister cells have an increased expression of *yoeB* (Shah et al. 2006) and Hha influence persistence in *E. coli* BW25113 (Kim and Wood 2010).

As mentioned above, several type II toxins are cross-correlated (Kasari et al. 2013). Furthermore, the type II toxin MqsR activates the type V toxin GhoT (discussed below) by degrading *ghoS* mRNA (Wang et al. 2013). A schematic representation of this TA network is depicted in Fig. 7.1. For clarity, only TA modules that are implicated in persistence are shown.

7.7.3   Type V TA Modules

In type V TA modules, the antitoxin is a protein that directly degrades the toxin mRNA, thereby preventing translation (Page and Peti 2016). GhoT/GhoS is the only type V TA system known to date. After expression of *ghoT*, 60% of the cells lose their membrane integrity and show ghost morphology. In addition, expression of *ghoT* increases survival following ampicillin treatment (Wang et al. 2012).

7.8   Energy Metabolism

In general, nutrients are channeled through glycolysis, the tricarboxylic acid (TCA) pathway and the pentose phosphate pathway (PPP) to yield metabolites, ATP, and reduced cofactors (NADH, FADH$_2$, NADPH) (Cohen 2014). Electrons from NADH and FADH$_2$ are used to produce energy via the electron transport chain (ETC), a cluster of enzyme complexes that transfer electrons from donors to acceptors via a series of redox reactions. The ETC in *E. coli* is strongly branched, giving the cells the opportunity to respond to changing environments (Steinsiek et al. 2014). The ETC consist of two NADH dehydrogenases (I and II), and three terminal oxidases (cytochrome bo3, cytochrome bd-I, and cytochrome bd-II) (Borisov et al. 2011). In aerobic conditions, ubiquinone accepts electrons from NADH dehydrogenase I and transports them to one of the terminal oxidases (Cox et al. 1970). During electron transport, protons are transported across the membrane, creating an electrochemical proton gradient, which drives ATP synthesis (Unden and Bongaerts 1997).

A long-standing hypothesis states that persisters are transiently dormant, rendering them tolerant to antibiotics that target metabolically active cells (Lewis 2010). However, recent literature shows that dormancy does not explain the persister phenotype of all persister cells (Orman and Brynildsen 2013). Indeed, stationary-phase persisters are metabolically active (Orman and Brynildsen 2015) and persister cells treated with fluoroquinolones acquired DNA damage, indicative of an active target (Völzing and Brynildsen 2015). In addition, persister levels of a single population vary depending on the used antibiotic, casting the idea of a homogeneous dormant subpopulation (Amato and Brynildsen 2015; Allison et al. 2011). Nevertheless, a link between persistence and energy metabolism has been reported by several research groups, although findings are often contradictory (Table 7.7).

Several enzymes of the TCA cycle have been implicated in persistence. Deletion of *sdhC, mdh, and sucB* or inactivation by transposon insertion of several genes (*acnA, acnB, icdA,* and *sdhA*) was shown to result in a decreased persister fraction in a stationary phase (Wu et al. 2015; Liu et al. 2017; Shan et al. 2015; Luidalepp et al. 2011; Orman and Brynildsen 2015; Ma et al. 2010; Leatham-Jensen et al. 2016). In contrast, inactivation by transposon insertion of *sucAB, sucCD, sdhABCD, fumB, gltA, acnA,* and *acnB* resulted in an increased persister fraction in stationary phase (Shan et al. 2015; Kim et al. 2016). However, these transposon mutants require further confirmation by clean knockout mutations before strong conclusions can be drawn. Furthermore, the effect of the deletion on cellular energy should be investigated.

Several lines of evidence suggest that the induction of persistence is linked with decreased respiration. For example, perturbing the *nuo* genes (encoding the NADH dehydrogenase complex I) by deletion (*nuoG, nuoL*) or via a mutation (*nuoN*) as well as deleting cytochrome bd-I oxidase (*cydAB*) and cytochrome bd-o oxidase (cyo) results in an increased persister fraction (Shan et al. 2015; Kim et al. 2016; Van den Bergh et al. 2016). Furthermore, a triple knockout mutant with deletions in all three terminal oxidases (*cyoA, cydB, appB*) shows lower respiration and a higher persister fraction. In addition, deletion of *atpA*, encoding for ATP synthase subunit alpha, causes higher respiration and a lower persister fraction (Lobritz et al. 2015). However, deletion of genes encoding other parts of the ATP synthase (*atpC* and *atpF*) increases the persister fraction (Girgis et al. 2012; Kiss 2000). In addition, bacterial cultures treated with salicylate, which amongst others, represses genes

Table 7.7 Genetic determinants of persistence involved in the energy metabolism

	Gene	Protein	Genetic background	Mutation	Persister fraction	Growth phase	Medium	Antibiotic	References
TCA cycle	acnA	Aconitate hydratase	MG1655	Transposon	Decrease	Stat	MOPS + 0.2% Glc + 0.2% CAA	Gm	Shan et al. (2015)
	acnB	Aconitate hydratase	MG1655	Transposon	Decrease	Stat	MOPS + 0.2% Glc + 0.2% CAA	Gm	Shan et al. (2015)
			BW25113	Deletion	Decrease	Stat*	Lennox LB	Ap	Li and Zhang (2007)
			MG1655	Deletion	Decrease	Stat	LB	Ap, Of	Orman and Brynildsen (2015)
			MG1655	Deletion	Increase	Exp	LB	Ap, Km, Nor	Kohanski et al. (2007)
	FRD	Fumarate reductase	BW25113	Overexpression	Increase	Exp	LB	Ap, Nor	Kim et al. (2016)
	fumB	Fumarate hydratase	MG1655	Transposon insertion	Increase	Stat	MOPS + 0.2% Glc + 0.2% CAA	Gm	Shan et al. (2015)
	gltA	Citrate synthase	MG1655	Transposon insertion	Increase	Stat	MOPS + 0.2% Glc + 0.2% CAA	Gm	Shan et al. (2015)
	icdA	Isocitrate dehydrogenase	MG1655	Transposon insertion	Decrease	Stat	MOPS + 0.2% Glc + 0.2% CAA	Gm	Shan et al. (2015)
			MG1655	Deletion	Increase	Exp	LB	Ap, Km, Nor	Kohanski et al. (2007)
	mdh	Malate dehydrogenase	MG1655	Deletion	Decrease	Stat	LB	Ap, Of	

(continued)

Table 7.7 (continued)

Gene	Protein	Genetic background	Mutation	Persister fraction	Growth phase	Medium	Antibiotic	References
								Orman and Brynildsen (2015)
		BW25113	Deletion	Decrease	Stat*	Lennox LB	Ap	Li and Zhang (2007)
		MG1655	Deletion	Increase	Exp	LB	Km	Kohanski et al. (2007)
SDH	Succinate dehydrogenase	BW25113	Deletion	Increase	Stat	LB	Nor	Kim et al. (2016)
sdhA	Succinate dehydrogenase	MG1655	Transposon insertion	Increase	Stat	MOPS + 0.2% Glc + 0.2% CAA	Gm	Shan et al. (2015)
		CFT073	Transposon insertion	Decrease	Stat	M9 + 0.2% Glc and LB	Ap	Leatham-Jensen et al. (2016)
sdhB	Succinate dehydrogenase	MG1655	Transposon insertion	Increase	Stat	MOPS + 0.2% Glc + 0.2% CAA	Gm	Shan et al. (2015)
sdhC	Succinate dehydrogenase	MG1655	Transposon insertion	Increase	Stat	MOPS + 0.2% Glc + 0.2% CAA	Gm	Shan et al. (2015)
		MG1655	Deletion	Decrease	Exp	LB	Ap, Of	Lobritz et al. (2015)
		MG1655	Deletion	Decrease	Stat	LB	Ap, Of	Orman and Brynildsen (2015)
sdhD	Succinate dehydrogenase	MG1655	Transposon insertion	Increase	Stat	MOPS + 0.2% Glc + 0.2% CAA	Gm	Shan et al. (2015)

	Gene	Protein	Strain	Mutation	Effect	Phase	Medium	Antibiotic	Reference
	sucACD	2-Oxoglutarate dehydrogenase	MG1655	Transposon insertion	Increase	Stat	MOPS + 0.2% Glc + 0.2% CAA	Gm	Shan et al. (2015)
	sucB	2-Oxoglutarate dehydrogenase	W3110	Deletion	Decrease	Stat	LB	Ap, Gm, Tmp	Hong et al. (2012)
			W3110 (ΔrelA)	Deletion	Decrease	Stat	LB	Ap, Gm, Nor	Liu et al. (2017)
			BW25113	Deletion	Decrease	Stat*	Lennox LB	Ap	Li and Zhang (2007)
			MG1655	Deletion	Decrease	Stat	LB	Ap, Of	Orman and Brynildsen (2015)
			MG1655	Transposon insertion	Increase	Stat	MOPS + 0.2% Glc + 0.2% CAA	Gm	Shan et al. (2015)
			BW25113	Deletion	Decrease	Stat, exp	LB	Ap, Gm	Ma et al. (2010)
			MG1655	Deletion	Increase	Exp	LB	Ap, Km	Kohanski et al. (2007)
Respiratory chain	appB	Cytochrome bd-II ubiquinol oxidase	MG1655 ΔcyoA ΔcydB	Deletion	Increase	Exp	M9 + 0.2% CAA + 10 mM Glc	Ap, Gm, Nor	Lobritz et al. (2015)
	atpF	Fo/F1 ATP synthase	MG1655	Transposon insertion	Increase	Plates	LB	Ap	Girgis et al. (2012)
	atpC	Fo/F1 ATP synthase	MG1655	Deletion	Increase	Exp	LB	Ap, Of	Lobritz et al. (2015)
			MG1655	Deletion	Increase	Exp	LB	Km	Kohanski et al. (2007)
			MG1655	Deletion	Decrease	Stat	LB	Ap, Of	Orman and Brynildsen (2015)

(continued)

Table 7.7 (continued)

Gene	Protein	Genetic background	Mutation	Persister fraction	Growth phase	Medium	Antibiotic	References
CYD	Cytochrome bd-I ubiquinol oxidase	BW25113	Deletion	Increase	Exp, Stat	LB	Nor	Kim et al. (2016)
cydB	Cytochrome bd-I ubiquinol oxidase	MG1655 ΔcyoA ΔappB	Deletion	Increase	Exp	M9 + 0.2% CAA + 10 mM Glc	Ap, Gm, Nor	Lobritz et al. (2015)
CYO	Cytochrome bo ubiquinol oxidase	BW25113	Deletion	Decrease	Stat	LB	Nor	Kim et al. (2016)
cyoA	Cytochrome bo ubiquinol oxidase	MG1655 ΔappB ΔcydB	Deletion	Increase	Exp	M9 + 0.2% CAA + 10 mM Glc	Ap, Gm, Nor	Lobritz et al. (2015)
		MG1655	Deletion	Decrease	Exp	LB	Ap, Of	Lobritz et al. (2015)
menA	1,4-Dihydroxy-2-naphthoate octaprenyltransferase	BW25113	Deletion	Decrease	Stat	LB	Nor	Kim et al. (2016)
ndh	NADH dehydrogenase	BW25113	Deletion	Decrease	Stat	LB	Nor	Kim et al. (2016)
		BW25113	Deletion	Increase	Exp	LB	Nor	Kim et al. (2016)
NUO	NADH-quinone oxidoreductase	BW25113	Deletion	Decrease	Exp, Stat	LB	Nor	Kim et al. (2016)
nuoG	NADH-quinone oxidoreductase	MG1655	Deletion	Decrease	Exp	LB	Ap, Of	Lobritz et al. (2015)
nuoL	NADH-quinone oxidoreductase	MG1655	Deletion	Increase	Stat	MOPS + 0.2% Glc + 0.2% CAA	Gm	Shan et al. (2015)

	Gene	Description	Strain	Mutation	Effect	Phase	Media	Antibiotics	Reference
	nuoN	NADH-quinone oxidoreductase	BW25993	Point mutation (G402R)	Increase	Stat	MHB	Amk, Of	Van den Bergh et al. (2016)
	ubiF	2-Octaprenyl-3-methyl-6-methoxy-1,4-benzoquinol hydroxylase	BW25113	Deletion	Decrease	Exp, Stat	LB	Ap, Gm	Ma et al. (2010)
			MG1655	Deletion	Decrease	Stat	LB	Ap, Of	Orman and Brynildsen (2015)
PPP	gnd	6-Phosphogluconate dehydrogenase	BW25113 Δzwf	Deletion	Decrease	Stat	LB and M9 salts	Gm	Wang et al. (2014), Girgis et al. (2012)
			MG1655	Deletion	Increase	Exp	LB	Ap, Of	Lobritz et al. (2015)
	talA	Transaldolase A	BW25113	Deletion	Decrease	Stat	LB and M9 salts	Gm	Wang et al. (2014)
	tktA	Transketolase	MG1655	Null mutation	Increase	Plates	LB	Ap	Girgis et al. (2012)
	zwf	Glucose-6-phosphate 1-dehydrogenase	BW25113 Δgnd	Deletion	Decrease	Stat	LB and M9 salts	Gm	Wang et al. (2014)
			MG1655	Deletion	Increase	Exp	LB	Of	Lobritz et al. (2015), Hansen et al. (2008)
Transport	pntA	NAD (P) transhydrogenase subunit	MG1655 (ΔrelA ΔspoT)	Overexpression	Increase	Exp	LB	Ap, Cip	Chowdhury et al. (2016), Hansen et al. (2008)
			MG1655	Deletion	Increase	Exp	LB	Ap, Km	Kohanski et al. (2007)

(continued)

Table 7.7 (continued)

	Gene	Protein	Genetic background	Mutation	Persister fraction	Growth phase	Medium	Antibiotic	References
	yigB	5-amino-6-(5-phospho-D-ribitylamino)uracil phosphatase	BW25113	Deletion	Decrease	Exp, Stat	MOPS + 0.1% Suc + 0.05% CAA	Of, Cip, Strep, Ap, BZK	Hansen et al. (2008)
			BW25113	Overexpression	Increase	Stat	MOPS + 0.1% Suc + 0.05% CAA	Of	Hansen et al. (2008)
NAD+ biosynthesis	nadA	Quinolinate synthase A	MG1655	Transposon insertion	Decrease	Stat	MOPS + 0.2% Glc + 0.2% CAA	Gm	Shan et al. (2015)
	nadB	L-Aspartate oxidase	MG1655	Transposon insertion	Decrease	Stat	MOPS + 0.2% Glc + 0.2% CAA	Gm	Shan et al. (2015)
	nadC	Nicotinate-nucleotide pyrophosphorylase	MG1655	Transposon insertion	Decrease	Stat	MOPS + 0.2% Glc + 0.2% CAA	Gm	Shan et al. (2015)
Other	focA	Probable formate transporter	MG1655 (ΔrelA ΔspoT)	Overexpression	Increase	Exp	LB	Ap, Cip	Chowdhury et al. (2016)
	pta	Phosphate acetyltransferase	MG1655	Deletion	Decrease	Exp	LB	Of	Lobritz et al. (2015)
	yihS	Sulfoquinovose isomerase	MG1655 (ΔrelA ΔspoT)	Overexpression	Increase	Exp	LB	Ap, Cip	Chowdhury et al. (2016)

Stat stationary, *Stat** stationary-phase cells treated after dilution, *Exp* exponential, *LB* lysogeny broth, *MHB* Mueller Hinton broth, *MOPS* (3-(N-morpholino) propanesulfonic acid), *Glc* glucose, *Suc* sucrose, *CAA* casamino acids, *Amk* amikacin, *Ap* ampicillin, *BZK* benzalkonium chloride, *Cip* ciprofloxacin, *Gm* gentamicin, *Km* kanamycin, *Nor* norfloxacin, *Strep* streptomycin

encoding ATP synthase subunits, also exhibit high-persister phenotypes (Wang et al. 2017).

Conversely, deletion of *ubiF* (ubiquinone biosynthesis) (Orman and Brynildsen 2015; Ma et al. 2010) and *nuoG* (Kiss 2000), both important for respiration in aerobic conditions, was reported to result in a decreased persister fraction (Orman and Brynildsen 2015). Moreover, inhibition of stationary-phase respiration chemically, via the addition of KCN, or via changing to anaerobic conditions inhibit the formation of persister cells in stationary phase (Orman and Brynildsen 2015). In addition, an observed rise in O_2 and CO_2 yields together with lower biomass yields suggest that persisters respire more than non-persisters, possibly resulting from the upregulation of persister-promoting genes and downregulation of growth-related genes (Radzikowski et al. 2016).

7.9   Other Mechanisms

Additional genes that are not directly related to stress responses or metabolism have been reported to affect persistence. For example, several screens have revealed the role of glycerol-3-phosphate dehydrogenase in the formation of persister cells. In the absence of glycerol, this enzyme is essential for the production of glycerol-3-phosphate. Overexpression of glycerol-3-phosphate dehydrogenase subunits (*glpABCD*) increases the persister fraction (Spoering et al. 2006), while deletion results in a decrease (Wu et al. 2015; Hansen et al. 2008; Spoering et al. 2006). Conversely, inactivation of *glpD* via transposon mutagenesis was reported to upregulate persistence (Girgis et al. 2012; Li et al. 2013). In addition to glycerol-3-phosphate dehydrogenase, some outer membrane components (mainly related to motility) have been linked to persistence as deletion of these genes decreases the persister fraction. Examples include genes involved in flagellar formation, specifically the basal body (*motAB, fliL, flhABD*) as well as the hook (*flgABCDEFGHIJKL, fliAEFGHIJKMNOPQR*) and the filament (*fliC*) (Shan et al. 2015). Furthermore, transposon insertion in *qseC*, coding for a membrane sensor kinase that activates type 1 pili, curli and flagella (Kostakioti et al. 2010), results in a decreased persister fraction, suggesting that flagellar formation and rotation affect persistence (Shan et al. 2015). Two genes related to chromosome segregation, *xerCD*, have also been linked to persistence. The site-specific recombinase XerCD recognizes the *dif* site located near the replication terminus and resolves chromosomal dimers. Inactivation of *xerCD* leads to the formation of chromosomal concatemers that are not lethal to the cell but rather inhibit proper septation and give rise to filamentous cells in a portion of the population. In *xerC* and *xerD* deletion mutants the persister level is diminished, suggesting that most persisters have undergone at least one successful recombination event (Dörr et al. 2009). Additional persister genes that are not directly related to the biological processes described above are listed in Table 7.8.

Table 7.8 Genetic determinants of persistence involved in other mechanisms

Gene	Protein	Genetic background	Mutation	Persister fraction	Growth phase	Medium	Antibiotic	References
appY	DNA-binding global transcriptional activator	MG1655	Transposon	Decrease	Stat	MOPS + 0.2% Glc + 0.2% CAA	Gm	Shan et al. (2015)
arcB	Aerobic respiration control sensor	MG1655	Transposon	Decrease	Stat	MOPS + 0.2% Glc + 0.2% CAA	Gm	Shan et al. (2015)
asmA	OM assembly protein	MG1655	Transposon insertion	Increase	Plates	LB	Ap	Girgis et al. (2012)
fis	DNA-binding protein	BW25113	Deletion	Decrease	Exp, Stat	MOPS + 0.1% Suc + 0.05% CAA and LB	Of, Cip, Strep, Ap, BZK	Hansen et al. (2008)
flgABCDEFGHIJKL[a]	Flagellar protein	MG1655	Transposon insertion	Decrease	Stat	MOPS + 0.2% Glc + 0.2% CAA	Gm	Shan et al. (2015)
flhABD[a]	Flagellar protein	MG1655	Transposon insertion	Decrease	Stat	MOPS + 0.2% Glc + 0.2% CAA	Gm	Shan et al. (2015)
flhC	Flagellar transcriptional regulator	MG1655	Transposon insertion and deletion	Decrease	Stat	MOPS + 0.2% Glc + 0.2% CAA	Gm	Shan et al. (2015)
fliAEFGHIJKMNOPQR[a]	Flagellar protein	MG1655	Transposon insertion	Decrease	Stat	MOPS + 0.2% Glc + 0.2% CAA	Gm	Shan et al. (2015)
fliC	Flagellar protein	MG1655	Transposon insertion and deletion	Decrease	Stat	MOPS + 0.2% Glc + 0.2% CAA	Gm	Shan et al. (2015)
fliL	Flagellar protein	MG1655	Transposon insertion and deletion	Decrease	Stat	MOPS + 0.2% Glc + 0.2% CAA	Gm	Shan et al. (2015)
galU	Glucose-1-phosphate uridylyltransferase	MG1655	Transposon insertion	Increase	Plates	LB	Ap	Girgis et al. (2012)

Gene	Function	Strain	Type	Change	Phase	Medium	Antibiotics	Reference
gdhA	Glutamate dehydrogenase	CFT073	Transposon insertion	Decrease	Stat	M9 + 0.2% glc and LB	Ap	Leatham-Jensen et al. (2016)
glpABC[a]	Anaerobic G3P dehydrogenase	EMG2	Deletion	Decrease	Stat	LB	Cip	Spoering et al. (2006)
glpD	Aerobic G3P dehydrogenase	MG1655	Transposon insertion	Increase	Plates	LB	Ap	Girgis et al. (2012)
		BW25113	Deletion	Decrease	Exp, Stat*	MOPS + 0.1% Suc + 0.05% CAA and LB	Of, Cip, Strep, Ap, BZK	Luidalepp et al. (2011)
		W3110	Deletion	Decrease	Stat	LB	Ap, Nor	Wu et al. (2015)
		EMG2	Deletion	Decrease	Stat	LB	Cip	Spoering et al. (2006)
		EMG2	Overexpression	Increase	Exp	LB	Ap, Of	Spoering et al. (2006)
greA	Transcript cleavage factor	MG1655	Transposon	Decrease	Stat	MOPS + 0.2% Glc + 0.2% CAA	Gm	Shan et al. (2015)
hns	DNA-binding protein	BW25113	Deletion	Decrease	Exp, Stat	MOPS + 0.1% Suc + 0.05% CAA and LB	Of, Cip, Strep, Ap, BZK	Hansen et al. (2008)
ihfAB	Nucleoid-binding protein	BW25113	Deletion	Increase	Stat	MOPS	Of	Hansen et al. (2008)
iscS	Cysteine desulfurase	MG1655	Deletion	Increase	Exp	LB	Ap, Km, Nor	Kohanski et al. (2007)
lpxK	lipid A 4' kinase	MG1655	Transposon insertion	Decrease	Stat	MOPS + 0.2% Glc + 0.2% CAA	Gm	Shan et al. (2015)
lysP	Lysine transporter	MG1655	Transposon insertion	Decrease	Stat	MOPS + 0.2% Glc + 0.2% CAA	Gm	Shan et al. (2015)

(continued)

Table 7.8 (continued)

Gene	Protein	Genetic background	Mutation	Persister fraction	Growth phase	Medium	Antibiotic	References
metG	Methionyl-tRNA synthetase	MG1655 (metG*)	Transposon insertion	Increase	Plates	LB	Ap	Girgis et al. (2012)
mnmE	GTPase required for protein folding	MG1655	Transposon insertion	Decrease	Stat	MOPS + 0.2% Glc + 0.2% CAA	Gm	Shan et al. (2015)
motA	Motility protein	MG1655	Transposon insertion	Decrease	Stat	MOPS + 0.2% Glc + 0.2% CAA	Gm	Shan et al. (2015)
motB	Motility protein	MG1655	Transposon insertion and deletion	Decrease	Stat	MOPS + 0.2% Glc + 0.2% CAA	Gm	Shan et al. (2015)
plsB	Acyltransferase	EMG2	Missense (plsB26)	Decrease	Stat	LB	Cip	Spoering et al. (2006)
pmrC	Phosphoethanolamine transferase	LMG194	Overexpression	Increase	Exp	M9, 2% CAA, 1% Glyc	Ap, Cip	Vázquez-Laslop et al. (2006)
pspA	Phage shock protein A	HM22 (hipA7)	Upregulated in persister cells		Exp	LB	Amp	Keren et al. (2004a)
		BW25113	Upregulated in persister cells		Exp	LB	Carb	Pu et al. (2016)
pspB	Phage shock protein B	HM22 (hipA7)	Upregulated in persister cells		Exp	LB	Amp	Keren et al. (2004a)
		BW25113	Upregulated in persister cells		Exp	LB	Carb	Pu et al. (2016)
pspF	Psp operon transcriptional activator	W3110	Deletion	Decrease	Stat	LB	Nor	Wu et al. (2015)
		W3110	Deletion	Decrease	Stat	LB	Nor	Liu et al. (2017)
		W3110 (ΔrelA)	Deletion	Decrease	Stat	LB	Ap, Gm, Nor	Liu et al. (2017)

qseC	Response regulator	MG1655	Transposon insertion	Decrease	Stat	MOPS + 0.2% Glc + 0.2% CAA	Gm	Shan et al. (2015)
rcnR	Transcriptional repressor	MG1655 (metG*)	Transposon insertion	Increase	Plates	LB	Ap	Girgis et al. (2012)
rfaQ	Lipopolysaccharide core heptosyltransferase	MG1655	Transposon insertion	Increase	Plates	LB	Ap	Girgis et al. (2012)
rffM	UDP-N-acetyl-D-mannosaminuronic acid transferase	MG1655	Transposon insertion	Increase	Plates	LB	Ap	Girgis et al. (2012)
rob	Right origin-binding protein	MG1655	Insertion	Decrease	Plates	LB	Ap	Girgis et al. (2012)
smpB	ssrA-binding protein	W3110	Deletion	Decrease	Stat	LB	Ap, Nor, Gm, Tmp, Tet, Strep	Li et al. (2013)
		W3110 (ΔrelA)	Deletion	Decrease	Stat	LB	Ap, Gm, Nor	Liu et al. (2017)
		W3110	Deletion	Decrease	Stat	LB	Gm, Tmp	Wu et al. (2015)
ssrA	tmRNA	W3110	Deletion	Decrease	Stat	LB	Ap, Nor	Liu et al. (2017)
		W3110 (ΔrelA)	Deletion	Decrease	Stat	LB	Ap, Gm, Nor	Liu et al. (2017)
		W3110	Deletion	Decrease	Stat	LB	Gm, Tmp	Wu et al. (2015)
		W3110	Deletion	Decrease	Stat	LB	Ap, Nor, Gm, Tmp, Tet, Strep	Li et al. (2013)

(continued)

Table 7.8 (continued)

Gene	Protein	Genetic background	Mutation	Persister fraction	Growth phase	Medium	Antibiotic	References
surA	Chaperone	BW25113	Deletion	Decrease	Exp, Stat	MOPS + 0.1% Suc + 0.05% CAA or LB	Of, Cip, Strep, Ap, BZK	Hansen et al. (2008)
		W3110	Deletion	Increase	Stat	LB	Ap	Liu et al. (2017)
ubiI	Ubiquitin-like protein	MG1655	Transposon insertion	Increase	Stat	MOPS + 0.2% Glc + 0.2% CAA	Gm	Shan et al. (2015)
visC	Unknown	MG1655	Transposon insertion	Increase	Plates	LB	Ap	Girgis et al. (2012)
xerC	Tyrosine recombinase	MG1655	Deletion	Decrease	Exp	MHB	Cip	Dörr et al. (2009)
xerD	Tyrosine recombinase	MG1655	Deletion	Decrease	Exp	MHB	Cip	Dörr et al. (2009)
yacC	Unknown	MG1655	Transposon insertion	Increase	Plates	LB	Ap	Girgis et al. (2012)
ybaZ	Unknown	MG1655	Transposon insertion	Increase	Plates	LB	Ap	Girgis et al. (2012)
ycfE	Unknown	MG1655 (metG*)	Transposon insertion	Decrease	Plates	LB	Ap	Girgis et al. (2012)
yeeY	Uncharacterized HTH-type transcriptional regulator	MG1655 (metG*)	Transposon insertion	Decrease	Plates	LB	Ap	Girgis et al. (2012)
yfcN	Unknown	MG1655	Transposon insertion	Decrease	Plates	LB	Ap	Girgis et al. (2012)
ygfA	5-Formyl tetrahydrofolate cyclo-ligase	BW25113	Deletion	Decrease	Exp, Stat	MOPS + 0.1% Suc + 0.05% CAA	Of, Cip, Strep, Ap, BZK	Hansen et al. (2008)

		BW25113	Overexpression	Increase	Stat	MOPS + 0.1% Suc + 0.05% CAA	Of	Hansen et al. (2008)
	Unknown	BW25113	Deletion	Decrease	Stat*	Lennox LB	Ap	Luidalepp et al. (2011)
yhaC	Unknown	MG1655	Transposon insertion	Decrease	Plates	LB	Ap	Girgis et al. (2012)
yiiS	Unknown	MG1655	Transposon insertion	Increase	Plates	LB	Ap	Girgis et al. (2012)
yjbE	Unknown	MG1655	Transposon insertion	Increase	Plates	LB	Ap	Girgis et al. (2012)
yjfI	Unknown	MG1655 (*metG**)	Transposon insertion	Increase	Plates	LB	Ap	Girgis et al. (2012)
yqeK	Unknown	MG1655 (*metG**)	Transposon insertion	Increase	Plates	LB	Ap	Girgis et al. (2012)
ygiE	Unknown	MG1655 (Δ*relA* Δ*spoT*)	Overexpression	Increase	Exp	LB	Ap, Cip	Chowdhury et al. (2016)
zur	Zinc uptake	MG1655 (Δ*relA* Δ*spoT*)	Overexpression	Increase	Exp	LB	Ap, Cip	Chowdhury et al. (2016)

G3P glyceraldehyde-3-phosphate, *metG** *metG* missing 7 amino acids at the C-terminus, *LPS* lipopolysaccharides, *OM* outer membrane, *QS* quorum sensing, *Stat* stationary, *Stat** stationary-phase cells treated after dilution, *Exp* exponential, *LB* lysogeny broth, *MHB* Mueller Hinton broth, *MOPS* (3-(*N*-morpholino) propanesulfonic acid), *Glc* glucose, *Glyc* glycerol, *Suc* sucrose, *CAA* casamino acids, *Ap* ampicillin, *BZK* benzalkonium chloride, *Cip* ciprofloxacin, *Gm* gentamicin, *Km* kanamycin, *Nor* norfloxacin, *Of* ofloxacin, *Strep* streptavidin, *Tet* tetracycline, *Tmp* trimethoprim

[a]Genes have been individually tested

7.10 Concluding Remarks

In the past few decades, there has been major progress in the field of bacterial persistence yielding valuable insights into the underlying mechanisms. A large number of persister genes involved in major global cellular processes have been uncovered and await more detailed investigation. While writing this chapter, we realized that persistence research is subjected to several constraints including the transient nature of the phenomenon as well as the low abundance of persister cells and aspects of redundancy and variability that make research in this domain both highly interesting and challenging. We also noticed that experimental conditions often differ between independent research studies, making direct comparisons of results difficult and a careful examination of experimental protocols highly appropriate. Nevertheless, our analysis of *E. coli* persistence genes clearly shows both the width and complexity of the genetic network underlying persistence. Research integrating this multilevel nature of persistence is needed and may offer new insights in this complex phenomenon.

References

Aizenman, E., Engelberg-Kulka, H., & Glaser, G. (1996). An *Escherichia coli* chromosomal "addiction module" regulated by guanosine [corrected] $3',5'$-bispyrophosphate: A model for programmed bacterial cell death. *Proceedings of the National Academy of Sciences, 93*, 6059–6063.

Allison, K. R., Brynildsen, M. P., & Collins, J. J. (2011). Heterogeneous bacterial persisters and engineering approaches to eliminate them. *Current Opinion in Microbiology, 14*, 593–598.

Amato, S. M., & Brynildsen, M. P. (2015). Persister heterogeneity arising from a single metabolic stress. *Current Biology, 25*, 2090–2098.

Amato, S. M., Orman, M. A., & Brynildsen, M. P. (2013). Metabolic control of persister formation in *Escherichia coli*. *Molecular Cell, 50*, 475–487.

An, G., Justesen, J., Watson, R. J., & Friesen, J. D. (1979). Cloning the *spoT* gene of *Escherichia coli*: Identification of the *spoT* gene product. *Journal of Bacteriology, 137*, 1100–1110.

Anders, S., McCarthy, D. J., Chen, Y. S., Okoniewski, M., Smyth, G. K., Huber, W., & Robinson, M. D. (2013). Count-based differential expression analysis of RNA sequencing data using R and bioconductor. *Nature Protocols, 8*, 1765–1786.

Balaban, N. Q., Merrin, J., Chait, R., Kowalik, L., & Leibler, S. (2004). Bacterial persistence as a phenotypic switch. *Science, 305*, 1622–1625.

Battesti, A., & Bouveret, E. (2006). Acyl carrier protein/SpoT interaction, the switch linking SpoT-dependent stress response to fatty acid metabolism. *Molecular Microbiology, 62*, 1048–1063.

Battesti, A., Majdalani, N., & Gottesman, S. (2011). The RpoS-mediated general stress response in *Escherichia coli*. *Annual Review of Microbiology, 65*, 189–213.

Behmardi, P., Grewal, E., Kim, Y., & Yang, H. N. (2009). RpoS-dependant mechanism is required for cross protection conferred to hyperosmolarity by heat shock. *Journal of Experimental Microbiology and Immunology, 13*, 18–21.

Bernier, S. P., Lebeaux, D., Defrancesco, A. S., Valomon, A., Ghigo, J., & Beloin, C. (2013). Starvation, together with the SOS response, mediates high biofilm-specific tolerance to the fluoroquinolone ofloxacin. *PLoS Genetics, 9*, e1003144.

Bokinsky, G., Baidoo, E. E. K., Akella, S., Burd, H., Weaver, D., Alonso-Gutierrez, J., García-Martín, H., Lee, T. S., & Keasling, J. D. (2013). HipA-triggered growth arrest and β-lactam tolerance in *Escherichia coli* are mediated by RelA-dependent ppGpp synthesis. *Journal of Bacteriology, 195*, 3173–3182.

Borisov, V. B., Gennis, R. B., Hemp, J., & Verkhovsky, M. I. (2011). The cytochrome bd respiratory oxygen reductases. *Biochimica et Biophysica Acta (BBA) – Bioenergetics, 1807*, 1398–1413.

Boutte, C. C., & Crosson, S. (2013). Bacterial lifestyle shapes stringent response activation. *Trends in Microbiology, 21*, 174–180.

Brent, R., & Ptashne, M. (1980). The *lexA* gene product represses its own promoter. *Proceedings of the National Academy of Sciences of the United States of America, 77*, 1932–1938.

Brielle, R., Pinel-Marie, M. L., & Felden, B. (2016). Linking bacterial type I toxins with their actions. *Current Opinion in Microbiology, 30*, 144–121.

Brown, L., Gentry, D., Elliott, T., & Cashel, M. (2002). DksA affects ppGpp induction of RpoS at a translational level. *Journal of Bacteriology, 184*, 4455–4465.

Chang, Z. (2016). The function of the DegP (HtrA) protein: Protease versus chaperone. *IUBMB Life, 68*, 904–907.

Chowdhury, N., Kwan, B. W., & Wood, T. K. (2016). Persistence increases in the absence of the alarmone guanosine tetraphosphate by reducing cell growth. *Scientific Reports, 6*, 20519.

Christensen, S. K., Mikkelsen, M., Pedersen, K., & Gerdes, K. (2001). RelE, a global inhibitor of translation, is activated during nutritional stress. *Proceedings of the National Academy of Sciences, 98*, 14328–14333.

Christensen, S. K., Maenhaut-Michel, G., Mine, N., Gottesman, S., Gerdes, K., & Van Melderen, L. (2004). Overproduction of the Lon protease triggers inhibition of translation in *Escherichia coli*: Involvement of the *yefM-yoeB* toxin-antitoxin system. *Molecular Microbiology, 51*, 1705–1717.

Christensen-Dalsgaard, M., Jørgensen, M. G., & Gerdes, K. (2010). Three new RelE-homologous mRNA interferases of *Escherichia coli* differentially induced by environmental stresses. *Molecular Microbiology, 75*, 333–348.

Cohen, G. N. (2014). *Microbial biochemistry*. New York: Springer International.

Courcelle, J., & Hanawalt, P. C. (2003). RecA-dependent recovery of arrested DNA replication forks. *Annual Review of Genetics, 37*, 611–646.

Cox, G. B., Newton, N. A., Gibson, F., Snoswell, A., & Hamilton, J. A. (1970). The function of ubiquinone in *Escherichia coli*. *The Biochemical Journal, 117*, 551–562.

Debbia, E. A., Roveta, S., Schito, A. M., Gualco, L., & Marchese, A. (2001). Antibiotic persistence: The role of spontaneous DNA repair response. *Microbial Drug Resistance, 7*, 335–342.

Dong, T., & Schellhorn, H. E. (2009). Control of RpoS in global gene expression of *Escherichia coli* in minimal media. *Molecular Genetics and Genomics, 281*, 19–33.

Dörr, T., Lewis, K., & Vulić, M. (2009). SOS response induces persistence to fluoroquinolones in *Escherichia coli*. *PLoS Genetics, 5*, e1000760.

Dörr, T., Vulić, M., & Lewis, K. (2010). Ciprofloxacin causes persister formation by inducing the TisB toxin in *Escherichia coli*. *PLoS Biology, 8*, e1000317.

English, B. P., Hauryliuk, V., Sanamrad, A., Tankov, S., Dekker, N. H., & Elf, J. (2011). Single-molecule investigations of the stringent response machinery in living bacterial cells. *Proceedings of the National Academy of Sciences, 108*, 365–373.

Fung, D. K. C., Chan, E. W. C., Chin, M. L., & Chan, R. C. Y. (2010). Delineation of a bacterial starvation stress response network which can mediate antibiotic tolerance development. *Antimicrobial Agents and Chemotherapy, 54*, 1082–1093.

Garbe, T. R., Kobayashi, M., & Yukawa, H. (2000). Indole-inducible proteins in bacteria suggest membrane and oxidant toxicity. *Archives of Microbiology, 173*, 78–82.

Gentry, D. R., Hernandez, V. J., Nguyen, L. H., Jensen, D. B., & Cashel, M. (1993). Synthesis of the stationary-phase sigma factor σs is positively regulated by ppGpp. *Journal of Bacteriology, 175*, 7892–7989.

Gerdes, K., Rasmussen, P. B., & Molin, S. (1986). Unique type of plasmid maintenance function: Postsegregational killing of plasmid-free cells. *Proceedings of the National Academy of Sciences of the United States of America, 83*, 3116–3120.

Germain, E., Castro-Roa, D., Zenkin, N., & Gerdes, K. (2013). Molecular mechanism of bacterial persistence by HipA. *Molecular Cell, 52*, 248–254.

Germain, E., Roghanian, M., Gerdes, K., & Maisonneuve, E. (2015). Stochastic induction of persister cells by HipA through (p)ppGpp-mediated activation of mRNA endonucleases. *Proceedings of the National Academy of Sciences of the United States of America, 112*, 5171–5176.

Giese, K. C., Michalowski, C. B., & Little, J. W. (2008). RecA-dependent cleavage of LexA dimers. *Journal of Molecular Biology, 377*, 148–161.

Girard, M. E., Gopalkrishnan, S., Grace, E. D., Halliday, J. A., Gourse, R. L., & Herman, C. (2018). DksA and ppGpp regulate the σS stress response by activating promoters for the small RNA DsrA and the anti-adapter protein IraP. *Journal of Bacteriology, 200*, e00463–e00417.

Girgis, H. S., Harris, K., & Tavazoie, S. (2012). Large mutational target size for rapid emergence of bacterial persistence. *Proceedings of the National Academy of Sciences, 109*, 12740–12745.

Giudice, E., Mac, K., & Gillet, R. (2014). *Trans*-translation exposed: Understanding the structures and functions of tmRNA-SmpB. *Frontiers in Microbiology, 5*, 1–11.

Goldfless, S. J., Morag, A. S., Belisle, K. A., Sutera, V. A., & Lovett, S. T. (2006). DNA repeat rearrangements mediated by DnaK-dependent replication fork repair. *Molecular Cell, 21*, 595–604.

Goltermann, L., Good, L., & Bentin, T. (2013). Chaperonins fight aminoglycoside-induced protein misfolding and promote short-term tolerance in *Escherichia coli*. *The Journal of Biological Chemistry, 288*, 10483–10489.

Gragerov, A. I., Martin, E. S., Krupenko, M. A., Kashlev, M. V., & Nikiforov, V. G. (1991). Protein aggregation and inclusion body formation in *Escherichia coli rpoH* mutant defective in heat shock protein induction. *FEBS Letters, 291*, 222–224.

Grudniak, A. M., Kuć, M., & Wolska, K. I. (2005). Role of *Escherichia coli* DnaK and DnaJ chaperones in spontaneous and induced mutagenesis and their effect on UmuC stability. *FEMS Microbiology Letters, 242*, 361–366.

Gupta, A., Venkataraman, B., Vasudevan, M., & Gopinath, B. K. (2017). Co-expression network analysis of toxin-antitoxin loci in *Mycobacterium tuberculosis* reveals key modulators of cellular stress. *Scientific Reports, 7*, 5868.

Gur, E. (2013). The Lon AAA+ protease. *Sub-Cellular Biochemistry, 66*, 35–51.

Gurnev, P. A., Ortenberg, R., Dörr, T., Lewis, K., & Bezrukov, S. M. (2012). Persister-promoting bacterial toxin TisB produces anion-selective pores in planar lipid bilayers. *FEBS Letters, 586*, 2529–2534.

Hansen, S., Lewis, K., & Vulić, M. (2008). Role of global regulators and nucleotide metabolism in antibiotic tolerance in *Escherichia coli*. *Antimicrobial Agents and Chemotherapy, 52*, 2718–2726.

Harms, A., Fino, C., Sørensen, M. A., Semsey, S., & Gerdes, K. (2017). Prophages and growth dynamics confound experimental results with antibiotic-tolerant persister cells. *mBio, 8*, e01964-17.

Harms, A., Brodersen, D. E., Mitarai, N., & Gerdes, K. (2018). Toxins, targets, and triggers: An overview of toxin-antitoxin biology. *Molecular Cell, 70*, 768–784.

Harrison, J. J., Wade, W. D., Akierman, S., Vacchi-Suzzi, C., Stremick, C. A., Turner, R. J., & Ceri, H. (2009). The chromosomal toxin gene *yafQ* is a determinant of multidrug tolerance for *Escherichia coli* growing in a biofilm. *Antimicrobial Agents and Chemotherapy, 53*, 2253–2258.

Harshman, R. B., & Yamazaki, H. (1971). Formation of ppGpp in a relaxed and stringent strain of *Escherichia coli* during diauxie lag. *Biochemistry, 10*, 3980–3982.

Harshman, R. B., & Yamazakif, H. (1972). MSI accumulation induced by sodium chloride. *Biochemistry, 11*, 615–618.

Haseltine, W. A., & Block, R. (1973). Synthesis of guanosine tetra- and pentaphosphate requires the presence of a codon-specific, uncharged transfer ribonucleic acid in the acceptor site of ribosomes. *Proceedings of the National Academy of Sciences, 70*, 1564–1568.

Helaine, S., Cheverton, A. M., Watson, K. G., Faure, L. M., Matthews, S. A., & Holden, D. W. (2014). Internalization of Salmonella by macrophages induces formation of nonreplicating persisters. *Science, 343*, 204–208.

Hengge-Aronis, R. (2002). Signal transduction and regulatory mechanisms involved in control of the σS (RpoS) subunit of RNA polymerase. *Microbiology and Molecular Biology Reviews, 66*, 373–395.

Hirakawa, H., Inazumi, Y., Masaki, T., Hirata, T., & Yamaguchi, A. (2005). Indole induces the expression of multidrug exporter genes in *Escherichia coli*. *Molecular Microbiology, 55*, 1113–1126.

Hong, S. H., Wang, X., O'Connor, H. F., Benedik, M. J., & Wood, T. K. (2012). Bacterial persistence increases as environmental fitness decreases. *Microbial Biotechnology, 5*, 509–522.

Hu, Y., Kwan, B. W., Osbourne, D. O., Benedik, M. J., & Wood, T. K. (2015). Toxin YafQ increases persister cell formation by reducing indole signalling. *Environmental Microbiology, 17*, 1275–1285.

Jenkins, D. E., Auger, E. A., & Matin, A. (1991). Role of RpoH, a heat shock regulator protein, in *Escherichia coli* carbon starvation protein synthesis and survival. *Journal of Bacteriology, 173*, 1992–1996.

Kamenšek, S., Podlesek, Z., Gillor, O., & Žgur-Bertok, D. (2010). Genes regulated by the *Escherichia coli* SOS repressor LexA exhibit heterogenous expression. *BMC Microbiology, 10*, 283.

Kasari, V., Mets, T., Tenson, T., & Kaldalu, N. (2013). Transcriptional cross-activation between toxin-antitoxin systems of *Escherichia coli*. *BMC Microbiology, 13*, 45.

Kaspy, I., Rotem, E., Weiss, N., Ronin, I., Balaban, N. Q., & Glaser, G. (2013). HipA-mediated antibiotic persistence via phosphorylation of the glutamyl-tRNA-synthetase. *Nature Communications, 4*, 3001.

Keren, I., Shah, D., Spoering, A., Kaldalu, N., & Lewis, K. (2004a). Specialized persister cells and the mechanism of multidrug tolerance in *Escherichia coli*. *Journal of Bacteriology, 186*, 8172–8180.

Keren, I., Kaldalu, N., Spoering, A., Wang, Y., & Lewis, K. (2004b). Persister cells and tolerance to antimicrobials. *FEMS Microbiology Letters, 230*, 13–18.

Kim, Y., & Wood, T. K. (2010). Toxins Hha and CspD and small RNA regulator Hfq are involved in persister cell formation through MqsR in *Escherichia coli*. *Biochemical and Biophysical Research Communications, 391*, 209–213.

Kim, J., Cho, D., Heo, P., Jung, S., Park, M., Oh, E., Sung, J., & Kim, P. (2016). Fumarate-mediated persistence of *Escherichia coli* against antibiotics. *Antimicrobial Agents and Chemotherapy, 60*, 2232–2240.

Kiss, P. (2000). Results concerning products and sums of the terms of linear recurrences. *Annales Mathematicae et Informaticae, 27*, 1–7.

Kohanski, M. A., Dwyer, D. J., Hayete, B., Lawrence, C. A., & Collins, J. J. (2007). A common mechanism of cellular death induced by bactericidal antibiotics. *Cell, 130*, 797–810.

Korch, S. B., & Hill, T. M. (2006). Ectopic overexpression of wild-type and mutant *hipA* genes in *Escherichia coli*: Effects on macromolecular synthesis and persister formation. *Journal of Bacteriology, 188*, 3826–3836.

Korch, S. B., Henderson, T. A., & Hill, T. M. (2003). Characterization of the *hipA7* allele of *Escherichia coli* and evidence that high persistence is governed by (p)ppGpp synthesis. *Molecular Microbiology, 50*, 1199–1213.

Kostakioti, M., Hadjifrangiskou, M., Pinkner, J. S., & Hultgren, S. J. (2010). QseC-mediated dephosphorylation of QseB is required for expression of genes associated with virulence in uropathogenic *Escherichia coli*. *Molecular Microbiology, 73*, 1020–1031.

Kreuzer, K. N. (2013). DNA damage responses in prokaryotes: Regulating gene expression, modulating growth patterns, and manipulating replication forks. *Cold Spring Harbor Perspectives in Biology, 5*, a012674.

Kuczyńska-Wiśnik, D., Kędzierska, S., Matuszewska, E., Lund, P., Taylor, A., Lipińska, B., & Laskowska, E. (2002). The *Escherichia coli* small heat-shock proteins IbpA and IbpB prevent the aggregation of endogenous proteins denatured *in vivo* during extreme heat shock. *Microbiology, 148*, 1757–1765.

Lacour, S., & Landini, P. (2004). σS-dependent gene expression at the onset of stationary phase in *Escherichia coli*: Function of σS-dependent genes and identification of their promoter sequences. *Society, 186*, 7186–7195.

Landini, P., Egli, T., Wolf, J., & Lacour, S. (2014). sigmaS, a major player in the response to environmental stresses in *Escherichia coli*: Role, regulation and mechanisms of promoter recognition. *Environmental Microbiology Reports, 6*, 1–13.

Langklotz, S., & Narberhaus, F. (2011). The *Escherichia coli* replication inhibitor CspD is subject to growth-regulated degradation by the Lon protease. *Molecular Microbiology, 80*, 1313–1325.

Leatham-Jensen, M. P., Mokszycki, M. E., Rowley, D. C., Robert, D., Camberg, J. L., Sokurenko, E. V., Tchesnokova, V. L., Frimodt-Møller, J., Krogfelte, K. A., Nielsen, K. L., Frimodt-Møller, N., Sun, G., & Cohen, P. S. (2016). Uropathogenic *Escherichia coli* metabolite-dependent quiescence and persistence may explain antibiotic tolerance during urinary tract infection. *MSphere, 1*, e00055-15.

Leszczynska, D., Matuszewska, E., Kuczynska-Wisnik, D., Furmanek-Blaszk, B., & Laskowska, E. (2013). The formation of persister cells in stationary-phase cultures of *Escherichia coli* is associated with the aggregation of endogenous proteins. *PLoS One, 8*, e54737.

Lewis, K. (2010). Persister cells. *Annual Review of Microbiology, 64*, 357–372.

Li, Y., & Zhang, Y. (2007). PhoU is a persistence switch involved in persister formation and tolerance to multiple antibiotics and stresses in *Escherichia coli*. *Antimicrobial Agents and Chemotherapy, 51*, 2092–2099.

Li, X., Yagi, M., Morita, T., & Aiba, H. (2008). Cleavage of mRNAs and role of tmRNA system under amino acid starvation in *Escherichia coli*. *Molecular Microbiology, 68*, 462–473.

Li, J., Ji, L., Shi, W., Xie, J., & Zhang, Y. (2013). Trans-translation mediates tolerance to multiple antibiotics and stresses in *Escherichia coli*. *The Journal of Antimicrobial Chemotherapy, 68*, 2477–2481.

Lindner, A. B., Madden, R., Demarez, A., Stewart, E. J., & Taddei, F. (2008). Asymmetric segregation of protein aggregates is associated with cellular aging and rejuvenation. *Proceedings of the National Academy of Sciences of the United States of America, 105*, 3076–3081.

Little, J. W. (1991). Mechanism of specific LexA cleavage: Autodigestion and the role of RecA coprotease. *Biochimie, 73*, 411–421.

Liu, S., Wu, N., Zhang, S., Yuan, Y., Zhang, W., & Zhang, Y. (2017). Variable persister gene interactions with (p)ppGpp for persister formation in *Escherichia coli*. *Frontiers in Microbiology, 8*, 1795.

Lobritz, M. A., Belenky, P., Porter, C. B. M., Gutierrez, A., Yang, J. H., Schwarz, E. G., Dwyer, D. J., Khalil, A. S., & Collins, J. J. (2015). Antibiotic efficacy is linked to bacterial cellular respiration. *Proceedings of the National Academy of Sciences, 112*, 8173–8180.

Luidalepp, H., Jõers, A., Kaldalu, N., & Tenson, T. (2011). Age of inoculum strongly influences persister frequency and can mask effects of mutations implicated in altered persistence. *Journal of Bacteriology, 193*, 3598–3605.

Luo, Y., Pfuetzner, R. A., Mosimann, S., Paetzel, M., Frey, E. A., Cherney, M., Kim, B., Little, J. W., & Strynadka, N. C. J. (2001). Crystal structure of LexA: A conformational switch for regulation of self-cleavage. *Cell, 106*, 585–594.

Ma, C., Sim, S., Shi, W., Du, L., Xing, D., & Zhang, Y. (2010). Energy production genes *sucB* and *ubiF* are involved in persister survival and tolerance to multiple antibiotics and stresses in *Escherichia coli*. *FEMS Microbiology Letters, 303*, 33–40.

Michiels, J. E., Van den Bergh, B., Verstraeten, N., & Michiels, J. (2016). Molecular mechanisms and clinical implications of bacterial persistence. *Drug Resistance Updates, 29*, 76–89.

Miller, C., Thomsen, L. E., Gaggero, C., Mosseri, R., Ingmer, H., & Cohen, S. N. (2004). SOS response induction by beta-lactams and bacterial defense against antibiotic lethality. *Science, 305*, 1629–1631.

Mok, W. W. K., & Brynildsen, M. P. (2018). Timing of DNA damage responses impacts persistence to fluoroquinolones. *Proceedings of the National Academy of Sciences of the United States of America, 115*, e6301–e6309.

Moyed, H. S., & Bertrand, K. P. (1983). *hipA*, a newly recognized gene of *Escherichia coli* K-12 that affects frequency of persistence after inhibition of murein synthesis. *Journal of Bacteriology, 155*, 768–775.

Muffler, A., Fischer, D., Altuvia, S., Storz, G., & Hengge-Aronis, R. (1996). The response regulator RssB controls stability of the sigma(S) subunit of RNA polymerase in *Escherichia coli*. *The EMBO Journal, 15*, 1333–1339.

Muthuramalingam, M., White, J. C., & Bourne, C. R. (2016). Toxin-antitoxin modules are pliable switches activated by multiple protease pathways. *Toxins, 8*, 214–230.

Nichols, R. J., Sen, S., Choo, Y. J., Beltrao, P., Zietek, M., Chaba, R., Lee, S., Kazmierczak, K. M., Lee, K. J., Wong, A., Shales, M., Lovett, S., Winkler, M. E., Krogan, N. J., Typas, A., & Gross, C. A. (2011). Phenotypic landscape of a bacterial cell. *Cell, 144*, 143–156.

Norton, J. P., & Mulvey, M. A. (2012). Toxin-antitoxin systems are important for niche-specific colonization and stress resistance of uropathogenic *Escherichia coli*. *PLoS Pathogens, 8*, e1002954.

Opperman, T., Murli, S., Smith, B. T., & Walker, G. C. (1999). A model for a *umuDC*-dependent prokaryotic DNA damage checkpoint. *Proceedings of the National Academy of Sciences of the United States of America, 96*, 9218–9223.

Orman, M. A., & Brynildsen, M. P. (2013). Dormancy is not necessary or sufficient for bacterial persistence. *Antimicrobial Agents and Chemotherapy, 57*, 3230–3239.

Orman, M. A., & Brynildsen, M. P. (2015). Inhibition of stationary phase respiration impairs persister formation in *E. coli*. *Nature Communications, 6*, 7983.

Page, R., & Peti, W. (2016). Toxin-antitoxin systems in bacterial growth arrest and persistence. *Nature Chemical Biology, 12*, 208–214.

Pandey, D. P., & Gerdes, K. (2005). Toxin-antitoxin loci are highly abundant in free-living but lost from host-associated prokaryotes. *Nucleic Acids Research, 33*, 966–976.

Parsons, C. A., & West, S. C. (1993). Formation of a RuvAB-holliday junction complex *in vitro*. *Journal of Molecular Biology, 232*, 397–405.

Pedersen, K., Zavialov, A. V., Pavlov, M. Y., Elf, J., Gerdes, K., & Ehrenberg, M. (2003). The bacterial toxin RelE displays codon-specific cleavage of mRNAs in the ribosomal A site. *Cell, 112*, 131–140.

Petit, M. A., Bedale, W., Osipiuk, J., Lu, C., Rajagopalant, M., McInerney, P., Goodman, M. F., & Echols, H. (1994). Sequential folding of UmuC by the Hsp70 and Hsp60 chaperone complexes of *Escherichia coli*. *The Journal of Biological Chemistry, 269*, 23824–23829.

Potrykus, K., Murphy, H., Philippe, N., & Cashel, M. (2011). ppGpp is the major source of growth rate control in *E. coli*. *Environmental Microbiology, 13*, 563–575.

Prysak, M. H., Mozdzierz, C. J., Cook, A. M., Zhu, L., Zhang, Y., Inouye, M., & Woychik, N. A. (2009). Bacterial toxin YafQ is an endoribonuclease that associates with the ribosome and blocks translation elongation through sequence-specific and frame-dependent mRNA cleavage. *Molecular Microbiology, 71*, 1071–1087.

Pu, Y., Zhao, Z., Li, Y., Zou, J., Ma, Q., Zhao, Y., Ke, Y., Zhu, Y., Chen, H., Baker, M. A. B., Ge, H., Sun, Y., Xie, X. S., & Bai, F. (2016). Enhanced efflux activity facilitates drug tolerance in dormant bacterial cells. *Molecular Cell, 62*, 284–294.

Pu, Y., Li, Y., Jin, X., Tian, T., Ma, Q., Zhao, Z., Lin, S., Chen, Z., Li, B., Yao, G., Leake, M. C., Lo, C.-J., & Bai, F. (2018). ATP-dependent dynamic protein aggregation regulates bacterial dormancy depth critical for antibiotic tolerance. *Molecular Cell, 73*, 143–156.

Radzikowski, J. L., Vedelaar, S., Siegel, D., Ortega, Á. D., Schmidt, A., & Heinemann, M. (2016). Bacterial persistence is an active σS stress response to metabolic flux limitation. *Molecular Systems Biology, 12,* 1–12.

Raivio, T. L. (2005). Envelope stress responses and Gram-negative bacterial pathogenesis. *Molecular Microbiology, 56,* 1119–1128.

Ramisetty, B. C. M., Ghosh, D., Chowdhury, M. R., & Santhosh, R. S. (2017). What is the link between stringent response, endoribonuclease encoding type II toxin-antitoxin systems and persistence? *Frontiers in Microbiology, 7,* 1882.

Rao, N. N., Liu, S., & Kornberg, A. (1998). Inorganic polyphosphate in *Escherichia coli*: The phosphate regulon and the stringent response. *Journal of Bacteriology, 180,* 2186–2193.

Rice, C. D., Pollard, J. E., Lewis, Z. T., & McCleary, W. R. (2009). Employment of a promoter-swapping technique shows that PhoU modulates the activity of the PstSCAB2ABC transporter in *Escherichia coli*. *Applied and Environmental Microbiology, 75,* 573–582.

Rotem, E., Loinger, A., Ronin, I., Levin-Reisman, I., Gabay, C., Shoresh, N., Biham, O., & Balaban, N. Q. (2010). Regulation of phenotypic variability by a threshold-based mechanism underlies bacterial persistence. *Proceedings of the National Academy of Sciences of the United States of America, 107,* 12541–12546.

Rowe, M. T., & Kirk, R. (1999). An investigation into the phenomenon of cross-protection in *Escherichia coli* O157:H7. *Food Microbiology, 16,* 157–164.

Runyon, G. T., Bear, D. G., & Lohman, T. M. (1990). *Escherichia coli* helicase II (UvrD) protein initiates DNA unwinding at nicks and blunt ends. *Proceedings of the National Academy of Sciences of the United States of America, 87,* 6386–6393.

Sakoh, M., Ito, K., & Akiyama, Y. (2005). Proteolytic activity of HtpX, a membrane-bound and stress-controlled protease from *Escherichia coli*. *The Journal of Biological Chemistry, 280,* 33305–33310.

Santos-Beneit, F. (2015). The Pho regulon: A huge regulatory network in bacteria. *Frontiers in Microbiology, 6,* 1–13.

Sat, B., Hazan, R., Fisher, T., Khaner, H., Glaser, G., & Engelberg-Kulka, H. (2001). Programmed cell death in *Escherichia coli*: Some antibiotics can trigger *mazEF* lethality. *Journal of Bacteriology, 183,* 2041–2045.

Schröder, H., Langer, T., Hartl, F. U., & Bukau, B. (1993). DnaK, DnaJ and GrpE form a cellular chaperone machinery capable of repairing heat-induced protein damage. *The EMBO Journal, 12,* 4137–4144.

Seong, I. S., Oh, J. Y., Lee, J. W., Tanaka, K., & Chung, C. H. (2000). The HslU ATPase acts as a molecular chaperone in prevention of aggregation of SulA, an inhibitor of cell division in *Escherichia coli*. *FEBS Letters, 477,* 224–229.

Shah, D., Zhang, Z., Khodursky, A., Kaldalu, N., Kurg, K., & Lewis, K. (2006). Persisters: A distinct physiological state of *E. coli*. *BMC Microbiology, 6,* 53.

Shan, Y., Lazinski, D., Rowe, S., Camilli, A., & Lewis, K. (2015). Genetic basis of persister tolerance to aminoglycosides in *Escherichia coli*. *mBio, 6,* e00078-15.

Shan, Y., Gandt, A. B., Rowe, S. E., Deisinger, J. P., Conlon, B. P., & Lewis, K. (2017). ATP-dependent persister formation in *Escherichia coli*. *mBio, 8,* e02267-16.

Simmons, L. A., Foti, J. J., Cohen, S. E., & Walker, G. C. (2008). *The SOS regulatory network*. EcoSal Plus.

Spira, B., Silberstein, N., & Yagil, E. (1995). Guanosine 3′,5′-bispyrophosphate (ppGpp) synthesis in cells of *Escherichia coli* starved for P(i). *Journal of Bacteriology, 177,* 4053–4058.

Spoering, A. L., Vulić, M., & Lewis, K. (2006). GlpD and PlsB participate in persister cell formation in *Escherichia coli*. *Journal of Bacteriology, 188,* 5136–5144.

Steed, P. M., & Wanner, B. L. (1993). Use of the rep technique for allele replacement to construct mutants with deletions of the pstSCAB-phoU operon: Evidence of a new role for the PhoU protein in the phosphate regulon. *Journal of Bacteriology, 175,* 6797–6809.

Steinsiek, S., Stagge, S., & Bettenbrock, K. (2014). Analysis of *Escherichia coli* mutants with a linear respiratory chain. *PLoS One, 9,* e87307.

Stewart, E. J., Madden, R., & Paul, G. (2005). Aging and death in an organism that reproduces by morphologically symmetric division. *PLoS Biology, 3*, e45.

Tashiro, Y., Kawata, K., Taniuchi, A., Kakinuma, K., May, T., & Okabe, S. (2012). RelE-mediated dormancy is enhanced at high cell density in *Escherichia coli*. *Journal of Bacteriology, 194*, 1169–1176.

Theodore, A., Lewis, K., & Vulić, M. (2013). Tolerance of *Escherichia coli* to fluoroquinolone antibiotics depends on specific components of the SOS response pathway. *Genetics, 195*, 1265–1276.

Tramonti, A., Visca, P., De Canio, M., De Biase, D., & Falconi, M. (2002). Functional character-ization and regulation of *gadX*, a gene encoding an AraC/XylS-like transcriptional activator of the *Escherichia coli* glutamic acid decarboxylase system. *Journal of Bacteriology, 184*, 2306–2613.

Tripathi, A., Dewan, P. C., Siddique, S. A., & Varadarajan, R. (2014). MazF-induced growth inhibition and persister generation in *Escherichia coli*. *The Journal of Biological Chemistry, 289*, 4191–4205.

Tuteja, N., & Tuteja, R. (2004). Prokaryotic and eukaryotic DNA helicases: Essential molecular motor proteins for cellular machinery. *European Journal of Biochemistry, 271*, 1835–1848.

Unden, G., & Bongaerts, J. (1997). Alternative respiratory pathways of *Escherichia coli*: Energetics and transcriptional regulation in response to electron acceptors. *Biochimica et Biophysica Acta (BBA) – Bioenergetics, 1320*, 217–234.

Van den Bergh, B., Michiels, J. E., Wenseleers, T., Windels, E. M., Vanden, B. P., Kestemont, D., De Meester, L., Verstrepen, K. J., Verstraeten, N., Fauvart, M., & Michiels, J. (2016). Fre-quency of antibiotic application drives rapid evolutionary adaptation of *Escherichia coli* persistence. *Nature Microbiology, 1*, 16020.

Vázquez-Laslop, N., Lee, H., & Neyfakh, A. A. (2006). Increased persistence in *Escherichia coli* caused by controlled expression of toxins or other unrelated proteins. *Journal of Bacteriology, 188*, 3494–3497.

Vega, N. M., Allison, K. R., Khalil, A. S., & Collins, J. J. (2012). Signaling-mediated bacterial persister formation. *Nature Chemical Biology, 8*, 431–433.

Verstraeten, N., Knapen, W. J., Kint, C. I., Liebens, V., Van den Bergh, B., Dewachter, L., Michiels, J. E., Fu, Q., David, C. C., Fierro, A. C., Marchal, K., Beirlant, J., Versées, W., Hofkens, J., Jansen, M., Fauvart, M., & Michiels, J. (2015). Obg and membrane depolarization are part of a microbial bet-hedging strategy that leads to antibiotic tolerance. *Molecular Cell, 59*, 9–21.

Vinella, D., Albrecht, C., Cashel, M., & D'Ari, R. (2005). Iron limitation induces SpoT-dependent accumulation of ppGpp in *Escherichia coli*. *Molecular Microbiology, 56*, 958–970.

Völzing, K. G., & Brynildsen, M. P. (2015). Stationary-phase persisters to ofloxacin sustain DNA damage and require repair systems only during recovery. *mBio, 6*, e00731–e00746.

Wang, X., Lord, D. M., Cheng, H. Y., Osbourne, D. O., Hong, S. H., Sanchez-Torres, V., Quiroga, C., Zheng, K., Herrmann, T., Peti, W., Benedik, M. J., Page, R., & Wood, T. K. (2012). A new type V toxin-antitoxin system where mRNA for toxin GhoT is cleaved by antitoxin GhoS. *Nature Chemical Biology, 8*, 855–861.

Wang, X., Lord, D. M., Hong, S. H., Peti, W., Benedik, M. J., Page, R., & Wood, T. K. (2013). Type II toxin/antitoxin MqsR/MqsA controls type V toxin/antitoxin GhoT/GhoS. *Environmen-tal Microbiology, 15*, 1734–1744.

Wang, J. H., Singh, R., Benoit, M., Keyhan, M., Sylvester, M., Hsieh, M., Thathireddy, A., Hsieh, Y. J., & Matin, A. C. (2014). Sigma S-dependent antioxidant defense protects stationary-phase *Escherichia coli* against the bactericidal antibiotic gentamicin. *Antimicrobial Agents and Che-motherapy, 58*, 5964–5975.

Wang, T., El Meouche, I., & Dunlop, M. J. (2017). Bacterial persistence induced by salicylate via reactive oxygen species. *Scientific Reports, 7*, 43839.

Weber, H. H., Polen, T. T., Heuveling, J. J., Wendisch, V. F. V. F., & Hengge-Aronis, R. (2005). Genome-wide analysis of the general stress response network in *Escherichia coli*: SigmaS-dependent genes, promoters, and sigma factor selectivity. *Journal of Bacteriology, 187,* 1591–1603.

Wessner, F., Lacoux, C., Goeders, N., Fouquier d'Hérouel, A., Matos, R., Serror, P., Van Melderen, L., & Repoila, F. (2015). Regulatory crosstalk between type I and type II toxin-antitoxin systems in the human pathogen *Enterococcus faecalis. RNA Biology, 12,* 1099–1108.

Wilmaerts, D., Bayoumi, M., Dewachter, L., Knapen, W., Mika, J. T., Hofkens, J., Dedecker, P., Maglia, G., Verstraeten, N., & Michiels, J. (2018). The persistence-inducing toxin HokB forms dynamic pores that cause ATP leakage. *mBio, 9,* e00744-18.

Wout, P., Pu, K., Sullivan, S. M., Reese, V., Zhou, S., Lin, B., & Maddock, J. R. (2004). The *Escherichia coli* GTPase CgtAE cofractionates with the 50S ribosomal subunit and interacts with SpoT, a ppGpp synthetase/hydrolase. *Journal of Bacteriology, 186,* 5249–5257.

Wu, Y., Vulić, M., Keren, I., & Lewis, K. (2012). Role of oxidative stress in persister tolerance. *Antimicrobial Agents and Chemotherapy, 56,* 4922–4926.

Wu, N., He, L., Cui, P., Wang, W., Yuan, Y., Liu, S., Xu, T., Zhang, S., Wu, J., Zhang, W., & Zhang, Y. (2015). Ranking of persister genes in the same *Escherichia coli* genetic background demonstrates varying importance of individual persister genes in tolerance to different antibiotics. *Frontiers in Microbiology, 6,* 1003.

Xiao, H., Kalman, M., Ikehara, K., Zemel, S., Glaser, G., & Cashel, M. (1991). Residual guanosine 3′,5′-bispyrophosphate synthetic activity of *relA* null mutants can be eliminated by *spoT* null mutations. *The Journal of Biological Chemistry, 266,* 5980–5990.

Yamaguchi, Y., Park, J. H., & Inouye, M. (2009). MqsR, a crucial regulator for quorum sensing and biofilm formation, is a GCU-specific mRNA interferase in *Escherichia coli. The Journal of Biological Chemistry, 284,* 28746–28753.

Yamanaka, K., & Inouye, M. (1997). Growth-phase-dependent expression of *cspD*, encoding a member of the CspA family in *Escherichia coli. Journal of Bacteriology, 176,* 5126–5130.

Yamanaka, K., Zheng, W., Crooke, E., Wang, Y. H., & Inouye, M. (2001). CspD, a novel DNA replication inhibitor induced during the stationary phase in *Escherichia coli. Molecular Microbiology, 39,* 1572–1584.

Yim, H. H., Brems, R. L., & Villarejo, M. (1994). Molecular characterization of the promoter of osmY, an rpoS-dependent gene. *Journal of Bacteriology, 176,* 100–107.

Zhang, Y., & Inouye, M. (2011). RatA (YfjG), an *Escherichia coli* toxin, inhibits 70S ribosome association to block translation initiation. *Molecular Microbiology, 79,* 1418–1429.

Zhang, Y., Zhang, J., Hara, H., Kato, I., & Inouye, M. (2005). Insights into the mRNA cleavage mechanism by MazF, an mRNA interferase. *The Journal of Biological Chemistry, 280,* 3143–3150.

Zolkiewski, M. (1999). ClpB cooperates with DnaK, DnaJ, and GrpE in suppressing protein aggregation. A novel multi-chaperone system from *Escherichia coli. Journal of Biological Chemistry, 274,* 28083–28086.

Chapter 8
Toxin-Antitoxin Systems and Persistence

Nathan Fraikin, Frédéric Goormaghtigh, and Laurence Van Melderen

Abstract Toxin-antitoxin (TA) systems are small genetic modules comprising a stable toxic protein and an antitoxin preventing the toxin activity. In type II TA systems, antitoxins are unstable proteins that are degraded by host ATP-dependent proteases. In steady-state conditions, the antitoxin forms a complex with the toxin in which the toxic activity is inactivated, this complex also being responsible for negative autoregulation of the system. Environmental or physiological conditions generating a imbalanced toxin:antitoxin ratio should induce TA systems and halt cell growth. Persistence has been linked to type II TA systems activation in *Escherichia coli* K-12 via a complex regulatory cascade involving antitoxin degradation by the Lon protease, polyphosphate, and (p)ppGpp. However, this model has been recently disproved questioning the involvement of type II TA systems in persistence, at least in the *E. coli* K-12 model. In this chapter, we discuss the relevant data linking type II TA systems and persistence in *E. coli* and other bacterial species.

8.1 Introduction

In the last two decades, there has been an increasing amount of publications linking bacterial persistence with toxin-antitoxin (TA) systems in various bacterial species. TA systems are small genetic modules composed of a toxic protein and an antitoxin that neutralizes its cognate toxin. They can be classified in up to six different types, depending on the nature and the mode of action of the antitoxin (Harms et al. 2018). Type I and II TA systems, in which antitoxins are antisense RNAs or proteins, respectively, are the most abundant of these systems, with predicted type II systems

---

Nathan Fraikin and Frédéric Goormaghtigh contributed equally with all other contributors.

N. Fraikin · F. Goormaghtigh · L. Van Melderen (✉)
Cellular and Molecular Microbiology, Faculté des Sciences, Université Libre de Bruxelles (ULB), Gosselies, Belgium
e-mail: lvmelder@ulb.ac.be

© Springer Nature Switzerland AG 2019   181
K. Lewis (ed.), *Persister Cells and Infectious Disease*,
https://doi.org/10.1007/978-3-030-25241-0_8

constituting up to 3.7% of the open reading frames (ORFs) in some bacterial isolates (Leplae et al. 2011). The present chapter discusses the data linking type II TA systems and persistence in various bacterial species. Recent developments in the field lead to an increasingly growing controversy on the relationship between TA systems and persistence in *E. coli* K-12 (Goormaghtigh et al. 2018b; Harms et al. 2017a; Holden and Errington 2018; Ramisetty et al. 2016; Shan et al. 2017; Van Melderen and Wood 2017), which we will discuss in this chapter. We will review how type II TA systems came to be linked with persistence in different bacterial species and whether the past and current evidence of this relationship are still relevant today.

8.2   Type II TA Systems: A General Overview

Type II TA systems are commonly composed of two proteins, although examples of three-component systems have been described (Bordes et al. 2011; de la Hoz et al. 2000; Hallez et al. 2010). The corresponding genes are organized in operons, with the antitoxin gene preceding that of the toxin in most cases. In the classical type II TA systems, antitoxins are composed of two domains. Antitoxins bind and neutralize their cognate toxin through an intrinsically disordered domain. This unfolded region is thought to make antitoxins susceptible to degradation by ATP-dependent proteases such as Lon or ClpXP (Lehnherr and Yarmolinsky 1995; Van Melderen et al. 1994), conferring them their unstable nature. The second domain of antitoxins is a structured DNA-binding domain that binds operator sequences upstream of the operon and thus transcriptionally represses the expression of the TA system (Salmon et al. 1994; Tsuchimoto and Ohtsubo 1993). Toxins can act as co-regulators when bound to their cognate antitoxin: unsaturated concentrations of toxin in regards to the antitoxin greatly enhances binding to operator sequences while an excess of toxin displaces the antitoxin from the operator, leading to the derepression of the operon (Afif et al. 2001; Garcia-Pino et al. 2010; Overgaard et al. 2008). As antitoxins are translated more abundantly than the toxin (Deter et al. 2017; Ruiz-Echevarría et al. 1995), this mechanism, dubbed "conditional cooperativity," could allow rapid synthesis of antitoxin should the antitoxin be depleted due to stress or transcriptional noise.

Translation inhibition is, by far, the most widespread activity found in type II toxins, whether it is accomplished by ribosome-dependent (Christensen-Dalsgaard et al. 2010; Pedersen et al. 2003; Prysak et al. 2009) or independent (Muñoz-Gómez et al. 2005; Zhang et al. 2003) mRNA cleavage, tRNA acetylation (Cheverton et al. 2016; Jurenas et al. 2017; Rycroft et al. 2018), tRNA cleavage (Winther and Gerdes 2011), rRNA cleavage (Culviner and Laub 2018; Mets et al. 2017; Winther et al. 2013), phosphorylation of the translation elongation factor EF-Tu (Castro-Roa et al. 2013; Kaspy et al. 2013) or glutamyl tRNA-synthetase GltX (Germain et al. 2013; Kaspy et al. 2013).

Type II TA systems were first identified on plasmids, which they stabilize due to their addictive properties. As antitoxins are less stable than toxins, loss of a TA-encoding plasmid will lead to depletion of the antitoxin and activation of the toxin, intoxicating and killing daughter cells that did not inherit a plasmid copy during cell division (Jaffé et al. 1985). Numerous type II TA systems were subsequently discovered in bacterial chromosomes (Anantharaman and Aravind 2003; Gerdes 2000; Guglielmini et al. 2008; Leplae et al. 2011; Pandey and Gerdes 2005; Ramage et al. 2009; Ramisetty and Santhosh 2016; Shao et al. 2010). Two striking features rapidly stemmed from these bioinformatics studies. First, TA systems are detected among nearly every genome that has been sequenced. In some genomes of microorganism such as *Mycobacterium tuberculosis* and *Microcystis aeruginosa*, 76 and 113 TA systems, respectively, have been predicted (Shao et al. 2010). Second, the distribution of TA systems tends to vary between different isolates of the same species, indicating that these systems move by horizontal gene transfer (Hayes and Van Melderen 2011). These systems are often found in genomic islands such as prophages, ICEs, and transposons, thus, being part of the accessory genome (Escudero et al. 2015; Huguet et al. 2016; Leplae et al. 2011; Wozniak and Waldor 2009; Yao et al. 2015).

While the role of plasmid-encoded TA systems appears quite clear, the function of their chromosomal counterparts remains elusive to this day. Several roles have been attributed to chromosomal TA system such as protection against phage infections (Hazan and Engelberg-Kulka 2004; Koga et al. 2011), neutralization of the addictive properties of homologous plasmid-encoded systems (Saavedra De Bast et al. 2008), stabilization of superintegrons (Szekeres et al. 2007) and accessory chromosomes (Yuan et al. 2011), reservoir of effectors and immunities for secretion systems (Harms et al. 2017b) and persistence to antibiotics (Harms et al. 2016). An interesting postulate which can be considered as a null hypothesis is that TA systems are "junk DNA." TA systems can be inherited from mobile genetic elements and, due to their addictive nature, be maintained in genomes despite providing no competitive advantage. A previous study from our group showed that the *ccdAB* chromosomal system in *E. coli* is under neutral selection, indicating that it is devoid of biological function (Mine et al. 2009).

8.3   Toxin-Antitoxin Systems and Persistence in *Escherichia coli K-12*

8.3.1   The hipA7 *Allele*

The first study linking TA systems and persistence was conducted by Moyed and Bertrand in the 1980s (Moyed and Bertrand 1983). The authors subjected *Escherichia coli* K-12 to multiple rounds of ampicillin treatment after EMS mutagenesis to isolate *high-persistence* (*hip*) mutants. Two mutations, *hipA7* and *hipA9*, were mapped at 33.8 min of the chromosome to a yet uncharacterized locus: *hipA*. Subsequent work by Moyed and collaborators demonstrated that *hipA* was the toxic component of the *hipBA* type II TA system (Black et al. 1991, 1994). The *hipA7* gain-of-function phenotype was also shown to be the result of two point mutations in the *hipA* open reading frame (G22S and D291A) and to be dependent on the (p) ppGpp alarmone (Korch et al. 2003). Biochemical studies first characterized HipA as a kinase phosphorylating Elongation factor Tu (EF-Tu) (Schumacher et al. 2009). However, this was contested by two subsequent and independent studies showing that HipA phosphorylates glutamyl-tRNA synthetase GltX, preventing glutamate charging on its cognate tRNA (Germain et al. 2013; Kaspy et al. 2013). This would lead to incorporation of uncharged tRNA in the ribosomal A site, a condition well known to activate (p)ppGpp synthesis by the ribosome-bound RelA enzyme (Potrykus and Cashel 2008).

In 2004, Balaban et al. laid the foundation for single-cell analysis of bacterial persistence using the *hipA7* mutant as a model. They showed that *hipA7* persisters are stationary phase cells originating from the dilution of the overnight inoculum used in their experimental setup (Balaban et al. 2004). These persisters were classified as "type I," and are cells in a non-growing state induced by a trigger which was, in this case, stationary phase-induced starvation. On the other hand, type II persisters were defined as slow-growing cells generated stochastically in exponential phase (Balaban et al. 2004). Further work showed that upon inoculation from stationary phase to fresh medium, a subpopulation of the *hipA7* mutant had an abnormally long lag phase during which it can survive ampicillin treatment (Rotem et al. 2010). This study proposed that HipA could induce dormancy above a certain threshold of expression, threshold which can be reached stochastically in a fraction of the population due to the noisy nature of *hipBA* autoregulation. The increased lag of the *hipA7* persisters was attributed to a reduced binding of HipA7 for the HipB antitoxin, which partially alleviated autorepression of the TA operon, increasing *hipA* expression closer to the threshold required for dormancy (Rotem et al. 2010). Biochemical and structural studies of HipBA–DNA complexes revealed that the four *hipBA* operator–HipBA complexes formed higher-order complexes, which tighten the autorepression of the system. These higher-order complexes were found to be disrupted by the amino acid substitutions present in the HipA7 variant, thus, leading to reduced autorepression (Schumacher et al. 2015).

One could wonder whether the *hipA7* mutant, isolated in a test tube, is clinically relevant. To test this hypothesis, Schumacher et al. screened a library of 477 clinical isolates of commensal and uropathogenic *E. coli*. Noticeably, 23 of these clones possessed the *hipA7* allele (G22S and D291A) and showed a high-persistence phenotype dependent on this allele, indicating this *hipA7* could be important for multidrug tolerance in vivo (Schumacher et al. 2015).

Later on, the Balaban group performed experimental evolution under intermittent ampicillin treatment to isolate tolerant and resistant mutants (Levin-Reisman et al. 2017). Interestingly, mutations in the DNA-binding domains of the *vapB* and *yafN* antitoxins were detected in tolerant mutants, indicating that modification of TA systems other than *hipBA* can also be selected for hyper-persistent or tolerant phenotypes.

8.3.2 Toxin-Antitoxin Genetics

The advent of transcriptomics in the early 2000s due to the democratization of microarrays allowed to describe the first bacterial transcriptomes (Bernstein et al. 2002; Khodursky et al. 2000). The Lewis group first characterized the transcriptome of persistence by enriching persisters using ampicillin to lyse non-persisters (Keren et al. 2004). They then used the $rrnB_{P1}$-gfp_{ASV} fusion, a fluorescent reporter based on a ribosomal promoter, and observed a small subpopulation of non-fluorescent cells enriched in persisters, which they sorted from the bulk of the population (Shah et al. 2006). The authors were able to report increased expression of various TA systems (*dinJ-yafQ*, *relBE*, *yefM-yoeB*, *mazEF*, and *mqsRA*) in these persister-enriched sorted subpopulations, kickstarting the hypothesis that TA system upregulation could lead to persistence. Several follow-up studies found that TA systems were overexpressed in conditions where persisters are more abundant such as intracellular *Salmonella* (Helaine et al. 2014) or hypoxic *Mycobacteria* (Ramage et al. 2009) (see Sects. 8.4.1 and 8.4.2).

Since genetics has always been a powerful tool to study gene function, several studies deleted and overexpressed TA systems to identify their potential roles in various processes, including persistence. It was shown that the deletion of the *mqsR* toxin gene and that of the *mqsRA* system reduced persistence to ampicillin (Kim and Wood 2010). Deleting *relBE* or *hipBA* systems also reduced persistence to ofloxacin and mitomycin C (Keren et al. 2004). The *hipBA* deletion was also shown to reduce persistence to these two antibiotics in biofilms (Keren et al. 2004). In another study, deletion of the *yafQ* toxin gene reduced persistence of *E. coli* biofilms to cefazoline and tobramycin without significantly altering biofilm structure (Harrison et al. 2009). The authors also observed no effect of *yafQ* deletion on persistence to doxycycline and rifampicin in a biofilm setting as well as no effect of this deletion on persistence to the four tested antibiotics (cefazoline, tobramycin, doxycycline, and rifampicin) in a planktonic setting (Harrison et al. 2009).

However, the effect of *mqsRA*, *hipBA*, and *dinJ-yafQ* deletions on persistence was contested by three separate follow-up studies. The effect of the *mqsR* deletion on persister formation was found to be poorly reproducible and heavily dependent on inoculum age (Luidalepp et al. 2011). The *hipBA* deletion mutant previously used by the Lewis group (Keren et al. 2004) was showed by the same authors to have an extended deletion in the *dif* region, a noncoding locus pivotal in chromosome partitioning (Hansen et al. 2008). The same group constructed a strain with a more precise deletion of *hipBA* and observed no decrease in persistence compared to a wild-type strain (Hansen et al. 2008). A third study showed that biofilms formed by a *dinJ-yafQ* strain did not produce significantly fewer persisters to ofloxacin than the corresponding wild-type strain (Bernier et al. 2013). Moreover, we and others showed that the deletion of 10 TA systems in *E. coli*, comprising *mqsRA* and *dinJ-yafQ*, did not affect persistence to ampicillin, ofloxacin, and ciprofloxacin (Goormaghtigh et al. 2018a; Harms et al. 2017a), casting doubts on the involvement of TA systems in persistence, at least under the conditions tested (see Sect. 8.3.3).

Another common and widely accessible way to assess the role of TA systems in persistence is to ectopically overexpress a toxin of interest and assess its effect on persistence. Previously mentioned studies also used this overexpression approach: YafQ overexpression increased persistence of *E. coli* biofilms to cefazolin and tobramycin (Harrison et al. 2009), RelE overexpression increased persistence to cefotaxime, mitomycin C, ofloxacin, and tobramycin (Keren et al. 2004), HipA overexpression increased persistence to ampicillin and ofloxacin (Falla and Chopra 1998; Korch and Hill 2006) and MazF overexpression increased persistence to cefotaxime, mitomycin C, ciprofloxacin, tobramycin (Tripathi et al. 2014), and ofloxacin (Mok and Brynildsen 2018). It is worth to note that many authors cite a study by Neyfakh and colleagues as an evidence of TA implication in persistence (Vázquez-Laslop et al. 2006). In this study, the authors overexpressed the MazF and HipA toxins showing a drastic increase in persistence to ampicillin and ciprofloxacin. However, the authors also overexpressed unrelated proteins such as the DnaJ chaperone or the heterologous PmrC protein. Overexpression of these proteins turned out to inhibit cell growth and to increase persistence frequency substantially (100- to 1000-fold), indicating that overexpression approaches are not appropriate to study persistence (Vázquez-Laslop et al. 2006). Similar increases in persister levels can be achieved by artificially arresting growth by using bacteriostatic antibiotics (Kwan et al. 2013; Ocampo et al. 2014). Concomitantly, toxin overexpression has been dismissed as a reliable way to study persistence by several groups (Goormaghtigh et al. 2018b; Kaldalu et al. 2016; Ramisetty et al. 2016), despite still being used as of today (Dufour et al. 2018; Mok and Brynildsen 2018; Muthuramalingam et al. 2018; Rycroft et al. 2018).

8.3.3 Controversy Surrounding a Unifying Model Linking TA Systems and Persistence in E. coli K-12

In *E. coli* K-12, there are eleven *bona fide* type II TA systems, ten of which encode endoribonuclease toxins (Harms et al. 2018). For some of the systems, growth inhibition by ectopic overexpression of toxins has been shown to be reversible upon rescue by antitoxin overexpression (Christensen and Gerdes 2003) leading to the appealing idea that TA activation could lead to dormancy and transiently protect cells against stress (Gerdes 2000). In 2013, a model linking TA systems with the stochastic generation of persister cells in exponential phase (a.k.a. type II persisters) was published by the Gerdes group (Fig. 8.1), raising considerable attention on the relationship between TA systems and persistence (Maisonneuve and Gerdes 2014). In a first, now retracted, study published in 2011, it was observed that successive deletions of 10 TA systems in *E. coli* progressively reduces persistence to ampicillin and ciprofloxacin, showing that TA systems were involved in the persistence phenomenon. This phenomenon was dependent on the Lon protease as deletion of the *lon* gene reduced persistence to levels comparable to the strain deleted for the

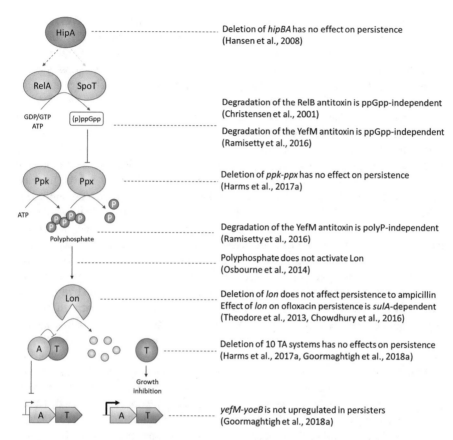

Fig. 8.1 The controversial model unifying persistence and toxin-antitoxin systems. The signaling cascade described in Germain et al. (2015) is represented on the left while contradictory results for each step are shown on the right. Note: The paper Germain et al. (2015) has been retracted

10 TA systems (Δ10TA). Moreover, *lon* overexpression drastically increased persistence in wild-type *E. coli* but not in the $\Delta 10TA$ strain (Maisonneuve et al. 2011).

The same authors published a follow-up study (also retracted) in which they described a signaling cascade leading to the stochastic induction of TA systems and the formation of persister cells (Maisonneuve et al. 2013). The authors showed that persistence was dependent on (p)ppGpp and polyphosphate since deletion of the genes responsible for polyphosphate synthesis and degradation (*ppk-ppx*) and for (p)ppGpp synthesis and degradation (*relA spoT*) reduced persistence to levels similar to the $\Delta 10TA$ strain (Maisonneuve et al. 2013). Involvement of (p)ppGpp was further confirmed by overexpressing *relA* that encodes a (p)ppGpp synthetase or by reducing (p)ppGpp hydrolysis through the *spoT1* allele (Maisonneuve et al. 2013). Moreover, overexpression of the *ppk* gene, which encodes the polyphosphate kinase responsible for polyphosphate synthesis, increased persister levels as did the deletion of the *ppx* gene, encoding the polyphosphatase responsible for polyphosphate hydrolysis (Maisonneuve et al. 2013). Epistasis analysis showed that the persistence-enhancing effects of *relA* and *ppk* overexpression were absent in the Δ*lon* and Δ*10TA* strains (Maisonneuve et al. 2013). The authors were thus able to reconstruct a signaling cascade by linking these data to the current literature: (p)ppGpp has been reported to prevent polyphosphate hydrolysis by inhibiting the Ppx exopolyphosphatase (Kuroda et al. 1997) while another study reported an activating effect of polyphosphate on Lon (Kuroda et al. 2001).

The authors postulated that the (p)ppGpp synthetase activity of RelA could be stochastically activated in a subset of cells within an isogenic population. This increase of (p)ppGpp levels would inhibit the Ppx exopolyphosphatase and lead to polyphosphate accumulation which would, in turn, activate the Lon protease (Maisonneuve et al. 2013). Since Lon is known to degrade several antitoxins (Christensen et al. 2001, 2003, 2004; Christensen-Dalsgaard et al. 2010; Jorgensen et al. 2009; Prysak et al. 2009), activation of Lon could lead to the degradation of antitoxin, release of their cognate toxins and growth arrest (Maisonneuve et al. 2013). To confirm the requirement for (p)ppGpp for antitoxin degradation, the authors ectopically expressed His-tagged RelB and YefM antitoxins and monitored the turnover of these proteins after inducing (p)ppGpp synthesis by serine hydroxamate (SHX) (Maisonneuve et al. 2013). The authors showed that SHX treatment induces rapid degradation of His-RelB and His-YefM in wild-type *E. coli* but not in a Δ*lon* or a Δ*ppk-ppx* strain, demonstrating that (p)ppGpp induces antitoxin proteolysis in a polyphosphate and Lon-dependent manner (Maisonneuve et al. 2013). Note that polyphosphate-dependency was not assessed for the other eight antitoxins.

The authors used live imaging coupled with fluorescence microscopy to visualize persistence at the single-cell level. Two fluorescent reporters were used, RpoS-mCherry and *yefM-yoeB:gfp*. The *rpoS* locus was translationally fused to *mCherry*, serving as the sole form of RpoS in this strain (Maisonneuve et al. 2013). This fusion was used as a proxy for (p)ppGpp levels as (p)ppGpp both induces transcription of *rpoS* and inhibits RpoS degradation (Battesti et al. 2011). The *yefM-yoeB:gfp* transcriptional fusion was constructed by inserting the *gfp* gene downstream of the *yefM-yoeB* locus, serving as a third cistron for the TA system. Since proteolysis of an antitoxin derepresses its cognate promoter (Christensen et al. 2001; Christensen-Dalsgaard et al. 2010), this fusion was particularly amenable to report antitoxin degradation and toxin activation at the single-cell level. Studying these two reporters independently, the authors found that a small number ($\sim 10^{-4}$) of non-growing cells showed high fluorescence for these reporters. Exponentially growing cultures of these strains were challenged with a short (60 min) ampicillin treatment and regrown afterward. For each reporter, one instance of a high-fluorescence and non-growing cell able to regrow after ampicillin removal was shown, demonstrating that (p) ppGpp and TA systems are induced in persisters (Maisonneuve et al. 2013).

In a last study, the same authors determined that the HipA toxin, which was not included in the previously 10 deleted TA systems, was the factor inducing stochastic (p)ppGpp synthesis in persister cells, thus placing this TA system as the master regulator of persistence in *E. coli* (Germain et al. 2015). This study showed that ectopic overexpression of HipA induces persistence in a polyphosphate, Lon, (p) ppGpp, and 10 TA-dependent manner (Germain et al. 2015). Moreover, it was shown that the *hipA7* allele increased the fraction of cells with high RpoS-mCherry fluorescence and that these RpoS-mCherry "ON" cells required the 10 previously deleted TA systems to survive antibiotic treatment (Germain et al. 2015).

This model was widely accepted since its publication. However, several studies questioned the legitimacy of this model (Fig. 8.1). First, deleting *lon* was shown to have no effect on persistence to ampicillin (Chowdhury et al. 2016). Moreover, the reduced survival to ciprofloxacin in the *lon* mutant was shown to be dependent on the *sulA* gene, which encodes a SOS-controlled division inhibitor that accumulates during ciprofloxacin treatment (Theodore et al. 2013). Second, using transcriptional upregulation as a proxy for YefM degradation, it was shown that (p)ppGpp and polyphosphate had no effect on the SHX-induced upregulation of *yefM-yoeB* transcripts, thus, suggesting that YefM degradation is (p)ppGpp and polyphosphate-independent (Ramisetty et al. 2016). Similar experiments performed earlier by the Gerdes group have shown that the RelE antitoxin is also upregulated by SHX in a (p)ppGpp-independent manner as well as by chloramphenicol treatment, which does not induce (p)ppGpp production (Christensen et al. 2001). Third, polyphosphate was shown to inhibit Lon in vitro rather than activate it (Osbourne et al. 2014). Also, the low-persistence phenotype of the Δ10TA strain was shown to be medium and antibiotic-dependent: Δ10TA cells grown in LB medium showed reduced persistence to both ampicillin and ciprofloxacin while the same strain was grown in MOPS minimal medium only showed reduced persistence to ciprofloxacin (Shan et al. 2017). Ramisetty et al. reported reduced persistence rates for the Δ10TA strain in LB medium to ampicillin and ciprofloxacin but not to chloramphenicol, erythromycin, or kanamycin (Ramisetty et al. 2016). Finally, deletion of the *hipBA* system has no effect on persistence, disproving the role of wild-type HipA as the master regulator of persistence (Hansen et al. 2008).

This suite of contradictory reports culminated in a publication of the Gerdes group disproving their previous claims (Harms et al. 2017a, b). This new study showed that deletion mutants generated during in the previous studies, including the Δ10TA strain, were contaminated by lambdoid prophages, namely lambda and phi80. The authors concluded that these phage contaminations combined with technical drawbacks inherent to antibiotic killing assays lead to a misinterpretation of the results obtained in the previous studies (Harms et al. 2017a, b). This lead to the retraction of the three previous studies of the group supporting the role of TA systems in persistence (Maisonneuve et al. 2018a, b; Germain et al. 2015). A recent study from our group and that of T. Tenson confirmed the lysogenization of the Δ*10TA* strain by three phi80 prophages (Goormaghtigh et al. 2018a). Using an independently constructed Δ*10TA* strain and defined growth conditions, we showed that TA deletion had no effect on persistence. Moreover, we investigated the validity of the RpoS-mCherry and *yefM-yoeB:gfp* fluorescent reporters used by (Maisonneuve et al. 2013). Our results showed that the RpoS-mCherry did not report type II persister cells as stated by the authors but rather stationary phase cells with an extended lag time. On the other hand, we showed that the *yefM-yoeB:gfp* fusion was nonfunctional and it is likely that the authors tracked autofluorescence rather than a GFP signal (Goormaghtigh et al. 2018a).

8.4   Toxin-Antitoxin Systems and Persistence Outside of *E. coli K-12* Lab Strain

TA systems are highly abundant in several major human pathogens: 79 total and 37 confirmed systems were identified in *M. tuberculosis* (Sala et al. 2014), 26 type II TAs in *Pseudomonas aeruginosa* (Andersen et al. 2017), 27 total and 18 confirmed in *Salmonella enterica* serovar Typhimurium (Lobato-Marquez et al. 2015), 16 in *Burkholderia cenocepacia* (Van Acker et al. 2014), 5 confirmed in *Acinetobacter baumanii* (Jurėnaitė et al. 2013). Bearing a large number of TA system is not a general rule for pathogenic bacteria as shown by the very low number of TA modules found in some pathogenic strains, for example, three in *Staphylococcus aureus* (Conlon et al. 2016), three in *Clostridium difficile* (Shao et al. 2010) and none at all in obligate intracellular pathogens such as *Rickettsia conorii* (Pandey and Gerdes 2005).

8.4.1   Mycobacterium tuberculosis

Perhaps the two most striking features of *M. tuberculosis* are its ability to persist in its host and as mentioned above, the outrageous amount of TA systems encoded in its chromosome. Patients infected with *M. tuberculosis* are treated with a combination of four antibiotics (isoniazid, rifampicin, pyrazinamide, and ethambutol) for up to 9 months, after which a persistent population of pathogens often survives and causes infection relapse of multidrug-resistant tuberculosis (Singh et al. 2010). To this day, 79 type II TA systems were identified in *M. tuberculosis* H_{37}Rv, which represents ~4% of its ORFs (Sala et al. 2014). Importantly, the large number of TA systems present in the *M. tuberculosis* genome (most of them located on genomic islands) is widely conserved within the MTBC (*M. tuberculosis* complex), but largely absent from close relatives such as *Mycobacterium marinum* and *Mycobacterium smegmatis*, suggesting an important role for these genes in the evolution of *M. tuberculosis* (Ramage et al. 2009).

Ramage and colleagues showed that four TA systems were specifically upregulated in response to stresses encountered by *M. tuberculosis* during the infective process, that is, hypoxia and internalization by macrophages (Ramage et al. 2009). At the same time, Singh et al. found that exposure to rifampicin, gentamycin, levofloxacin (but not isoniazid), and 4-weeks infection of mice lungs lead to the upregulation of three *relE* homologs in *M. tuberculosis* (Singh et al. 2010). However, while deletion of *relE2* led to a defect in survival to rifampicin in liquid cultures, this was not the case in a murine model as no difference in lung or spleen mycobacterial load was observed in the *relE2* mutant compared to the wild type (Singh et al. 2010). The authors, thus, concluded that these systems were unlikely to play a role in persistence (Singh et al. 2010). In a later study, transcriptomic analysis of a population of *M. tuberculosis* challenged in vitro with

D-cycloserine led to a similar observation, that is, the upregulation of a set of 10 TA systems (Keren et al. 2011). However, as we previously discussed, this does not constitute evidence of TA role in persistence (see Sect. 8.3.2).

8.4.2 Salmonella enterica

The *Salmonella* genus is the causative agent of a wide range of infectious diseases, from food poisoning to typhoid fever. *Salmonella enterica* subsp. *enterica* serovar *Typhimurium* (*S. typhimurium* hereafter), a close relative of *E. coli* is a widely studied pathogen, which induces typhoid-like symptoms in mice. In this model where *S. typhimurium* proliferates in macrophages (Richter-Dahlfors et al. 1997), antibiotic treatment (e.g., enrofloxacin) reduces bacterial load below detectable levels (Griffin et al. 2011). However, a relapse in the infection is observed when the treatment is interrupted (Griffin et al. 2011). Griffin et al. observed that *S. typhimurium* was still present in mesenteric lymph nodes, suggesting that macrophages from these nodes are reservoirs for *S. typhimurium* persisters (Griffin et al. 2011).

Similarly to *M. tuberculosis*, TA acquisition seems to be favored in pathogenic strains as shown by the absence of 17 TAs from *S. typhimurium* in two non-pathogenic *Salmonella bongori* isolates (Lobato-Marquez et al. 2015). In an attempt to better understand the genetic basis of persistence in *Salmonella*, Slattery and colleagues identified a new TA system related to the ParE/RelE superfamily named *shpAB* (*Salmonella high persistence*) (Slattery et al. 2013). A nonsense mutation resulting in truncation of the last four residues of the antitoxin ShpB conferred a three- to four-orders of magnitude increase in survival after ampicillin exposure, without affecting the MIC or the growth rate (Slattery et al. 2013). Similarly to the *hipA7* mutant, this point mutant showed an extended lag when inoculated on fresh solid medium (Slattery et al. 2013). However, deletion of the entire *shpAB* operon did not result in any significant defect in survival to ampicillin in liquid culture, similarly to what is observed in a Δ*hipBA* mutant in *E. coli* (Hansen et al. 2008).

An influential study by Helaine et al. showed that TA systems-dependent *S. typhimurium* persisters are formed inside macrophages after phagocytosis (Helaine et al. 2014). Helaine and colleagues found that 14 type II TA systems were upregulated upon phagocytosis by bone marrow-derived macrophages in vitro and that deletion of any of those 14 TA systems (including *shpAB*) resulted in a significant (although modest for several systems) drop in the formation of macrophage-induced persisters (Helaine et al. 2014). This upregulation was found to be (p)ppGpp- and Lon-dependent. It was, thus, concluded that macrophage internalization activates the (p)ppGpp-Lon cascade leading to antitoxin degradation, toxin liberation and growth arrest (Helaine et al. 2014). In another paper, using a different experimental setup, Lobato-Marquez et al. showed that the expression level of 4 type II and 3 type I TA systems are increased in *S. typhimurium* internalized by human fibroblasts (Lobato-Marquez et al. 2015). However, only deletion of a specific type II TA system (*vapBC2*) led to decreased survival in human HeLa epithelial cells and fibroblasts (Lobato-Marquez et al. 2015). Note that a recently published paper showed that TA modules are dispensable for Salmonella persister formation in vitro, confirming the data obtained in *E. coli* (Pontes and Groisman, 2019, https://stke.sciencemag.org/content/12/592/eaax3938.long).

Claudi and colleagues designed a single-cell growth reporter (TIMER[bac]) and used it in a different infection/treatment model, that is, mouse typhoid fever, allowing them to monitor *S. typhimurium* growth rates in host tissues. Cells were then sorted by FACS on the basis of their growth rates and proteomic analyses revealed differences in the proteome of slow-growing cells as compared to moderate- and fast-growing cells (Claudi et al. 2014). The authors detected increased production of only one type II toxin (*ecnB*). A mutant deleted for three TA systems (*ecnB*, *shpAB*, and *phd-doc*), shown to influence both growth rate and persistence level in macrophage cultures, had an unchanged growth rate and almost normal virulence in the mouse typhoid fever model (Claudi et al. 2014). Importantly, they showed that infection relapse after enrofloxacin treatment was mostly due to a subpopulation of *S. typhimurium* with moderate growth rates and partial tolerance, which outcompeted the very small subpopulation of non-dividing/persistent *S. typhimurium* (Claudi et al. 2014). Accordingly, two transposition mutagenesis studies coupled to DNA microarrays failed to identify TA systems as essential for survival in a murine model (Chan et al. 2005; Lawley et al. 2006).

This body of data points out that what we perceive as persistence and its potential mechanisms can vary greatly, whether *S. typhimurium* cells are treated in vitro, inside of a macrophage or in a murine model. In the case of TA systems, their role in *S. typhimurium* persistence remains ambiguous.

8.4.3 Pseudomonas aeruginosa

Pseudomonas aeruginosa, an opportunistic pathogen often associated with nosocomial infections and late-stage cystic fibrosis, is listed as a critical pathogen new antibiotics are needed for (Tacconelli et al. 2018). Unlike *E. coli* or *M. tuberculosis*, TA systems remain poorly characterized in *P. aeruginosa* on the functional level.

In *P. aeruginosa*, early screening for high-/low-persistent mutants did not lead to the identification of any transposon-insertion mutants in TA operons (De Groote et al. 2009). Later work performed by Vogwill and colleagues revealed a slight correlation ($R^2 = 0.629$) between the number of chromosome-encoded type II TA systems and persistence (but not resistance, $R^2 = 0.229$) (Vogwill et al. 2016). Similarly to *M. tuberculosis* and *S. typhimurium* (Lobato-Marquez et al. 2015), some TA systems are preferentially found in clinical isolates of *P. aeruginosa* and *Pseudomonas putida*, as compared to environmental isolates (Andersen et al. 2017; Molina et al. 2016). In a recent study conducted by Andersen and colleagues, the authors used a bioinformatics approach to explore the distribution and evolution of 26 type II TA systems within *P. aeruginosa* strains isolated from cystic fibrosis patients over a certain period of time (Andersen et al. 2017). Most type II TA systems (22 out of 26) were found to be within genomic islands (GIs). Interestingly, even though some of these GIs were shown to be partially lost over time, the remnants of these GIs tended to contain the portions encoding TA systems (Andersen et al. 2017). Andersen and colleagues, therefore, suggested that GI-encoded TA modules may serve to stabilize pathogenicity-related GIs rather than to play a central role in bacterial persistence (Andersen et al. 2017).

8.4.4 *Uropathogenic* Escherichia coli

Seven TA systems present in the MG1655 *E. coli* lab strain were detected in the CFT073 uropathogenic *E. coli* strain. Single deletions mutants were tested in competition with the wild-type strain in a mice urinary tract infection model. While the majority of the mutants behaved like the wild-type strain, deletion mutants of the *yefM-yoeB* TA system were outcompeted by the wild-type CFT073 during infection of the bladder (but not the kidneys) in a murine infection model (Norton and Mulvey 2012). Interestingly, deletion of the *pasTI* (*P*ersistence *A*nd *S*tress-resistance *T*oxin and *I*mmunity, previously dubbed *ratAB*) locus had an opposite effect: mutants were defective for infecting kidneys but not the bladder, indicating that different TA systems might provide significant advantages to UPEC in specific host environments (Norton and Mulvey 2012). Furthermore, a *pasTI* deleted mutant forms 100-fold fewer persisters to ampicillin or ciprofloxacin in vitro in LB medium, but deletion of that same locus in the *E. coli* MG1655 laboratory strain did not result in any survival defect (Norton and Mulvey 2012).

8.4.5 *Other Bugs*

The relationship between TA systems and persistence was also studied in a few other bacterial species. Van Acker and colleagues identified 16 putative TAs in *B. cenocepacia*, among which 9 were upregulated after treatment with tobramycin, but none after treatment with ciprofloxacin (Van Acker et al. 2014). Another study in *Burkholderia pseudomallei* revealed that deletion of the entire *hicAB* locus reduced persistence to ciprofloxacin, but not to ceftazidime (Butt et al. 2014). Finally, and worthy of mention, deletion of the three known type II TA modules in *S. aureus* does not impact persistence to rifampicin, vancomycin, or oxacillin in liquid cultures (Conlon et al. 2016). Similar observations were made in *Streptococcus mutans*. A tripartite TA system called *smuATR* is thought to be induced by the CSP-ComDE system in response to adverse environmental conditions such as acid shock, amino acid starvation, or heat shock (Dufour et al. 2018). However, deletion of the *smuATR* locus had no effect on persistence to ofloxacin, oxacillin, vancomycin, or cefotaxime (Dufour et al. 2018).

8.5   Conclusions

The first link between persistence and type II TA systems stemmed from the isolation of hyper-persistent mutants in the *E. coli* laboratory strain in the 1980s (Moyed and Bertrand 1983). The hyper-persistent *hipA7* allele was shown to map in the toxin gene of a type II TA system (Black et al. 1991, 1994). Subsequently, attempts to isolate *E. coli* persisters and to decipher their transcriptomes indicated that TA systems were in general upregulated (Keren et al. 2004; Shah et al. 2006). Since the mainstream hypothesis at the time was that persister cells are slow- or non-growing cells, the idea that type II TA systems could be activated in persister cells was quite appealing. However, in *E. coli* K-12, in a substantial number of cases, single or multiple deletions of TA systems did not show any phenotype (Bernier et al. 2013; Goormaghtigh et al. 2018a; Hansen et al. 2008; Harms et al. 2017a, b; Luidalepp et al. 2011; Norton and Mulvey 2012). For other bacterial species, such as *S. enterica* and *M. tuberculosis*, the role of TA systems remains quite ambiguous with some TA being overexpressed upon internalization in macrophages or other cell types and the corresponding deletion mutants showing in specific cases some persistence defects. However, in general, when tested in mice models, the TA deletion mutants did not display any phenotypes.

Finding phenotypes associated with TA systems have been a quest for the last 30 years for many research groups. What appears to be clear is that the TA field should go back to the basic questions, which concerns the regulation of these systems. As mentioned above, although transcription activation of these systems is observed in persister cells, the causality is not established as in most of the cases, activation of transcription is not corroborated by the phenotype of deletion mutants. As antitoxins are unstable and carrying the DNA-binding activity, every condition or treatment that will prevent antitoxin (and toxin) synthesis will de facto lead to the derepression of the system as evidenced by a transcription increase. Whether this leads to a phenotype remains to be shown. Moreover, it remains to be shown how TA systems are activated in such a small subset of the population and how do cells resume their growth should the toxin be activated. Nevertheless gain of function mutations conferring a hyper-persistent or tolerant phenotypes can be selected during experimental evolution indicating that indeed, under specific conditions, activation of TA systems might confer a selective advantage (Levin-Reisman et al. 2017; Moyed and Bertrand 1983). This suggests that wild-type TA systems, while not being directly responsible for persistence, can constitute a malleable reservoir of growth-inhibiting activities to be used as a canvas for the ontogenesis of new functions.

Acknowledgements Research in the Van Melderen lab is supported by the *Fonds National de la Recherche Scientifique* (FNRS, T.0147.15F PDR and J.0061.16F CDR), the *Fonds Jean Brachet* and the *Fondation Van Buuren*.

References

Afif, H., Allali, N., Couturier, M., & Van Melderen, L. (2001). The ratio between CcdA and CcdB modulates the transcriptional repression of the ccd poison-antidote system. *Molecular Microbiology, 41*, 73–82.

Anantharaman, V., & Aravind, L. (2003). New connections in the prokaryotic toxin-antitoxin network: Relationship with the eukaryotic nonsense-mediated RNA decay system. *Genome Biology, 4*, R81. https://doi.org/10.1186/gb-2003-4-12-r81

Andersen, S. B., Ghoul, M., Griffin, A. S., Petersen, B., Johansen, H. K., & Molin, S. (2017). Diversity, prevalence, and longitudinal occurrence of type II toxin-antitoxin systems of *Pseudomonas aeruginosa* infecting cystic fibrosis lungs. *Frontiers in Microbiology, 8*, 1180. https://doi.org/10.3389/fmicb.2017.01180

Balaban, N. Q., Merrin, J., Chait, R., Kowalik, L., & Leibler, S. (2004). Bacterial persistence as a phenotypic switch. *Science, 305*, 1622–1625. https://doi.org/10.1126/science.1099390

Battesti, A., Majdalani, N., & Gottesman, S. (2011). The RpoS-mediated general stress response in *Escherichia coli*. *Annual Review of Microbiology, 65*, 189–213. https://doi.org/10.1146/annurev-micro-090110-102946

Bernier, S. P., Lebeaux, D., DeFrancesco, A. S., Valomon, A., Soubigou, G., Coppée, J.-Y., Ghigo, J.-M., & Beloin, C. (2013). Starvation, together with the SOS response, mediates high biofilm-specific tolerance to the fluoroquinolone ofloxacin. *PLoS Genetics, 9*, e1003144. https://doi.org/10.1371/journal.pgen.1003144

Bernstein, J. A., Khodursky, A. B., Lin, P.-H., Lin-Chao, S., & Cohen, S. N. (2002). Global analysis of mRNA decay and abundance in *Escherichia coli* at single-gene resolution using two-color fluorescent DNA microarrays. *Proceedings of the National Academy of Sciences, 99*, 9697. https://doi.org/10.1073/pnas.112318199

Black, D. S., Kelly, A. J., Mardis, M. J., & Moyed, H. S. (1991). Structure and organization of hip, an operon that affects lethality due to inhibition of peptidoglycan or DNA synthesis. *Journal of Bacteriology, 173*, 5732. https://doi.org/10.1128/jb.173.18.5732-5739.1991

Black, D. S., Irwin, B., & Moyed, H. S. (1994). Autoregulation of hip, an operon that affects lethality due to inhibition of peptidoglycan or DNA synthesis. *Journal of Bacteriology, 176*, 4081. https://doi.org/10.1128/jb.176.13.4081-4091.1994

Bordes, P., Cirinesi, A.-M., Ummels, R., Sala, A., Sakr, S., Bitter, W., & Genevaux, P. (2011). SecB-like chaperone controls a toxin–antitoxin stress-responsive system in *Mycobacterium tuberculosis*. *Proceedings of the National Academy of Sciences, 108*, 8438. https://doi.org/10.1073/pnas.1101189108

Butt, A., Higman, V. A., Williams, C., Crump, M. P., Hemsley, C. M., Harmer, N., & Titball, R. W. (2014). The HicA toxin from *Burkholderia pseudomallei* has a role in persister cell formation. *The Biochemical Journal, 459*, 333. https://doi.org/10.1042/BJ20140073

Castro-Roa, D., Garcia-Pino, A., De Gieter, S., van Nuland, N. A. J., Loris, R., & Zenkin, N. (2013). The fic protein doc uses an inverted substrate to phosphorylate and inactivate EF-Tu. *Nature Chemical Biology, 9*, 811–817. https://doi.org/10.1038/nchembio.1364

Chan, K., Kim, C. C., & Falkow, S. (2005). Microarray-based detection of *Salmonella enterica* Serovar typhimurium transposon mutants that cannot survive in macrophages and mice. *Infection and Immunity, 73*, 5438. https://doi.org/10.1128/IAI.73.9.5438-5449.2005

Cheverton, A. M., Gollan, B., Przydacz, M., Wong, C. T., Mylona, A., Hare, S. A., & Helaine, S. (2016). A Salmonella toxin promotes persister formation through acetylation of tRNA. *Molecular Cell, 63*, 86–96. https://doi.org/10.1016/j.molcel.2016.05.002

Chowdhury, N., Kwan, B. W., & Wood, T. K. (2016). Persistence increases in the absence of the alarmone guanosine tetraphosphate by reducing cell growth. *Scientific Reports, 6*, 20519. https://doi.org/10.1038/srep20519

Christensen, S. K., & Gerdes, K. (2003). RelE toxins from bacteria and archaea cleave mRNAs on translating ribosomes, which are rescued by tmRNA. *Molecular Microbiology, 48*, 1389–1400. https://doi.org/10.1046/j.1365-2958.2003.03512.x

Christensen, S. K., Mikkelsen, M., Pedersen, K., & Gerdes, K. (2001). RelE, a global inhibitor of translation, is activated during nutritional stress. *Proceedings of the National Academy of Sciences of the United States of America, 98*, 14328–14333. https://doi.org/10.1073/pnas. 251327898

Christensen, S. K., Pedersen, K., Hansen, F. G., & Gerdes, K. (2003). Toxin-antitoxin loci as stress-response-elements: ChpAK/MazF and ChpBK cleave translated RNAs and are counteracted by tmRNA. *Journal of Molecular Biology, 332*, 809–819.

Christensen, S. K., Maenhaut-Michel, G., Mine, N., Gottesman, S., Gerdes, K., & Van Melderen, L. (2004). Overproduction of the Lon protease triggers inhibition of translation in *Escherichia coli*: Involvement of the yefM-yoeB toxin-antitoxin system. *Molecular Microbiology, 51*, 1705–1717.

Christensen-Dalsgaard, M., Jorgensen, M. G., & Gerdes, K. (2010). Three new RelE-homologous mRNA interferases of *Escherichia coli* differentially induced by environmental stresses. *Molecular Microbiology, 75*, 333–348. https://doi.org/10.1111/j.1365-2958.2009.06969.x

Claudi, B., Spröte, P., Chirkova, A., Personnic, N., Zankl, J., Schürmann, N., Schmidt, A., & Bumann, D. (2014). Phenotypic variation of Salmonella in host tissues delays eradication by antimicrobial chemotherapy. *Cell, 158*, 722–733. https://doi.org/10.1016/j.cell.2014.06.045

Conlon, B. P., Rowe, S. E., Gandt, A. B., Nuxoll, A. S., Donegan, N. P., Zalis, E. A., Clair, G., Adkins, J. N., Cheung, A. L., & Lewis, K. (2016). Persister formation in *Staphylococcus aureus* is associated with ATP depletion. *Nature Microbiology, 1*, 16051.

Culviner, P. H., & Laub, M. T. (2018). Global analysis of the *E. coli* toxin MazF reveals widespread cleavage of mRNA and the inhibition of rRNA maturation and ribosome biogenesis. *Molecular Cell, 70*, 868–880.e10. https://doi.org/10.1016/j.molcel.2018.04.026

De Groote, V. N., Verstraeten, N., Fauvart, M., Kint, C. I., Verbeeck, A. M., Beullens, S., Cornelis, P., & Michiels, J. (2009). Novel persistence genes in *Pseudomonas aeruginosa* identified by high-throughput screening. *FEMS Microbiology Letters, 297*, 73–79. https://doi.org/10.1111/j. 1574-6968.2009.01657.x

de la Hoz, A. B., Ayora, S., Sitkiewicz, I., Fernandez, S., Pankiewicz, R., Alonso, J. C., & Ceglowski, P. (2000). Plasmid copy-number control and better-than-random segregation genes of pSM19035 share a common regulator. *Proceedings of the National Academy of Sciences of the United States of America, 97*, 728–733.

Deter, S. H., Jensen, V. R., Mather, H. W., & Butzin, C. N. (2017). Mechanisms for differential protein production in toxin–antitoxin systems. *Toxins, 9*. https://doi.org/10.3390/toxins9070211

Dorr, T., Vulic, M., & Lewis, K. (2010). Ciprofloxacin causes persister formation by inducing the TisB toxin in *Escherichia coli*. *PLoS Biology, 8*, e1000317. https://doi.org/10.1371/journal. pbio.1000317

Dufour, D., Mankovskaia, A., Chan, Y., Motavaze, K., Gong, S.-G., & Lévesque, C. M. (2018). A tripartite toxin-antitoxin module induced by quorum sensing is associated with the persistence phenotype in *Streptococcus mutans*. *Molecular Oral Microbiology, 33*, 420–429. https://doi. org/10.1111/omi.12245

Escudero, J. A., Loot, C., Nivina, A., & Mazel, D. (2015). The integron: Adaptation on demand. *Microbiology Spectrum, 3*, MDNA3-0019-2014. https://doi.org/10.1128/microbiolspec. MDNA3-0019-2014

Falla, T. J., & Chopra, I. (1998). Joint tolerance to β-lactam and fluoroquinolone antibiotics in *Escherichia coli* results from overexpression of *hipA*. *Antimicrobial Agents and Chemotherapy, 42*, 3282. https://doi.org/10.1128/AAC.42.12.3282

Garcia-Pino, A., Balasubramanian, S., Wyns, L., Gazit, E., De Greve, H., Magnuson, R. D., Charlier, D., van Nuland, N. A. J., & Loris, R. (2010). Allostery and intrinsic disorder mediate transcription regulation by conditional cooperativity. *Cell, 142*, 101–111. https://doi.org/10. 1016/j.cell.2010.05.039

Gerdes, K. (2000). Toxin-antitoxin modules may regulate synthesis of macromolecules during nutritional stress. *Journal of Bacteriology, 182*, 561–572.

Germain, E., Castro-Roa, D., Zenkin, N., & Gerdes, K. (2013). Molecular mechanism of bacterial persistence by HipA. *Molecular Cell, 52*, 248–254. https://doi.org/10.1016/j.molcel.2013.08.045

Germain, E., Roghanian, M., Gerdes, K., & Maisonneuve, E. (2015). Stochastic induction of persister cells by HipA through (p)ppGpp-mediated activation of mRNA endonucleases. *Proceedings of the National Academy of Sciences of the United States of America, 112*, 5171–5176. https://doi.org/10.1073/pnas.1423536112

Goormaghtigh, F., Fraikin, N., Putrinš, M., Hallaert, T., Hauryliuk, V., Garcia-Pino, A., Sjödin, A., Kasvandik, S., Udekwu, K., Tenson, T., Kaldalu, N., & Van Melderen, L. (2018a). Reassessing the role of type II toxin-antitoxin systems in formation of *Escherichia coli* type II Persister cells. *mBio, 9*. https://doi.org/10.1128/mBio.00640-18

Goormaghtigh, F., Fraikin, N., Putrinš, M., Hauryliuk, V., Garcia-Pino, A., Udekwu, K., Tenson, T., Kaldalu, N., & Van Melderen, L. (2018b). Reply to Holden and Errington, Type II toxin-antitoxin systems and persister cells. *mBio, 9*. https://doi.org/10.1128/mBio.01838-18

Griffin, A. J., Li, L.-X., Voedisch, S., Pabst, O., & McSorley, S. J. (2011). Dissemination of persistent intestinal bacteria via the mesenteric lymph nodes causes typhoid relapse. *Infection and Immunity, 79*, 1479. https://doi.org/10.1128/IAI.01033-10

Guglielmini, J., Szpirer, C., & Milinkovitch, M. C. (2008). Automated discovery and phylogenetic analysis of new toxin-antitoxin systems. *BMC Microbiology, 8*, 104. https://doi.org/10.1186/1471-2180-8-104

Hallez, R., Geeraerts, D., Sterckx, Y., Mine, N., Loris, R., & Van Melderen, L. (2010). New toxins homologous to ParE belonging to three-component toxin-antitoxin systems in *Escherichia coli* O157:H7. *Molecular Microbiology, 76*, 719–732. https://doi.org/10.1111/j.1365-2958.2010.07129.x

Hansen, S., Lewis, K., & Vulić, M. (2008). Role of global regulators and nucleotide metabolism in antibiotic tolerance in *Escherichia coli*. *Antimicrobial Agents and Chemotherapy, 52*, 2718. https://doi.org/10.1128/AAC.00144-08

Harms, A., Maisonneuve, E., & Gerdes, K. (2016). Mechanisms of bacterial persistence during stress and antibiotic exposure. *Science, 354*. https://doi.org/10.1126/science.aaf4268

Harms, A., Fino, C., Sorensen, M. A., Semsey, S., & Gerdes, K. (2017a). Prophages and growth dynamics confound experimental results with antibiotic-tolerant Persister cells. *MBio, 8*. https://doi.org/10.1128/mBio.01964-17

Harms, A., Liesch, M., Körner, J., Québatte, M., Engel, P., & Dehio, C. (2017b). A bacterial toxin-antitoxin module is the origin of inter-bacterial and inter-kingdom effectors of Bartonella. *PLoS Genetics, 13*, e1007077. https://doi.org/10.1371/journal.pgen.1007077

Harms, A., Brodersen, D. E., Mitarai, N., & Gerdes, K. (2018). Toxins, targets, and triggers: An overview of toxin-antitoxin biology. *Molecular Cell, 70*, 768–784. https://doi.org/10.1016/j.molcel.2018.01.003

Harrison, J. J., Wade, W. D., Akierman, S., Vacchi-Suzzi, C., Stremick, C. A., Turner, R. J., & Ceri, H. (2009). The chromosomal toxin gene *yafQ* is a determinant of multidrug tolerance for *Escherichia coli* growing in a biofilm. *Antimicrobial Agents and Chemotherapy, 53*, 2253. https://doi.org/10.1128/AAC.00043-09

Hayes, F., & Van Melderen, L. (2011). Toxins-antitoxins: Diversity, evolution and function. *Critical Reviews in Biochemistry and Molecular Biology, 46*, 386–408. https://doi.org/10.3109/10409238.2011.600437

Hazan, R., & Engelberg-Kulka, H. (2004). *Escherichia coli* mazEF-mediated cell death as a defense mechanism that inhibits the spread of phage P1. *Molecular Genetics and Genomics, 272*, 227–234. https://doi.org/10.1007/s00438-004-1048-y

Helaine, S., Cheverton, A. M., Watson, K. G., Faure, L. M., Matthews, S. A., & Holden, D. W. (2014). Internalization of Salmonella by macrophages induces formation of nonreplicating persisters. *Science, 343*, 204–208. https://doi.org/10.1126/science.1244705

Holden, D. W., & Errington, J. (2018). Type II toxin-antitoxin systems and persister cells. *mBio, 9*. https://doi.org/10.1128/mBio.01574-18

Huguet, K. T., Gonnet, M., Doublet, B., & Cloeckaert, A. (2016). A toxin antitoxin system promotes the maintenance of the IncA/C-mobilizable Salmonella Genomic Island 1. *Scientific Reports, 6*, 32285. https://doi.org/10.1038/srep32285

Jaffé, A., Ogura, T., & Hiraga, S. (1985). Effects of the ccd function of the F plasmid on bacterial growth. *Journal of Bacteriology, 163*, 841.

Jorgensen, M. G., Pandey, D. P., Jaskolska, M., & Gerdes, K. (2009). HicA of *Escherichia coli* defines a novel family of translation-independent mRNA interferases in bacteria and archaea. *Journal of Bacteriology, 191*, 1191–1199. https://doi.org/10.1128/JB.01013-08

Jurėnaitė, M., Markuckas, A., & Sužiedėlienė, E. (2013). Identification and characterization of type II toxin-antitoxin systems in the opportunistic pathogen *Acinetobacter baumannii*. *Journal of Bacteriology, 195*, 3165. https://doi.org/10.1128/JB.00237-13

Jurenas, D., Chatterjee, S., Konijnenberg, A., Sobott, F., Droogmans, L., Garcia-Pino, A., & Van Melderen, L. (2017). AtaT blocks translation initiation by N-acetylation of the initiator tRNAfMet. *Nature Chemical Biology, 13*, 640–646. https://doi.org/10.1038/nchembio.2346

Kaldalu, N., Hauryliuk, V., & Tenson, T. (2016). Persisters-as elusive as ever. *Applied Microbiology and Biotechnology, 100*, 6545–6553. https://doi.org/10.1007/s00253-016-7648-8

Kaspy, I., Rotem, E., Weiss, N., Ronin, I., Balaban, N. Q., & Glaser, G. (2013). HipA-mediated antibiotic persistence via phosphorylation of the glutamyl-tRNA-synthetase. *Nature Communications, 4*, 3001. https://doi.org/10.1038/ncomms4001

Keren, I., Shah, D., Spoering, A., Kaldalu, N., & Lewis, K. (2004). Specialized persister cells and the mechanism of multidrug tolerance in *Escherichia coli*. *Journal of Bacteriology, 186*, 8172–8180. https://doi.org/10.1128/JB.186.24.8172-8180.2004

Keren, I., Minami, S., Rubin, E., & Lewis, K. (2011). Characterization and transcriptome analysis of *Mycobacterium tuberculosis* Persisters. *mBio, 2*. https://doi.org/10.1128/mBio.00100-11

Khodursky, A. B., Peter, B. J., Cozzarelli, N. R., Botstein, D., Brown, P. O., & Yanofsky, C. (2000). DNA microarray analysis of gene expression in response to physiological and genetic changes that affect tryptophan metabolism in *Escherichia coli*. *Proceedings of the National Academy of Sciences, 97*, 12170. https://doi.org/10.1073/pnas.220414297

Kim, Y., & Wood, T. K. (2010). Toxins Hha and CspD and small RNA regulator Hfq are involved in persister cell formation through MqsR in *Escherichia coli*. *Biochemical and Biophysical Research Communications, 391*, 209–213. https://doi.org/10.1016/j.bbrc.2009.11.033

Koga, M., Otsuka, Y., Lemire, S., & Yonesaki, T. (2011). *Escherichia coli* rnlA and rnlB compose a novel toxin-antitoxin system. *Genetics, 187*, 123–130. https://doi.org/10.1534/genetics.110.121798

Korch, S. B., & Hill, T. M. (2006). Ectopic overexpression of wild-type and mutant *hipA* genes in *Escherichia coli*: Effects on macromolecular synthesis and persister formation. *Journal of Bacteriology, 188*, 3826. https://doi.org/10.1128/JB.01740-05

Korch, S. B., Henderson, T. A., & Hill, T. M. (2003). Characterization of the hipA7 allele of *Escherichia coli* and evidence that high persistence is governed by (p)ppGpp synthesis. *Molecular Microbiology, 50*, 1199–1213. https://doi.org/10.1046/j.1365-2958.2003.03779.x

Kuroda, A., Murphy, H., Cashel, M., & Kornberg, A. (1997). Guanosine tetra- and pentaphosphate promote accumulation of inorganic polyphosphate in *Escherichia coli*. *The Journal of Biological Chemistry, 272*, 21240–21243. https://doi.org/10.1074/jbc.272.34.21240

Kuroda, A., Nomura, K., Ohtomo, R., Kato, J., Ikeda, T., Takiguchi, N., Ohtake, H., & Kornberg, A. (2001). Role of inorganic polyphosphate in promoting ribosomal protein degradation by the Lon protease in *E. coli*. *Science, 293*, 705. https://doi.org/10.1126/science.1061315

Kwan, B. W., Valenta, J. A., Benedik, M. J., & Wood, T. K. (2013). Arrested protein synthesis increases persister-like cell formation. *Antimicrobial Agents and Chemotherapy, 57*, 1468–1473. https://doi.org/10.1128/AAC.02135-12

Lawley, T. D., Chan, K., Thompson, L. J., Kim, C. C., Govoni, G. R., & Monack, D. M. (2006). Genome-wide screen for Salmonella genes required for long-term systemic infection of the mouse. *PLoS Pathogens, 2*, e11. https://doi.org/10.1371/journal.ppat.0020011

Lehnherr, H., & Yarmolinsky, M. B. (1995). Addiction protein Phd of plasmid prophage P1 is a substrate of the ClpXP serine protease of *Escherichia coli*. *Proceedings of the National Academy of Sciences of the United States of America, 92*, 3274–3277.

Leplae, R., Geeraerts, D., Hallez, R., Guglielmini, J., Dreze, P., & Van Melderen, L. (2011). Diversity of bacterial type II toxin-antitoxin systems: A comprehensive search and functional analysis of novel families. *Nucleic Acids Research, 39*, 5513–5525. https://doi.org/10.1093/nar/gkr131

Levin-Reisman, I., Ronin, I., Gefen, O., Braniss, I., Shoresh, N., & Balaban, N. Q. (2017). Antibiotic tolerance facilitates the evolution of resistance. *Science, 355*, 826. https://doi.org/10.1126/science.aaj2191

Lobato-Marquez, D., Moreno-Cordoba, I., Figueroa, V., Diaz-Orejas, R., & Garcia-del Portillo, F. (2015). Distinct type I and type II toxin-antitoxin modules control Salmonella lifestyle inside eukaryotic cells. *Scientific Reports, 5*, 9374. https://doi.org/10.1038/srep09374

Luidalepp, H., Joers, A., Kaldalu, N., & Tenson, T. (2011). Age of inoculum strongly influences persister frequency and can mask effects of mutations implicated in altered persistence. *Journal of Bacteriology, 193*, 3598–3605. https://doi.org/10.1128/JB.00085-11

Maisonneuve, E., & Gerdes, K. (2014). Molecular mechanisms underlying bacterial persisters. *Cell, 157*, 539–548. https://doi.org/10.1016/j.cell.2014.02.050

Maisonneuve, E., Shakespeare, L. J., Jorgensen, M. G., & Gerdes, K. (2011). Bacterial persistence by RNA endonucleases. *Proceedings of the National Academy of Sciences of the United States of America, 108*, 13206–13211. https://doi.org/10.1073/pnas.1100186108

Maisonneuve, E., Castro-Camargo, M., & Gerdes, K. (2013). (p)ppGpp controls bacterial persistence by stochastic induction of toxin-antitoxin activity. *Cell, 154*, 1140–1150. https://doi.org/10.1016/j.cell.2013.07.048

Maisonneuve, E., Castro-Camargo, M., & Gerdes, K. (2018a). Retraction: (p)ppGpp controls bacterial persistence by stochastic induction of toxin-antitoxin activity. *Cell, 172*, 1135. https://doi.org/10.1016/j.cell.2018.02.023

Maisonneuve, E., Shakespeare, L. J., Jorgensen, M. G., & Gerdes, K. (2018b). Retraction: Bacterial persistence by RNA endonucleases. *Proceedings of the National Academy of Sciences of the United States of America.* https://doi.org/10.1073/pnas.1803278115

Mets, T., Lippus, M., Schryer, D., Liiv, A., Kasari, V., Paier, A., Maiväli, Ü., Remme, J., Tenson, T., & Kaldalu, N. (2017). Toxins MazF and MqsR cleave *Escherichia coli* rRNA precursors at multiple sites. *RNA Biology, 14*, 124–135. https://doi.org/10.1080/15476286.2016.1259784

Mine, N., Guglielmini, J., Wilbaux, M., & Van Melderen, L. (2009). The decay of the chromosomally encoded ccdO157 toxin-antitoxin system in the *Escherichia coli* species. *Genetics, 181*, 1557–1566. https://doi.org/10.1534/genetics.108.095190

Mok, W. W. K., & Brynildsen, M. P. (2018). Timing of DNA damage responses impacts persistence to fluoroquinolones. *Proceedings of the National Academy of Sciences, 115*, E6301. https://doi.org/10.1073/pnas.1804218115

Molina, L., Udaondo, Z., Duque, E., Fernández, M., Bernal, P., Roca, A., de la Torre, J., & Ramos, J. L. (2016). Specific gene loci of clinical *Pseudomonas putida* isolates. *PLoS One, 11*, e0147478. https://doi.org/10.1371/journal.pone.0147478

Moyed, H. S., & Bertrand, K. P. (1983). hipA, a newly recognized gene of *Escherichia coli* K-12 that affects frequency of persistence after inhibition of murein synthesis. *Journal of Bacteriology, 155*, 768–775.

Muñoz-Gómez, A. J., Lemonnier, M., Santos-Sierra, S., Berzal-Herranz, A., & Díaz-Orejas, R. (2005). RNase/anti-RNase activities of the bacterial *parD* toxin-antitoxin system. *Journal of Bacteriology, 187*, 3151. https://doi.org/10.1128/JB.187.9.3151-3157.2005

Muthuramalingam, M., White, J. C., Murphy, T., Ames, J. R., & Bourne, C. R. (2018). The toxin from a ParDE toxin-antitoxin system found in *Pseudomonas aeruginosa* offers protection to cells challenged with anti-gyrase antibiotics. *Molecular Microbiology.* https://doi.org/10.1111/mmi.14165

Norton, J. P., & Mulvey, M. A. (2012). Toxin-antitoxin systems are important for niche-specific colonization and stress resistance of uropathogenic *Escherichia coli*. *PLoS Pathogens, 8*, e1002954. https://doi.org/10.1371/journal.ppat.1002954

Ocampo, P. S., Lázár, V., Papp, B., & Arnoldini, M. (2014). Antagonism between bacteriostatic and bactericidal antibiotics is prevalent. *Antimicrobial Agents and Chemotherapy, 58*, 4573–4582.

Osbourne, D. O., Soo, V. W., Konieczny, I., & Wood, T. K. (2014). Polyphosphate, cyclic AMP, guanosine tetraphosphate, and c-di-GMP reduce in vitro Lon activity. *Bioengineered, 5*, 264–268. https://doi.org/10.4161/bioe.29261

Overgaard, M., Borch, J., Jørgensen, M. G., & Gerdes, K. (2008). Messenger RNA interferase RelE controls relBE transcription by conditional cooperativity. *Molecular Microbiology, 69*, 841–857. https://doi.org/10.1111/j.1365-2958.2008.06313.x

Pandey, D. P., & Gerdes, K. (2005). Toxin-antitoxin loci are highly abundant in free-living but lost from host-associated prokaryotes. *Nucleic Acids Research, 33*, 966–976. https://doi.org/10.1093/nar/gki201

Pedersen, K., Zavialov, A. V., Pavlov, M. Y., Elf, J., Gerdes, K., & Ehrenberg, M. (2003). The bacterial toxin RelE displays codon-specific cleavage of mRNAs in the ribosomal a site. *Cell, 112*, 131–140.

Potrykus, K., & Cashel, M. (2008). (p)ppGpp: Still magical? *Annual Review of Microbiology, 62*, 35–51. https://doi.org/10.1146/annurev.micro.62.081307.162903

Prysak, M. H., Mozdzierz, C. J., Cook, A. M., Zhu, L., Zhang, Y., Inouye, M., & Woychik, N. A. (2009). Bacterial toxin YafQ is an endoribonuclease that associates with the ribosome and blocks translation elongation through sequence-specific and frame-dependent mRNA cleavage. *Molecular Microbiology, 71*, 1071–1087. https://doi.org/10.1111/j.1365-2958.2008.06572.x

Ramage, H. R., Connolly, L. E., & Cox, J. S. (2009). Comprehensive functional analysis of *Mycobacterium tuberculosis* toxin-antitoxin systems: Implications for pathogenesis, stress responses, and evolution. *PLoS Genetics, 5*, e1000767. https://doi.org/10.1371/journal.pgen.1000767

Ramisetty, B. C., & Santhosh, R. S. (2016). Horizontal gene transfer of chromosomal type II toxin-antitoxin systems of *Escherichia coli*. *FEMS Microbiology Letters, 363*. https://doi.org/10.1093/femsle/fnv238

Ramisetty, B. C., Ghosh, D., Roy Chowdhury, M., & Santhosh, R. S. (2016). What is the link between stringent response, endoribonuclease encoding type II toxin-antitoxin systems and persistence? *Frontiers in Microbiology, 7*, 1882. https://doi.org/10.3389/fmicb.2016.01882

Richter-Dahlfors, A., Buchan, A. M. J., & Finlay, B. B. (1997). Murine salmonellosis studied by confocal microscopy: *Salmonella typhimurium* resides intracellularly inside macrophages and exerts a cytotoxic effect on phagocytes in vivo. *The Journal of Experimental Medicine, 186*, 569. https://doi.org/10.1084/jem.186.4.569

Rotem, E., Loinger, A., Ronin, I., Levin-Reisman, I., Gabay, C., Shoresh, N., Biham, O., & Balaban, N. Q. (2010). Regulation of phenotypic variability by a threshold-based mechanism underlies bacterial persistence. *Proceedings of the National Academy of Sciences, 107*, 12541. https://doi.org/10.1073/pnas.1004333107

Ruiz-Echevarría, M. J., de la Cueva, G., & Díaz-Orejas, R. (1995). Translational coupling and limited degradation of a polycistronic messenger modulate differential gene expression in the parD stability system of plasmid R1. *Molecular and General Genetics MGG, 248*, 599–609. https://doi.org/10.1007/BF02423456

Rycroft, J. A., Gollan, B., Grabe, G. J., Hall, A., Cheverton, A. M., Larrouy-Maumus, G., Hare, S. A., & Helaine, S. (2018). Activity of acetyltransferase toxins involved in Salmonella persister formation during macrophage infection. *Nature Communications, 9*, 1993. https://doi.org/10.1038/s41467-018-04472-6

Saavedra De Bast, M., Mine, N., & Van Melderen, L. (2008). Chromosomal toxin-antitoxin systems may act as antiaddiction modules. *Journal of Bacteriology, 190*, 4603–4609. https://doi.org/10.1128/JB.00357-08

Sala, A., Bordes, P., & Genevaux, P. (2014). Multiple toxin-antitoxin systems in *Mycobacterium tuberculosis*. *Toxins, 6*, 1002–1020.

Salmon, M. A., Van Melderen, L., Bernard, P., & Couturier, M. (1994). The antidote and autoregulatory functions of the F plasmid CcdA protein: A genetic and biochemical survey. *Molecular and General Genetics MGG, 244*, 530–538. https://doi.org/10.1007/BF00583904

Schumacher, M. A., Piro, K. M., Xu, W., Hansen, S., Lewis, K., & Brennan, R. G. (2009). Molecular mechanisms of HipA-mediated multidrug tolerance and its neutralization by HipB. *Science, 323*, 396. https://doi.org/10.1126/science.1163806

Schumacher, M. A., Balani, P., Min, J., Chinnam, N. B., Hansen, S., Vulić, M., Lewis, K., & Brennan, R. G. (2015). HipBA–promoter structures reveal the basis of heritable multidrug tolerance. *Nature, 524*, 59.

Shah, D., Zhang, Z., Khodursky, A., Kaldalu, N., Kurg, K., & Lewis, K. (2006). Persisters: A distinct physiological state of *E. coli*. *BMC Microbiol, 6*, 53. https://doi.org/10.1186/1471-2180-6-53

Shan, Y., Brown Gandt, A., Rowe, S. E., Deisinger, J. P., Conlon, B. P., & Lewis, K. (2017). ATP-dependent persister formation in *Escherichia coli*. *MBio, 8*. https://doi.org/10.1128/mBio.02267-16

Shao, Y., Harrison, E., Bi, D., Tai, C., He, X., Ou, H., Rajakumar, K., & Deng, Z. (2010). TADB: A web-based resource for type 2 toxin–antitoxin loci in bacteria and archaea. *Nucleic Acids Research, 39*, D606–D611. https://doi.org/10.1093/nar/gkq908

Singh, R., Barry, C. E., & Boshoff, H. I. M. (2010). The three RelE homologs of *Mycobacterium tuberculosis* have individual, drug-specific effects on bacterial antibiotic tolerance. *Journal of Bacteriology, 192*, 1279. https://doi.org/10.1128/JB.01285-09

Slattery, A., Victorsen, A. H., Brown, A., Hillman, K., & Phillips, G. J. (2013). Isolation of highly persistent mutants of *Salmonella enterica* Serovar typhimurium reveals a new toxin-antitoxin module. *Journal of Bacteriology, 195*, 647. https://doi.org/10.1128/JB.01397-12

Szekeres, S., Dauti, M., Wilde, C., Mazel, D., & Rowe-Magnus, D. A. (2007). Chromosomal toxin-antitoxin loci can diminish large-scale genome reductions in the absence of selection. *Molecular Microbiology, 63*, 1588–1605. https://doi.org/10.1111/j.1365-2958.2007.05613.x

Tacconelli, E., Carrara, E., Savoldi, A., Harbarth, S., Mendelson, M., Monnet, D. L., Pulcini, C., Kahlmeter, G., Kluytmans, J., Carmeli, Y., Ouellette, M., Outterson, K., Patel, J., Cavaleri, M., Cox, E. M., Houchens, C. R., Grayson, M. L., Hansen, P., Singh, N., Theuretzbacher, U., Magrini, N., Aboderin, A. O., Al-Abri, S. S., Awang Jalil, N., Benzonana, N., Bhattacharya, S., Brink, A. J., Burkert, F. R., Cars, O., Cornaglia, G., Dyar, O. J., Friedrich, A. W., Gales, A. C., Gandra, S., Giske, C. G., Goff, D. A., Goossens, H., Gottlieb, T., Guzman Blanco, M., Hryniewicz, W., Kattula, D., Jinks, T., Kanj, S. S., Kerr, L., Kieny, M.-P., Kim, Y. S., Kozlov, R. S., Labarca, J., Laxminarayan, R., Leder, K., Leibovici, L., Levy-Hara, G., Littman, J., Malhotra-Kumar, S., Manchanda, V., Moja, L., Ndoye, B., Pan, A., Paterson, D. L., Paul, M., Qiu, H., Ramon-Pardo, P., Rodríguez-Baño, J., Sanguinetti, M., Sengupta, S., Sharland, M., Si-Mehand, M., Silver, L. L., Song, W., Steinbakk, M., Thomsen, J., Thwaites, G. E., van der Meer, J. W., Van Kinh, N., Vega, S., Villegas, M. V., Wechsler-Fördös, A., Wertheim, H. F. L., Wesangula, E., Woodford, N., Yilmaz, F. O., & Zorzet, A. (2018). Discovery, research, and development of new antibiotics: The WHO priority list of antibiotic-resistant bacteria and tuberculosis. *The Lancet Infectious Diseases, 18*, 318–327. https://doi.org/10.1016/S1473-3099(17)30753-3

Theodore, A., Lewis, K., & Vulic, M. (2013). Tolerance of *Escherichia coli* to fluoroquinolone antibiotics depends on specific components of the SOS response pathway. *Genetics, 195*, 1265–1276. https://doi.org/10.1534/genetics.113.152306

Tripathi, A., Dewan, P. C., Siddique, S. A., & Varadarajan, R. (2014). MazF-induced growth inhibition and persister generation in *Escherichia coli*. *The Journal of Biological Chemistry, 289*, 4191–4205. https://doi.org/10.1074/jbc.M113.510511

Tsuchimoto, S., & Ohtsubo, E. (1993). Autoregulation by cooperative binding of the PemI and PemK proteins to the promoter region of the pem operon. *Molecular & General Genetics, 237*, 81–88.

Van Acker, H., Sass, A., Dhondt, I., Nelis, H. J., & Coenye, T. (2014). Involvement of toxin-antitoxin modules in *Burkholderia cenocepacia* biofilm persistence. *Pathogens and Disease, 71,* 326–335. https://doi.org/10.1111/2049-632X.12177

Van Melderen, L., & Wood, T. K. (2017). Commentary: What is the link between stringent response, endoribonuclease encoding type II toxin-antitoxin systems and persistence? *Frontiers in Microbiology, 8,* 191. https://doi.org/10.3389/fmicb.2017.00191

Van Melderen, L., Bernard, P., & Couturier, M. (1994). Lon-dependent proteolysis of CcdA is the key control for activation of CcdB in plasmid-free segregant bacteria. *Molecular Microbiology, 11,* 1151–1157.

Vázquez-Laslop, N., Lee, H., & Neyfakh, A. A. (2006). Increased persistence in *Escherichia coli* caused by controlled expression of toxins or other unrelated proteins. *Journal of Bacteriology, 188,* 3494–3497.

Verstraeten, N., Knapen, W. J., Kint, C. I., Liebens, V., Van den Bergh, B., Dewachter, L., Michiels, J. E., Fu, Q., David, C. C., Fierro, A. C., Marchal, K., Beirlant, J., Versées, W., Hofkens, J., Jansen, M., Fauvart, M., & Michiels, J. (2015). Obg and membrane depolarization are part of a microbial bet-hedging strategy that leads to antibiotic tolerance. *Molecular Cell, 59,* 9–21. https://doi.org/10.1016/j.molcel.2015.05.011

Vogwill, T., Comfort, A. C., Furió, V., & MacLean, R. C. (2016). Persistence and resistance as complementary bacterial adaptations to antibiotics. *Journal of Evolutionary Biology, 29,* 1223–1233. https://doi.org/10.1111/jeb.12864

Winther, K. S., & Gerdes, K. (2011). Enteric virulence associated protein VapC inhibits translation by cleavage of initiator tRNA. *Proceedings of the National Academy of Sciences of the United States of America, 108,* 7403–7407. https://doi.org/10.1073/pnas.1019587108

Winther, K. S., Brodersen, D. E., Brown, A. K., & Gerdes, K. (2013). VapC20 of *Mycobacterium tuberculosis* cleaves the sarcin-ricin loop of 23S rRNA. *Nature Communications, 4,* 2796. https://doi.org/10.1038/ncomms3796

Wozniak, R. A., & Waldor, M. K. (2009). A toxin-antitoxin system promotes the maintenance of an integrative conjugative element. *PLoS Genetics, 5,* e1000439. https://doi.org/10.1371/journal.pgen.1000439

Yao, X., Chen, T., Shen, X., Zhao, Y., Wang, M., Rao, X., Yin, S., Wang, J., Gong, Y., Lu, S., Le, S., Tan, Y., Tang, J., Fuquan, H., & Li, M. (2015). The chromosomal SezAT toxin-antitoxin system promotes the maintenance of the SsPI-1 pathogenicity island in epidemic *Streptococcus suis. Molecular Microbiology, 98,* 243–257. https://doi.org/10.1111/mmi.13116

Yuan, J., Yamaichi, Y., & Waldor, M. K. (2011). The three *Vibrio cholerae* chromosome II-encoded ParE toxins degrade chromosome I following loss of chromosome II. *Journal of Bacteriology, 193,* 611–619. https://doi.org/10.1128/JB.01185-10

Zhang, Y., Zhang, J., Hoeflich, K. P., Ikura, M., Qing, G., & Inouye, M. (2003). MazF cleaves cellular mRNAs specifically at ACA to block protein synthesis in *Escherichia coli. Molecular Cell, 12,* 913–923.

Chapter 9
Persister Resuscitation

Arvi Jõers, Marta Putrinš, Niilo Kaldalu, Hannes Luidalepp,
and Tanel Tenson

Abstract By definition, persister cells must resume growth after the bactericidal treatment. Growth resumption can also lead to the reoccurrence of the infections and is, therefore, the reason why persisters are considered clinically important. Furthermore, treatments that enforce the dormant bacteria to resuscitate during the antibiotic treatment might become a key for eradicating persistent infections. Unfortunately, resuscitation of dormant bacteria is still poorly studied and very little is known about resuscitation of persisters during infection.

In this chapter, we have summarized the knowledge of factors that affect growth resumption of bacterial cells in general, and more specifically, after antibiotic treatment. We also touch the potentially relevant field of Viable but nonculturable (VBNC) cells. To illustrate how different can be persister resuscitation in vivo compared to the in vitro conditions we draw an example from urinary tract infection. Understanding the mechanisms of bacterial growth resumption inside the host is one very promising direction where the field could move in order to find new therapeutic options against persistent infections.

9.1 Resuscitation of Dormant Bacteria

Persister cells survive antibiotic treatment in a non-proliferating form and switch back to proliferation only after the treatment is over. In this chapter, we focus on how bacteria transition from the non-growing state to growth and proliferation. While discussing these transitions, we use the terms "resuscitation," "growth resumption," and "regrowth" as synonyms.

Bacterial growth and metabolic activity depend on the external environment. Bacteria do not accumulate extensive reserves and their ability to grow relies on

---

A. Jõers · M. Putrinš · N. Kaldalu · T. Tenson (✉)
Insitute of Technology, University of Tartu, Tartu, Estonia
e-mail: tanel.tenson@ut.ee

H. Luidalepp
Quretec OÜ, Tartu, Estonia

© Springer Nature Switzerland AG 2019
K. Lewis (ed.), *Persister Cells and Infectious Disease*,
https://doi.org/10.1007/978-3-030-25241-0_9

nutrients they import. Once the nutrients run out, or waste products accumulate to intolerable levels, bacteria stop growing and enter a phase of decreased metabolic activity. Gram-positive bacteria form spores that are especially tolerant to adverse environmental conditions and can withstand long periods within inhospitable environments. Gram-negative bacteria also undergo extensive changes that, although morphologically less distinct, prepare them for long-term survival. There are two widespread dormancy phenotypes described in non-sporulating bacteria, persisters and viable but non-culturable (VBNC) cells.

Eventually cells may be exposed to a growth-supporting environment again—new nutrients become available in nature or cells are transferred to fresh medium in the laboratory. Bacteria must now (a) detect the nutrient availability; (b) restart their metabolism; (c) rearrange their gene expression pattern; and (d) start or resume cell growth and division. Failure in any of these steps prevents multiplication and colony formation; this often leads us to state that bacteria have lost their culturability or viability.

9.1.1 Heterogeneous Growth Resumption Timing

The period of no growth observed after transferring bacteria from a stationary phase culture to a fresh medium is termed the lag phase. Its length can vary depending on the culture conditions. Furthermore, even individual cells from a clonal population in the same environment can have quite different lag phase durations. *Escherichia coli* display significant phenotypic heterogeneity in lag phase durations when seeded from stationary phase cultures on agar plates (Levin-Reisman et al. 2010) or into flow chambers (Pin and Baranyi 2008). The distribution of lag phase durations typically exhibit a fat tail on the right side of the graph—the lag phases of many cells are very long and often exceed the experimental time window (Fig. 9.1). This leads to a situation where growing and non-growing cells are present at the same time.

Studies of growth resumption have shown that regrowth of individual bacteria depends on culture conditions both in the stationary phase culture (preculture) and during resuscitation (Figs. 9.1 and 9.2) (Joers et al. 2010; Luidalepp et al. 2011). In the rest of this chapter, we are using the term "preculture" to mark an initial stationary phase culture that was used as the source of the inoculated bacteria. Stresses experienced during the preculture phase typically delay growth resumption. One common stress that bacteria face is a lack of nutrients in the stationary phase. Longer stationary phase delays growth resumption and increases the number of non-growing bacteria. The preculture and outgrowth media also play a role. For reasons unknown, the outgrowth capacity is lost more rapidly in rich preculture medium (e.g., LB), when compared to minimal medium (Luidalepp et al. 2011). That is manifested in longer lag periods of the bacteria that resume growth and a larger fraction of the cells that remain non-growing until the end of the observation. The richness of the outgrowth medium has an opposite effect: bacteria resume growth slowly in poor media and have short individual lag times in rich media

Fig. 9.1 The time that bacteria have spent in a stationary state before inoculation affects their growth resumption kinetics. This schematic representation is based on the observations made by Levin-Reisman et al. (2010) and Luidalepp et al. (2011)

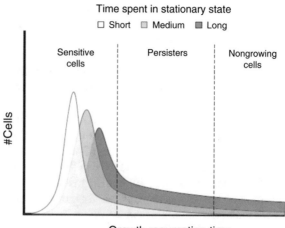

Fig. 9.2 Factors that affect bacteria during preculture and regrowth either facilitate or inhibit growth resumption

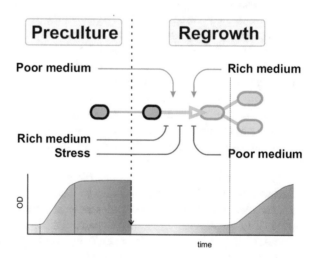

(Joers et al. 2010). A recent study found that delayed growth resumption of individual *E. coli* cells is often accompanied by the formation of protein aggresomes at the cell poles. These aggregates are cleared before resuscitation (Pu et al. 2018).

The rate of resuscitation is also influenced by the genetic background of the cells. This is clearly illustrated by the fact that it is possible to select mutants with increased lag phase lengths (Fridman et al. 2014). Remarkably, the selection can result in several *E. coli* strains with defined lag phase lengths—separate strains with average single-cell lag times of 3, 5, or 10 h can be obtained. This demonstrates that the length of the lag phase and its distribution is genetically controlled and was probably optimized during evolution. The wide distribution of lag times is also observed in environmental bacteria. Epstein and colleagues cultivated different bacteria isolated from the natural environment and found that the resuscitation times of individual cells of the same species varied over the time of weeks to months. Once cultured, most isolates grew without a long lag (Buerger et al. 2012).

Heterogeneous growth resumption timing of microbial populations in fresh growth-supporting media has been attributed to a bet-hedging strategy (de Jong et al. 2011). Cells with short lag phases can make the most of the new resource available, while the ones that remain dormant for longer act as "insurance" against possible disasters that could kill the growing cells. This is exactly what happens in the case of persister cells—antibiotics kill metabolically active cells while dormant cells with long lag phases survive. In this sense, these persisters are similar to the "superdormant" spores of *Bacillus* (Ghosh and Setlow 2009). The latter remain dormant under conditions where most of the spores germinate and are able to survive environmental shocks that kill both growing cells and germinated spores.

Another theoretical explanation for heterogeneous growth resumption timing under unknown environmental conditions is the "scout hypothesis" (Epstein 2009). According to this theory, a dormant population of bacteria in a nutrient-deprived environment must still monitor its surroundings for possible growth substrates. If cells miss a new resource and an opportunity to grow, they would be soon outcompeted by their more agile neighbors. However, monitoring the environment (staying alert) requires energy and can exhaust the modest reserves the dormant cells might have, leading to cell death. The scout hypothesis proposes that, from time to time, a cell recovers from dormancy and scans its surroundings for the opportunity to grow, while the rest of a population remains dormant. If the environment is supportive, the transiently active bacterium will quickly resume growth, if not, the cell perishes and the process is repeated after some time. In such a way, a population can survive for a long time while constantly monitoring its surroundings and being ready to resume growth quickly.

Heterogeneous growth resumption might not necessarily be an evolutionary selected survival strategy. Persisters may well occur without a dedicated mechanism, for example, as a result of irregularities in gene expression (Vázquez-Laslop et al. 2006). The persistence as Stuff Happens (PaSH) hypothesis suggests that the formation of persisters may be caused by unavoidable heterogeneous damage (Levin et al. 2014). The same can apply also for growth resumption where observed heterogeneity might be just inevitable and synchronized wake-up of dormant bacteria might not be physiologically possible due to different levels of damage.

9.1.2 Viable but Nonculturable Bacteria

Cells with exceptionally long lag phases might not resume growth during the observation time and thus are deemed nonculturable (Fig. 9.3). Cultivability has been a longstanding issue in environmental microbiology and microbiome studies. Comparison of bacterial counts under the microscope and colony-forming units (CFU) from the same samples have led to the conclusion that only a minority of bacteria can be cultivated (Rappé and Giovannoni 2003). Many bacteria in the

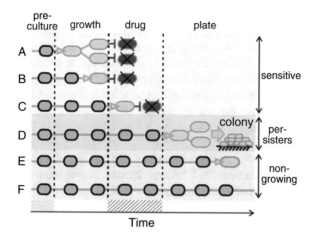

Fig. 9.3 Persister count reflects the heterogeneity of bacterial growth resumption. After dilution from a pre-culture into the growth medium, bacteria resuscitate at different times. Cells that resume growth before or during antibiotic treatment are killed and deemed antibiotic sensitive (**A–C**). Persister cells resume growth after the drug treatment but early enough to form a visible colony at the time of inspection (usually overnight incubation) (**D**). The bacteria, which resume growth very late (**E**) or not at all (**F**) are classified as nonculturable. Adapted from Joers et al. (2010)

"uncultured microbial majority" belong to uncultivable taxa. These microbes require unusual measures of cultivation and never grow under standard laboratory conditions (Stewart 2012). Uncultivable taxa remain out of the scope of this chapter. However, there are many bacteria from cultivable species that are able to grow in the medium used but still fail to do so (Epstein 2013). These cells have been labeled as Viable But Non Culturable (VBNC) (Oliver 2005). As stated in the definition, these bacteria do not proliferate but maintain a level of metabolism that sustains their viability. The viable state is detected through assays that employ metabolic conversion of model substrates (Zimmermann et al. 1978) or test for the intactness of the cell membrane (Porter et al. 1995). It has been demonstrated that, in the environment, bacteria can stay in the VBNC state for months or even years (Bunker et al. 2004). These cells become cultivable again after a change in growth conditions, for example, a change in temperature or nutrient supply (Oliver et al. 1995). Just like special media and methods of targeted culturing enable one to grow bacterial genera that have been considered uncultivable (Browne et al. 2016), studies of the VBNC state have shown that different growth media support growth with different efficiencies, resulting in different CFU counts (Azevedo et al. 2012; Pinto et al. 2011). Thus, swapping the media not only changes the list of culturable species, but also changes the resuscitation efficiency of the same species.

Environmental and foodborne VBNC evoke obvious public health concerns—if we cannot detect bacteria in drinking water by standard cultivation methods, can the resilient pathogenic bacteria still be a potential source of infection? It is indeed reported that *Vibrio cholerae* can regain cultivable state in the human intestine (Colwell et al. 1996). Similarly, *Campylobacter jejuni* in a VBNC state in water can cause infection in animal models (Jones et al. 1991).

The role of VBNC cells during infection and antibiotic treatment has not been studied. However, it has been shown that human serum induces the formation of both VBNC cells and persisters (Ayrapetyan et al. 2015). It has been suggested that they form a continuum of dormancy while persisters resume growth in the detection window, VBNC remains dormant for longer periods of time (Ayrapetyan et al. 2018; Kim et al. 2018; Matilla 2018). The different studies have used different definitions for the VBNC state and the results are sometimes not comparable between the reports. In some experimental systems, it has been reported that the apparent VBNC count actually reflects differences in survival of culturable bacteria in different culture conditions (Bogosian et al. 2000). Still, in some systems, the VBNC state seems to reflect "real" dormancy and, therefore, it is of interest for researchers studying persisters to follow the VBNC field.

9.1.3 Factors that Stimulate Resuscitation

In addition to direct uptake and use of a new growth substrate, cells can use specific signals and cues to evaluate the "goodness" of an environment. The first example of such signaling was the identification of a resuscitation-promoting factor (Rpf) in *Micrococcus luteus* (Mukamolova et al. 1998). Growing *M. luteus* cells secrete Rpf protein that was reported to stimulate growth resumption of dormant *M. luteus* cells. It was later shown that Rpf has a mucolytic activity and it is able to degrade cell wall peptidoglycan (Mukamolova et al. 2006). Proteins similar to Rpf were later discovered in many Gram-positive bacteria (Ravagnani et al. 2005) and some of these were reported to confer similar resuscitation activity (Nikitushkin et al. 2015). Meantime, several researchers have not been able to reproduce these results (Kim Lewis, personal communication).

Cell wall fragments (muropeptides) were identified as inducers of germination in *Bacillus* spores by Dworkin and coworkers (Shah et al. 2008). Muropeptides are generated and released into the medium during cell growth and division (Park and Uehara 2008), so their presence is a hallmark of a favorable environment. Interestingly, *Bacillus* spores respond not only to muropeptides from their own species, but also to, for example, *E. coli*-derived muropeptides (Shah et al. 2008). Muropeptides from different species can also induce growth resumption of dormant *E. coli* and *Pseudomonas aeruginosa* cells (Jõers et al, manuscript in preparation). These examples establish muropeptides as a universal cue of bacterial growth that many species have learned to associate with a growth-supporting environment.

Stimulating growth resumption by the addition of a negligible amount of a favorable carbon source can shorten a long lag phase. A 4-day *E. coli* stationary phase culture resumes growth slowly when transferred into fresh medium containing gluconate as a carbon source. However, supplementing the medium with a small amount of glucose (100 times less than gluconate) can speed up growth resumption significantly (Jõers and Tenson 2016). Here, glucose acts as a cue or signal for growth resumption while gluconate is metabolized to fuel the growth.

9.2   Resuscitation of Persisters

Non-growing bacteria can survive antibiotic treatment because they have entered into a dormant state, which may happen due to previous stress or a random phenotypic switch. After the treatment, persisters exit from dormancy, and thus their survival can be detected using cultivation. Some bacteria remain nondividing and standard cultivation does not indicate whether they were killed or are alive and able to regrow in the future (Fig. 9.3). If these cells are alive they correspond to the definition of VBNC. Resuscitation of persisters is distributed over time (between hours and days) and has been directly observed both in a liquid medium (Balaban et al. 2004; Goormaghtigh et al. 2018; Joers et al. 2010) and on agar plates (Levin-Reisman et al. 2010).

9.2.1   Factors that Affect Persister Resuscitation

9.2.1.1   Effects of Preculture

Generally, all factors that delay resuscitation and lengthen the lag time increase persistence, while resuscitation-stimulating factors enhance killing and decrease persistence. Antibiotic kill curves can be observed as biphasic exponential decay. The first phase of rapid decay in CFU count represents the killing of growing cells. The second phase represents the persister subpopulation and the slow decay in this phase can be explained by the resuscitation of some dormant cells during the antibiotic treatment (Dhar and McKinney 2007; Balaban et al. 2004; Joers et al. 2010) (Fig. 9.1). As with resuscitation in general, persister frequency depends on the preculture medium and increases with the time that the inoculated cells have spent in the stationary phase (Luidalepp et al. 2011). These findings can be fully explained by differences in bacterial resuscitation. Persister frequency depends also on the culture medium where the cells are during the treatment and is higher in a poorer medium (Joers et al. 2010). Once again, this can be explained by slower resuscitation and longer lag times of individual bacteria in the poor medium. Because of the sensitivity of experimental conditions on resuscitation and persistence, clarification and standardization of experimental procedures in persister research have only recently been agreed upon (Balaban et al. 2019).

9.2.1.2   Effects of Antibiotic Treatment Conditions

The influence of the carbon source on the resuscitation of *E. coli* persisters is illustrated by a study that uncovered that killing by aminoglycosides depends on membrane potential (Allison et al. 2011). In this study, stationary phase cultures were treated with ofloxacin. Surviving persisters were transferred into media containing an aminoglycoside antibiotic combined with different carbon sources. Some carbon sources, like glucose, were metabolized and enabled eradication of the ofloxacin-surviving cells because they induced a membrane potential that is required for the uptake of aminoglycosides. Other carbon sources, like arabinose, were not metabolized and did not facilitate killing by aminoglycosides (Allison et al. 2011). While both glucose and arabinose can be used by growing cells, only the former is able to create membrane potential in persisters (during the course of the experiment). Thus, the metabolism of resuscitating cells is different from that of growing cells.

9.2.1.3   Effects of Posttreatment Outgrowth Conditions

While the composition of the outgrowth medium has a large effect on cultivability (Lagier et al. 2012), as discussed above, the plating medium is also expected to influence the persister count. Until now, the possible effects of the resuscitation medium on cultivability of persisters have not been widely studied. Plating of ampicillin-treated *E. coli* samples on R2A agar plates resulted in ~tenfold fewer colonies compared to LB plates, while the same number of colonies formed after treatment with ofloxacin (Kaldalu et al. 2016). Interestingly, R2A agar (Reasoner and Geldreich 1985) allows one to culture many bacteria from environmental samples that do not readily grow on rich media. This shows that R2A agar is not universally superior for the resuscitation of damaged and dormant bacterial cells.

Under clinical settings, transient treatment with many antibiotics leads to suppression of bacterial growth for certain time periods after the antibiotic concentration in the medium decreases below the minimal inhibitory concentration. This posttreatment damage to bacteria is defined as the post-antibiotic effect (PAE) (MacKenzie and Gould 1993). PAE has been described for many antibiotics, including aminoglycosides (Zhanel and Craig 1994) and fluoroquinolones (Mizunaga et al. 2005; Athamna et al. 2004). The reasons for PAE involve the need to repair antibiotic-induced damage, reduction of the off-rate of the drug from its target, and reduction of the efflux rate of the antibiotic from the bacterial cell (Srimani et al. 2017). Besides the intracellular residual antibiotic, carry-over of the surface-bound drug may affect the viable count. Fluoroquinolones bind on the surface of bacteria and have low MIC values. Washing fluoroquinolone-treated bacteria or centrifugation through silicone oil before plating is required to avoid carry-over of the drug (Celesk and Robillard 1989). Washing of bacteria is not required after incubation with cell wall synthesis inhibitors when the residual drug is diluted below MIC upon plating. The PAE and carry-over of antibiotics can lead to the misinterpretation of the antibiotic effects on dormant cells. The decrease in the number of persisters during treatment with certain antibiotics might not show the killing of dormant bacteria but kill during growth resumption.

9.2.2 Persister Resuscitation During Infection

During infections, the bacterial populations are very complex. The outcome of antibiotic treatment reflects the drug pharmacokinetics, pharmacodynamics, and host immune factors among other things. In some cases, it has been observed that recurrent infection is caused by the resuscitation of dormant cells that survived antibiotic treatment.

Urinary tract infection (UTI) is an example of a common and recurrent disease where antibiotic treatment can fail to eradicate all bacterial cells (Foxman 2010). Many patients experience recurrent infections (rUTI) that are often caused by the same bacterial strain as in the first episode (Skjot-Rasmussen et al. 2011). Most of the knowledge of in vivo UTI persisters comes from different infection models, mostly from infected cell culture or mice.

There is clear evidence that uropathogenic *E. coli* (UPEC) can enter bladder epithelial cells in humans as well as mice (Mulvey et al. 2001; Rosen et al. 2007). This is one part of the uroinfection cycle where UPEC can invade both mature superficial/umbrella bladder epithelial cells and underlying non-differentiated cells. It has been shown that UPEC can reside in vacuoles and can replicate inside the cytosol of the host cells. In vacuoles, especially in underlying immature bladder epithelial cells, bacteria remain in a nonreplicating state forming a subpopulation termed "quiescent intracellular reservoirs"—QIRs (Mysorekar and Hultgren 2006). These cells are true persisters as they are tolerant to antibiotics and are able to resume growth after antibiotic treatment when transferred to rich media (Blango and Mulvey 2010). With unknown frequency, these quiescent cells can also resume growth in the host. It has been shown in mouse models that, after antibiotic treatment, mice can have negative urine cultures for several days or weeks yet still may develop a new infection episode (Mysorekar and Hultgren 2006).

Resuscitation of UPEC from the QIRs is most strongly associated with bladder epithelial turnover (Mysorekar and Hultgren 2006). Inside undifferentiated bladder cells, the bacteria-containing vacuoles are surrounded by actin filaments. Maturation of the epithelial cells induces rearrangement of the actin filaments and subsequent entry of the bacteria into the cytosol, where active replication can take place.

A recent study has elucidated the mechanisms that induce growth resumption of persistent UPEC in a mouse model. It was shown that after UPEC has established a persistent infection, a secondary infection with otherwise non-uropathogenic bacteria *Gardnerella vaginalis* is able to induce reactivation of UPEC (Gilbert et al. 2017). Bladder exposure to *G. vaginalis* results in apoptosis and exfoliation of superficial bladder epithelial cells and leads to maturation of the underlying epithelial cells and reactivation of QIRs within them.

One possibility to artificially induce maturation of underlying epithelial cells is forced resurgence of superficial epithelial cells. It has been shown in a mouse model that chitosan treatment causes exfoliation of superficial cells that in turn induces maturation of the underlying cells. Chitosan, in combination with antibiotics, efficiently eradicated bacteria and prevented persistent infection (Erman et al. 2017). This is an interesting example of an anti-persister strategy where host cells are targeted instead of persisters. Resuscitation of persisters by modulating host immunity has been suggested as a possible strategy also against other intracellular infections where the immune response is a major factor in restricting the regrowth of bacteria (Fisher et al. 2017).

9.2.3 Resuscitation of Persisters as a Treatment Strategy

Resuscitation of persisters might increase the efficiency of antibiotic treatment. A review of antipersister strategies was recently published (Defraine et al. 2018), yet most of the treatments presented do not attempt to directly inactivate persisters. However, attempts have also been made to screen for chemicals that induce metabolic activity and resuscitate persisters, thereby potentiating bactericidal antibiotics. For example, a compound that stimulates resuscitation and eradication of ampicillin and norfloxacin persisters in *E. coli* and *P. aeruginosa* was identified from a screen of a chemical library (Kim et al. 2011). The underlying molecular mechanisms by which the wake-up occurs remain to be elucidated, but stimulating cell metabolism is a probable scenario. Similarly, a fatty acid signaling molecule has been shown to eliminate *E. coli* and *P. aeruginosa* persisters by activating metabolism of the bacteria (Marques et al. 2014). Thus, induced activation of dormant bacteria might be a promising strategy to enhance the effectiveness of antibiotic treatments. Future studies must show if any of these findings will be applicable in drug development. Special efforts are required to target the dormant states of bacteria and growth resumption because current high-throughput screening assays are not being developed with the resuscitation process involved. Recently, antibiotic combinations and antibiotic potentiators are gaining increased attention as demonstrated by the pioneering work of Kim et al., which shows that resuscitation assays can open an avenue to new potentiators. To target persisters under more clinically relevant settings, the screening assays could also involve mammalian cells that model intracellular infections.

Acknowledgements This work was supported by Estonian Research Council (grant PRG335), and by the European Regional Development Fund (through the Centre of Excellence in Molecular Cell Engineering). We thank David Schryer for correcting the English language.

References

Allison, K. R., Brynildsen, M. P., & Collins, J. J. (2011). Metabolite-enabled eradication of bacterial persisters by aminoglycosides. *Nature, 473*(7346), 216–220. https://doi.org/10.1038/nature10069.

Athamna, A., Athamna, M., Medlej, B., Bast, D. J., & Rubinstein, E. (2004). In vitro post-antibiotic effect of fluoroquinolones, macrolides, -lactams, tetracyclines, vancomycin, clindamycin, linezolid, chloramphenicol, quinupristin/dalfopristin and rifampicin on *Bacillus anthracis*. *Journal of Antimicrobial Chemotherapy, 53*(4), 609–615. https://doi.org/10.1093/jac/dkh130.

Ayrapetyan, M., Williams, T. C., Baxter, R., & Oliver, J. D. (2015). Viable but nonculturable and persister cells coexist stochastically and are induced by human serum. *Infection and Immunity, 83*(11), 4194–4203. https://doi.org/10.1128/IAI.00404-15.

Ayrapetyan, M., Williams, T., & Oliver, J. D. (2018). Relationship between the viable but nonculturable state and antibiotic persister cells. *Journal of Bacteriology, 200*(20). https://doi.org/10.1128/JB.00249-18.

Azevedo, N. F., Bragança, S. M., Simões, L. C., Cerqueira, L., Almeida, C., Keevil, C. W., & Vieira, M. J. (2012). Proposal for a method to estimate nutrient shock effects in bacteria. *BMC Research Notes, 5*, 422. https://doi.org/10.1186/1756-0500-5-422.

Balaban, N. Q., Merrin, J., Chait, R., Kowalik, L., & Leibler, S. (2004). Bacterial persistence as a phenotypic switch. *Science (New York), 305*(5690), 1622–1625. https://doi.org/10.1126/science.1099390.

Balaban, N. Q., Helaine, S., Lewis, K., Ackermann, M., Aldridge, B., Andersson, D. I., Brynildsen, M. P., Bumann, D., Camilli, A., Collins, J. J., Dehio, C., Fortune, S., Ghigo, J. M., Hardt, W. D., Harms, A., Heinemann, M., Hung, D. T., Jenal, U., Levin, B. R., Michiels, J., Storz, G., Tan, M. W., Tenson, T., Van Melderen, L., Zinkernagel, A. (2019). A definitions and guidelines for research on antibiotic persistence. *Nature Review Microbiology, 17*(7), 441–448. (Erratum in: Nature Review Microbiology. 2019 Apr 29) https://doi.org/10.1038/s41579-019-0196-3.

Blango, M. G., & Mulvey, M. A. (2010). Persistence of uropathogenic *Escherichia coli* in the face of multiple antibiotics. *Antimicrobial Agents and Chemotherapy, 54*(5), 1855–1863. https://doi.org/10.1128/AAC.00014-10.

Bogosian, G., Aardema, N. D., Bourneuf, E. V., Morris, P. J., & O'Neil, J. P. (2000). Recovery of hydrogen peroxide-sensitive culturable cells of *Vibrio vulnificus* gives the appearance of resuscitation from a viable but nonculturable state. *Journal of Bacteriology, 182*(18), 5070–5075. http://www.ncbi.nlm.nih.gov/pubmed/10960089

Browne, H. P., Forster, S. C., Anonye, B. O., Kumar, N., Neville, B. A., Stares, M. D., Goulding, D., & Lawley, T. D. (2016). Culturing of 'unculturable' human microbiota reveals novel taxa and extensive sporulation. *Nature, 533*(7604), 543–546. https://doi.org/10.1038/nature17645.

Buerger, S., Spoering, A., Gavrish, E., Leslin, C., Ling, L., & Epstein, S. S. (2012). Microbial scout hypothesis, stochastic exit from dormancy, and the nature of slow growers. *Applied and Environmental Microbiology, 78*(9), 3221–3228. https://doi.org/10.1128/AEM.07307-11.

Bunker, S. T., Bates, T. C., & Oliver, J. D. (2004). Effects of temperature on detection of plasmid or chromosomally encoded Gfp- and lux-Labeled *pseudomonas fluorescens* in soil. *Environmental Biosafety Research, 3*(2), 83–90.

Celesk, R. A., & Robillard, N. J. (1989). Factors influencing the accumulation of ciprofloxacin in *Pseudomonas aeruginosa. Antimicrobial Agents and Chemotherapy, 33*(11), 1921–1926.

Colwell, R. R., Brayton, P., Herrington, D., Tall, B., Huq, A., & Levine, M. M. (1996). Viable but non-culturable *Vibrio cholerae* O1 revert to a cultivable state in the human intestine. *World Journal of Microbiology and Biotechnology, 12*(1), 28–31. https://doi.org/10.1007/BF00327795.

Defraine, V., Fauvart, M., & Michiels, J. (2018). Fighting bacterial persistence: Current and emerging anti-persister strategies and therapeutics. *Drug Resistance Updates, 38*, 12–26. https://doi.org/10.1016/J.DRUP.2018.03.002

Dhar, N., & McKinney, J. D. (2007). Microbial phenotypic heterogeneity and antibiotic tolerance. *Current Opinion in Microbiology, 10*(1), 30–38. https://doi.org/10.1016/J.MIB.2006.12.007.

Epstein, S. S. (2009). Microbial awakenings. *Nature, 457*(7233), 1083. https://doi.org/10.1038/4571083a.

Epstein, S. S. (2013). The phenomenon of microbial uncultivability. *Current Opinion in Microbiology, 16*(5), 636–642. https://doi.org/10.1016/j.mib.2013.08.003.

Erman, A., Hergouth, V. K., Blango, M. G., Kos, M. K., Mulvey, M. A., & Veranič, P. (2017). Repeated treatments with chitosan in combination with antibiotics completely eradicate uropathogenic *Escherichia coli* from infected mouse urinary bladders. *Journal of Infectious Diseases, 216*(3), jix023. https://doi.org/10.1093/infdis/jix023.

Fisher, R. A., Gollan, B., & Helaine, S. (2017). Persistent bacterial infections and persister cells. *Nature Reviews Microbiology.* https://doi.org/10.1038/nrmicro.2017.42

Foxman, B. (2010). The epidemiology of urinary tract infection. *Nature Reviews. Urology, 7*(12), 653–660 (Nature publishing group, a division of Macmillan publishers limited. *All Rights Reserved*). https://doi.org/10.1038/nrurol.2010.190

Fridman, O., Goldberg, A., Ronin, I., Shoresh, N., & Balaban, N. Q. (2014). Optimization of lag time underlies antibiotic tolerance in evolved bacterial populations. *Nature, 513*(7518), 418–421. https://doi.org/10.1038/nature13469.

Ghosh, S., & Setlow, P. (2009). Isolation and characterization of superdormant spores of Bacillus species. *Journal of Bacteriology, 191*(6), 1787–1797. https://doi.org/10.1128/JB.01668-08.

Gilbert, N. M., O'Brien, V. P., & Lewis, A. L. (2017). Transient microbiota exposures activate dormant *Escherichia coli* infection in the bladder and drive severe outcomes of recurrent disease. *PLOS Pathogens, 13*(3), e1006238. https://doi.org/10.1371/journal.ppat.1006238.

Goormaghtigh, F., Fraikin, N., Putrinš, M., Hallaert, T., Hauryliuk, V., Garcia-Pino, A., Sjödin, A., et al. (2018). Reassessing the role of type II toxin-antitoxin systems in formation of *Escherichia coli* type II persister cells. *MBio, 9*(3), e00640–e00618. https://doi.org/10.1128/mBio.00640-18.

Jõers, A., & Tenson, T. (2016). Growth resumption from stationary phase reveals memory in *Escherichia coli* cultures. *Scientific Reports, 6*(1), 24055. https://doi.org/10.1038/srep24055.

Joers, A., Kaldalu, N., & Tenson, T. (2010). The frequency of persisters in *Escherichia coli* reflects the kinetics of awakening from dormancy. *Journal of Bacteriology, 192*(13), 3379–3384. https://doi.org/10.1128/jb.00056-10.

Jones, D. M., Sutcliffe, E. M., & Curry, A. (1991). Recovery of viable but non-culturable *Campylobacter jejuni. Journal of General Microbiology, 137*(10), 2477–2482. https://doi.org/10.1099/00221287-137-10-2477.

Jong, d., Imke, G., Haccou, P., & Kuipers, O. P. (2011). Bet hedging or not? A guide to proper classification of microbial survival strategies. *BioEssays: News and Reviews in Molecular, Cellular and Developmental Biology, 33*(3), 215–223. https://doi.org/10.1002/bies.201000127.

Kaldalu, N., Jõers, A., Ingelman, H., & Tenson, T. (2016). A general method for measuring persister levels in *Escherichia coli* cultures. *Methods in Molecular Biology, 1333*. https://doi.org/10.1007/978-1-4939-2854-5_3

Kim, J.-S., Heo, P., Yang, T.-J., Lee, K.-S., Cho, D.-H., Kim, B. T., Suh, J.-H., et al. (2011). Selective killing of bacterial persisters by a single chemical compound without affecting normal antibiotic-sensitive cells. *Antimicrobial Agents and Chemotherapy, 55*(11), 5380–5383. https://doi.org/10.1128/AAC.00708-11.

Kim, J.-S., Chowdhury, N., Yamasaki, R., & Wood, T. K. (2018). Viable but non-culturable and persistence describe the same bacterial stress state. *Environmental Microbiology, 20*(6), 2038–2048. https://doi.org/10.1111/1462-2920.14075.

Lagier, J.-C., Armougom, F., Million, M., Hugon, P., Pagnier, I., Robert, C., Bittar, F., et al. (2012). Microbial culturomics: Paradigm shift in the human gut microbiome study. *Clinical Microbiology and Infection, 18*(12), 1185–1193. https://doi.org/10.1111/1469-0691.12023.

Levin, B. R., Concepción-Acevedo, J., & Udekwu, K. I. (2014). Persistence: A copacetic and parsimonious hypothesis for the existence of non-inherited resistance to antibiotics. *Current Opinion in Microbiology, 21*, 18–21. https://doi.org/10.1016/j.mib.2014.06.016.

Levin-Reisman, I., Gefen, O., Fridman, O., Ronin, I., Shwa, D., Sheftel, H., & Balaban, N. Q. (2010). Automated imaging with ScanLag reveals previously undetectable bacterial growth phenotypes. *Nature Methods, 7*(9), 737–739. https://doi.org/10.1038/nmeth.1485.

Luidalepp, H., Jõers, A., Kaldalu, N., & Tenson, T. (2011). Age of inoculum strongly influences persister frequency and can mask effects of mutations implicated in altered persistence. *Journal of Bacteriology, 193*(14), 3598–3605. https://doi.org/10.1128/JB.00085-11.

MacKenzie, F. M., & Gould, I. M. (1993). The post-antibiotic effect. *The Journal of Antimicrobial Chemotherapy, 32*(4), 519–537.

Marques, C. N. H., Morozov, A., Planzos, P., & Zelaya, H. M. (2014). The fatty acid signaling molecule Cis-2-decenoic acid increases metabolic activity and reverts persister cells to an antimicrobial-susceptible state. *Applied and Environmental Microbiology, 80*(22), 6976–6991. https://doi.org/10.1128/AEM.01576-14.

Matilla, M. A. (2018). Shedding light into the mechanisms of formation and resuscitation of persistent bacterial cells. *Environmental Microbiology, 20*(9), 3129–3131. https://doi.org/10.1111/1462-2920.14334.

Mizunaga, S., Kamiyama, T., Fukuda, Y., Takahata, M., & Mitsuyama, J. (2005). Influence of inoculum size of *Staphylococcus aureus* and *Pseudomonas aeruginosa* on in vitro activities and in vivo efficacy of fluoroquinolones and carbapenems. *Journal of Antimicrobial Chemotherapy, 56*(1), 91–96. https://doi.org/10.1093/jac/dki163.

Mukamolova, G. V., Kaprelyants, A. S., Young, D. I., Young, M., & Kell, D. B. (1998). A bacterial cytokine. *Proceedings of the National Academy of Sciences of the United States of America, 95*(15), 8916–8921. https://doi.org/10.1073/pnas.95.15.8916.

Mukamolova, G. V., Murzin, A. G., Salina, E. G., Demina, G. R., Kell, D. B., Kaprelyants, A. S., & Young, M. (2006). Muralytic activity of *Micrococcus luteus* Rpf and its relationship to physiological activity in promoting bacterial growth and resuscitation. *Molecular Microbiology, 59*(1), 84–98. https://doi.org/10.1111/j.1365-2958.2005.04930.x.

Mulvey, M. A., Schilling, J. D., & Hultgren, S. J. (2001). Establishment of a persistent *Escherichia coli* reservoir during the acute phase of a bladder infection. *Infection and Immunity, 69*(7), 4572–4579. https://doi.org/10.1128/IAI.69.7.4572-4579.2001.

Mysorekar, I. U., & Hultgren, S. J. (2006). Mechanisms of uropathogenic *Escherichia coli* persistence and eradication from the urinary tract. *Proceedings of the National Academy of Sciences of the United States of America, 103*(38), 14170–14175. https://doi.org/10.1073/pnas.0602136103.

Nikitushkin, V. D., Demina, G. R., Shleeva, M. O., Guryanova, S. V., Ruggiero, A., Berisio, R., & Kaprelyants, A. S. (2015). A product of {RpfB} and {RipA} joint enzymatic action promotes the resuscitation of dormant mycobacteria. *FEBS Journal, 282*(13), 2500–2511. https://doi.org/10.1111/febs.13292.

Oliver, J. D. (2005). The viable but nonculturable state in bacteria. *Journal of Microbiology (Seoul, Korea), 43*, 93–100.

Oliver, J. D., Hite, F., McDougal, D., Andon, N. L., & Simpson, L. M. (1995). Entry into, and resuscitation from, the viable but nonculturable state by *Vibrio vulnificus* in an estuarine environment. *Applied and Environmental Microbiology, 61*(7), 2624–2630.

Park, J. T., & Uehara, T. (2008). How bacteria consume their own exoskeletons (turnover and recycling of cell wall peptidoglycan). *Microbiology and Molecular Biology Reviews, 72*(2), 211–227. https://doi.org/10.1128/MMBR.00027-07.

Pin, C., & Baranyi, J. (2008). Single-cell and population lag times as a function of cell age. *Applied and Environmental Microbiology, 74*(8), 2534–2536. https://doi.org/10.1128/AEM.02402-07.

Pinto, D., Almeida, V., Almeida Santos, M., & Chambel, L. (2011). Resuscitation of *Escherichia coli* VBNC cells depends on a variety of environmental or chemical stimuli. *Journal of Applied Microbiology, 110*(6), 1601–1611. https://doi.org/10.1111/j.1365-2672.2011.05016.x.

Porter, J., Edwards, C., & Pickup, R. W. (1995). Rapid assessment of physiological status in *Escherichia coli* using fluorescent probes. *The Journal of Applied Bacteriology, 79*(4), 399–408.

Pu, Y., Li, Y., Jin, X., Tian, T., Qi, M., Zhao, Z., Lin, S.-Y., et al. (2018). ATP-dependent dynamic protein aggregation regulates bacterial dormancy depth critical for antibiotic tolerance. *Molecular Cell*. https://doi.org/10.1016/j.molcel.2018.10.022

Rappé, M. S., & Giovannoni, S. J. (2003). The uncultured microbial majority. *Annual Review of Microbiology, 57*, 369–394. https://doi.org/10.1146/annurev.micro.57.030502.090759.

Ravagnani, A., Finan, C. L., & Young, M. (2005). A novel firmicute protein family related to the actinobacterial resuscitation-promoting factors by non-orthologous domain displacement. TL - 6. *BMC Genomics, 6*, 39. https://doi.org/10.1186/1471-2164-6-39.

Reasoner, D. J., & Geldreich, E. E. (1985). A new medium for the enumeration and subculture of bacteria from potable water. *Applied and Environmental Microbiology, 49*(1), 1–7.

Rosen, D. A., Hooton, T. M., Stamm, W. E., Humphrey, P. A., & Hultgren, S. J. (2007). Detection of intracellular bacterial communities in human urinary tract infection. *PLoS Medicine, 4*(12), e329. https://doi.org/10.1371/journal.Pmed.0040329.

Shah, I. M., Laaberki, M.-H. H., Popham, D. L., & Dworkin, J. (2008). A eukaryotic-like {Ser/Thr} kinase signals bacteria to exit dormancy in response to peptidoglycan fragments. *Cell, 135*(3), 486–496. https://doi.org/10.1016/j.cell.2008.08.039.

Skjot-Rasmussen, L., Hammerum, A. M., Jakobsen, L., Lester, C. H., Larsen, P., & Frimodt-Moller, N. (2011). Persisting clones of *Escherichia coli* isolates from recurrent urinary tract infection in men and women. *Journal of Medical Microbiology, 60*(4), 550–554. https://doi.org/10.1099/jmm.0.026963-0.

Srimani, J. K., Huang, S., Lopatkin, A. J., & You, L. (2017). Drug detoxification dynamics explain the postantibiotic effect. *Molecular Systems Biology, 13*(10), 948–948. https://doi.org/10.15252/msb.20177723.

Stewart, E. J. (2012). Growing unculturable bacteria. *Journal of Bacteriology, 194*(16), 4151–4160. https://doi.org/10.1128/JB.00345-12.

Vázquez-Laslop, N., Lee, H., & Neyfakh, A. A. (2006). Increased persistence in *Escherichia coli* caused by controlled expression of toxins or other unrelated proteins. *Journal of Bacteriology, 188*(10), 3494–3497. https://doi.org/10.1128/JB.188.10.3494-3497.2006.

Zhanel, G. G., & Craig, W. A. (1994). Pharmacokinetic contributions to postantibiotic effects. *Clinical Pharmacokinetics, 27*(5), 377–392. https://doi.org/10.2165/00003088-199427050-00005.

Zimmermann, R., Iturriaga, R., & Becker-Birck, J. (1978). Simultaneous determination of the total number of aquatic bacteria and the number thereof involved in respiration. *Applied and Environmental Microbiology, 36*(6), 926–935.

Chapter 10
Host–Pathogen Interactions Influencing *Mycobacterium tuberculosis* Persistence and Drug Tolerance

Huiqing Zheng and Robert B. Abramovitch

Abstract *Mycobacterium tuberculosis* (Mtb) infection stimulates host immune responses that limit bacterial replication. During pathogenesis, the bacterium must sense and adapt to a variety of stressful environments including nutrient limitation, hypoxia, and acidification of the environment. These cues can drive the bacterium to establish a state of non-replicating persistence (NRP). NRP bacteria are tolerant to antibiotics and are thought to play a role in the months long course of tuberculosis (TB) therapy. Therefore, understanding the molecular mechanisms of Mtb establishment and maintenance of NRP will provide key insights into Mtb pathogenesis and present new drug targets that may shorten the course of TB therapy. In this chapter, we will examine host–pathogen dynamics that are associated with Mtb persistence and drug tolerance, including the use of in vitro and in vivo models to study Mtb persistence. Specific in vitro models of NRP will be examined, with a focus on nutrient starvation, hypoxia and acidic pH as host-relevant environments that promote NRP. Therapeutic strategies to control Mtb persistence will be also examined, with a focus on newly discovered compounds that target redox homeostasis, cell envelope integrity, respiration and ATP homeostasis, and the DosRST signaling pathway.

10.1 Introduction

During the golden era of antibiotic discovery in the mid-twentieth century, many new antibiotics were discovered that are still currently in use to treat infectious diseases. However, over time, antibiotics have become less effective at controlling bacterial infections. Treatment failure is due, in part, to the rise of drug-resistant strains that have acquired genetic elements to inactivate or efflux antibiotics or strains with mutations in drug targets that modulate drug–target interactions.

H. Zheng · R. B. Abramovitch (✉)
Department of Microbiology and Molecular Genetics, Michigan State University, East Lansing, MI, USA
e-mail: abramov5@msu.edu

© Springer Nature Switzerland AG 2019
K. Lewis (ed.), *Persister Cells and Infectious Disease*,
https://doi.org/10.1007/978-3-030-25241-0_10

Another factor driving treatment failure and the evolution of drug resistance is the phenomenon of bacterial persistence, which was first described by Hobby et al. (1942). At that time, scientists noticed that there existed a small fraction of a treated *Staphylococcus aureus* population that tolerated killing by penicillin. Pre-treatment of bacteria with a stressful condition, such as cold, or acidic pH, arrested bacterial replication and enhanced tolerance to antibiotics (Hobby et al. 1942; Bigger 1944). These populations of bacteria were referred to as persister cells.

Biphasic killing is often observed for bacterial cultures exposed to antibiotics under growth permissive conditions (Balaban et al. 2004). Treatment with antibiotics initiates rapid killing of the majority of bacteria in a population, however, a population of persister cells will often remain that are tolerant to the antibiotic. These persister cells are thought to be responsible, in part, for phenotypic tolerance to antibiotics. Persisters emerge through two general mechanisms (1) persisters may represent a small subpopulation of metabolically distinct bacteria ($<0.1\%$) in a replicating population that are naturally tolerant to antibiotics (Kint et al. 2012) and (2) persisters may emerge when the bacterial population responds to stressful conditions, such as hypoxia, acidic pH, or nutrient starvation (Nathan 2012). Persisters are also observed during infections where bacteria in the host are exposed to host immune pressures that trigger a population of bacteria to cease or limit replication. Both mechanisms of bacterial persistence promote antibiotic tolerance and treatment failure.

The focus of this chapter will be on the pathogen *Mycobacterium tuberculosis* (Mtb), where persistence plays an important role in both pathogenesis and antibiotic efficacy. Mtb requires a 6-month long course of multidrug therapy to achieve a cure. This long course of therapy and the requirement for multiple antibiotics with different mechanisms of action is motivated, in part, by the difficulty of killing all of the persistent, drug-tolerant bacteria that are naturally associated with tuberculosis (TB) infection. Mtb persistence can be induced by host-immune pressures that function to limit Mtb replication. These different immune pressures (e.g., hypoxia, nutrient restriction, or low pH) can exert their influence singly or in combination to place different metabolic constraints on bacterial physiology. Mtb has evolved mechanisms to alter its physiology to maintain viability, with limited or no replication, to overcome these challenging host immune obstacles. Recent studies have advanced our understanding of Mtb persistence. This chapter will survey host–pathogen interactions and environmental cues that drive Mtb into a state of non-replicating persistence (NRP), the biological consequences of persistence, models for studying persistence, and chemical biology approaches to define new strategies to control persisters.

10.2 Host–Pathogen Interactions that Promote Mtb NRP and Drug Tolerance

Mtb is an intracellular pathogen that during the initial phase of infection colonizes macrophages. Following phagocytosis, Mtb arrests phagosome maturation and resides in a vacuole where it is exposed to an initial burst of ROS from the NADPH oxidase, a mildly acidic pH and restricted access to nutrients, and metal ion cofactors (Rohde et al. 2007a; Sturgill-Koszycki et al. 1996). Genetic and chemical biology studies support that Mtb is particularly reliant on cholesterol and fatty acids as a nutrient source while residing in the macrophage phagosome (VanderVen et al. 2015; Pandey and Sassetti 2008; Daniel et al. 2011; McKinney et al. 2000). As infection progresses, the bacterium permeabilizes the phagosome membrane to gain access to the cytosol (Manzanillo et al. 2012; van der Wel et al. 2007), which will presumably neutralize the phagosome to the macrophage cytoplasm pH [~pH 7.0–7.3 (Swallow et al. 1989)] and provide access to a broader array of nutrients that are present in the host cytoplasm. Once established in macrophages, Mtb is capable of robust replication. Alternatively, in inflammatory environments, Mtb is trafficked to a more acidic phagosome or lysosomes, and experiences increased exposure to ROS and RNI, which would present additional stresses upon bacterial physiology. These stresses can function to kill Mtb or severely limit its growth.

Infected macrophages release cytokines and chemokines that initiate the formation of a granuloma around the infected macrophages (Russell 2007). The granuloma develops a fibrotic cuff around a collection of foamy macrophage and other immune cells. This structure limits the bacterium from disseminating in the body and also restricts its access to oxygen, as the core of the granuloma is not vascularized. Over time, the cells in the granuloma die, and the bacterium becomes encased in a dense matrix of caseum, composed of cholesterol, fatty acids, and other remnants of host cells. Mtb requires oxygen for growth and therefore, in response to the granuloma, it establishes a non-replicating persistent (NRP) state. Mtb has altered physiology and metabolism during NRP, including changes to its cell envelope (it loses its normal acid-fastness) and altered gene expression and metabolism (Galagan et al. 2013). Human granulomas have been shown to also be acidic environments (Kempker et al. 2017). Therefore, multiple host stresses in the granuloma can contribute to Mtb persistence including low oxygen, acidic pH, and nutrient availability, with the carbon sources enriched for cholesterol, fatty acids and proinflammatory lipids (Guerrini et al. 2018; Marakalala et al. 2016; Prideaux et al. 2015), and limited iron availability (Kurthkoti et al. 2017). Further complicating the impact on the bacterium, granulomas can exist in various stages of development during infection and this spectrum of disease will enable the bacterium to sample a variety of different environments with different combinations and intensities of immune pressures (Barry et al. 2009).

Interactions of Mtb with the host also drive the bacterium to develop phenotypic tolerance to antibiotics (Gold and Nathan 2017a). Drug tolerance can occur by multiple distinct mechanisms in both replicating and non-replicating Mtb. Shortly after macrophage infection and before granuloma formation, when Mtb is replicating, Mtb becomes tolerant to antibiotics such as isoniazid (INH) and rifampin (RIF) (Adams et al. 2011; Liu et al. 2016). Macrophage-induced resistance has been associated with the induction of bacterial efflux pumps (Adams et al. 2011) and tolerance has also associated with macrophage nitric oxide (NO) an acidic pH (Liu et al. 2016). It is not yet clear which cues are driving the induction of efflux pumps in the macrophage and if drug tolerance is due to a mechanism that may be independent of efflux pump induction. NO can poison the electron transport chain and reduce replication, which may function to promote drug tolerance independent of efflux. Mtb also exhibits drug tolerance during NRP in vitro and in vivo in granulomas. For example, it has been shown that in a rabbit infection model, intracaseum Mtb becomes highly tolerant to a broad array of antibiotics, where INH, kanamycin, and clofazamine are completely inactive, and other antibiotics such as RIF, bedaquiline, linezolid, and pyrazinamide (PZA) have significantly less potent activities (Sarathy et al. 2018). Furthermore, in non-human primate models [both macaques (Lin et al. 2012) and marmosets (Via et al. 2015)] it is shown that reduced sterilizing activity is associated with well-formed granulomas. This observation could be the combination of reduced drug penetration and the presence of persisters in the granuloma. As described below, Mtb becomes phenotypically drug tolerant in in vitro models and it is probable that this tolerance is translated to NRP bacteria in vivo. Thus, residence in the granuloma and NRP Mtb are associated with drug tolerance, supporting a role for NRP in both Mtb pathogenesis and antibiotic susceptibility.

10.3 In Vitro Models to Study NRP in Mtb

Mtb infection in animals generates a complex and heterogeneous immune environment, including the difficult to study granuloma environment. In vitro models of Mtb persistence are, thus, important tools to begin dissecting the genetic and biochemical foundations of Mtb persistence, with the caveat that each specialized model may not adequately reflect the more complex infection in vivo. Several well-characterized models of Mtb persistence have been developed and are reviewed in detail by Gibson et al. (2018). These models vary in their specifics but generally drive Mtb into NRP by culturing the bacteria in a stress-inducing conditions such as (1) starvation, (2) hypoxia, or (3) acidic pH. Other dormancy models have been developed including nitric oxide (Voskuil et al. 2003), vitamin C (Taneja et al. 2010) both of which likely function through modulating respiration and have shared adaptive pathways with hypoxia. Additionally, several variants of a multi-stress model that combine stresses such as nutrient starvation, hypoxia, and acidic pH, have been developed in an attempt to better mimic the mixture of stresses encountered in vivo (Deb et al. 2009; Rodrigues Felix et al. 2017; Warrier et al. 2015; Gold et al. 2015). A common theme of these dormancy models is a decrease in ATP levels and metabolic activity, where the bacterium is likely to have limited protein, DNA, or cell envelope synthesis (Bald et al. 2017). Drug tolerance is thus often seen for antibiotics targeting these less active pathways.

1. Nutrient Starvation

The Loebel model is a commonly employed model of starvation-induced NRP (Loebel et al. 1933). In this model, of which there are several variants, bacteria are grown in rich medium, pelleted, and resuspended in a medium without a nutrient source (e.g., phosphate-buffered saline). The bacteria are then cultured, usually without shaking, for a period of time (days to weeks) after which the bacteria cease replication and severely limit respiration (Betts et al. 2002; Gengenbacher et al. 2010). The bacteria, however, remain viable as they can be recovered when transferred to permissive growth conditions. NRP Mtb in this model become tolerant to diverse antibiotics, including INH, RIF, PZA, streptomycin, moxifloxacin, linezolid, kanamycin, clofazamine, and bedaquiline (Sarathy et al. 2018; Betts et al. 2002; Gengenbacher et al. 2010). In this state of NRP the bacterium still requires basic metabolic activities for survival, including ATP homeostasis and the metabolic enzyme isocitrate lyase (Gengenbacher et al. 2010). Additionally, the stringent response is required for Mtb to adapt to and survive sudden starvation, as a *relA* deletion mutant has significantly reduced survival as compared to the wild type when starved (Primm et al. 2000). Further evidence supports that starvation-induced NRP is an adaptive process because transcriptional profiling experiments show Mtb undergoes broad regulatory and metabolic remodeling (Betts et al. 2002). In common with other in vitro models of NRP, starved Mtb exhibits a downregulation of genes associated with growth (e.g., genes related to respiration and protein expression); however, the transcriptional profiles are sufficiently different from hypoxia and acidic pH, to support that nutrient starvation is a distinct adaptive state and NRP model.

2. Hypoxia

The interior of granulomas, even small granulomas, in diverse animal models including guinea pigs, rabbits, and non-human primates are highly hypoxic as evidenced by the use of oxygen sensors or hypoxia-detecting dyes such as pimonidazole (Mehra et al. 2015; Via et al. 2008). Hypoxia is thought to be a key player in driving Mtb into a state of NRP during infection, as oxygen is the primary terminal electron acceptor employed by Mtb for respiration during growth (Boshoff and Barry 2005). Alternative pathways may support basal respiration and maintenance of membrane potential during extended hypoxia-inducible NRP, such as nitrate reductase- and fumarate reductase-dependent respiration (Sohaskey 2008; Watanabe et al. 2011). In vitro models of Mtb hypoxia-dependent NRP have proven to be valuable tools for studying the key concepts in Mtb persistence.

The in vitro Wayne model has been widely employed to study hypoxia-driven NRP in Mtb (Wayne and Hayes 1996). In this model, bacteria are grown in a rich medium in a sealed screw cap tube with stirring. A defined head-space ratio, initial inoculum, and stirring rate, allows the slow and controlled decrease in oxygen levels as bacteria grow and consume oxygen. In the Wayne model, two distinct phases are observed in a time-dependent manner, including NRP1 (initiated at ~1% oxygen) and NRP2 (initiated at <0.06% oxygen). At NRP1, the bacilli cease replication and thicken their cell wall, while at NRP2 the bacilli become anaerobic-adapted bacteria and no longer increase in optical density (Chao and Rubin 2010). Notably, the bacteria exhibit distinct transcriptional responses during NRP1 and NRP2, which have been referred to as the initial and enduring hypoxic response, respectively (Rustad et al. 2008). NRP Mtb in the Wayne model become highly tolerant to diverse antibiotics, including near complete tolerance to INH (Sarathy et al. 2018; Gengenbacher et al. 2010).

The Wayne model represents a gradual reduction of oxygen and provides Mtb a window to adapt its physiology to the stress. Alternatively, Mtb can be driven into a state of NRP by more rapidly removing oxygen from the culture. Two such models include the Rapid Anaerobic Dormancy (RAD) model (Leistikow et al. 2010) and the hypoxic shiftdown model (Mak et al. 2012). In the RAD model, Mtb is cultured in sealed tubes similar to the Wayne model, however, the cultures are stirred more quickly with larger stir bars to promote aeration, growth, and an earlier onset of hypoxia. In the hypoxic shiftdown model, Mtb is cultured in Dubos medium and placed in an anaerobic chamber. The removal of the oxygen from the chamber combined with the consumption of the residual oxygen by Mtb in the medium, causes a rapid (~2 day) depletion of oxygen in the medium and promotes NRP. An advantage of the hypoxic shiftdown model is that it is amenable to high throughput screening methods (Mak et al. 2012), which are less practical in the Wayne or RAD models.

Using these models key physiological adaptations associated with hypoxia and NRP have been discovered, and have been reviewed in detail elsewhere (Peddireddy et al. 2017; Rustad et al. 2009; Gengenbacher and Kaufmann 2012). A key regulator of hypoxia-dependent adaptation was identified and named the DosRST (Boon and Dick 2002) or DevRST (Saini et al. 2004a, b; Malhotra et al. 2004) pathway (referred to by the DosRST nomenclature from here on). DosRST is a two-component regulatory systems that functions to establish and maintain NRP. It is composed of two histidine kinase sensors, DosS and DosT, and the cognate response regulator DosR (Park et al. 2003), which regulates expression of approximately 50 genes in the DosR regulon (Voskuil et al. 2003). Mtb can sense a variety of environmental cues, including nitric oxide, carbon monoxide, vitamin C, and oxygen, through DosS and DosT (Voskuil et al. 2003; Taneja et al. 2010; Vos et al. 2012; Kumar et al. 2007; Ohno et al. 2003; Roberts et al. 2004).

Upon receiving the environmental signals, DosS/T catalyzes an ATP-dependent autophosphorylation at a conserved histidine and transmits the signal by phosphorylating DosR at an aspartate residue (Roberts et al. 2004). Phosphorylated DosR is active and able to regulate transcription of the regulon (Park et al. 2003; Wisedchaisri et al. 2008). DosS and DosT share extensive amino acid sequence similarity, ~61%, and have structural homology. Each contains two N-terminal GAF domains (c*G*MP, *a*denylyl cyclase, *F*hlA), a HisKA domain (histidine kinase phospho-acceptor) where a phosphoryl group-accepting histidine is located, and a C-terminal HATPase domain (histidine kinase-like ATPase) that is the ATP-binding site (Sardiwal et al. 2005; Sivaramakrishnan and de Montellano 2013). The GAF domain functions as a small molecule binding regulatory domain that is present throughout prokaryotes and eukaryotes. Specifically, a *b*-type heme is embedded in the hydrophobic cavity of the GAF-A domain of DosS and DosT (Cho et al. 2009; Podust et al. 2008). Even though DosS and DosT are heme-based sensor proteins sharing a similar structure, their biochemical mechanism of signal sensing is different. For instance, DosS is a redox and oxygen sensor and autoxidizes quickly under aerobic conditions (Ioanoviciu et al. 2007). In contrast, DosT is a hypoxia sensor and has high affinity and sensitivity to O_2 (Cho et al. 2011). Both kinases sense O_2 or other ligands via heme, and are inactive when the heme group exists as either the Met (Fe^{3+}) form (DosS) or the oxy (Fe^{2+}–O_2) form (DosT) in the presence of O_2. However, hypoxic conditions induce the conversion of DosS to the ferrous form and DosT to the deoxy form, activating the kinases (Kumar et al. 2007; Cho et al. 2009; Podust et al. 2008; Ioanoviciu et al. 2007; Sousa et al. 2007). Therefore, DosS/T plays different roles in sensing the redox and oxygen status of the environment to turn on the DosR pathway.

The DosRST pathway plays important roles in vitro and in vivo to promote survival during NRP and virulence. For instance, in the Wayne, RAD and hypoxic shiftdown models, deletion of *dosR* causes a significant loss of viability as bacilli fail to establish NRP (Leistikow et al. 2010; Boon and Dick 2002; Zheng et al. 2017). In the RAD model, there is also a delay in the mutant in recovery after re-inoculating the NRP cells into aerobic conditions (Leistikow et al. 2010). These findings suggest that DosR plays a functional role for Mtb to enter, exit, and survive during NRP. The Δ*dosR* mutant during NRP shows sharply reduced intracellular ATP and NAD, ~10-fold and ~50%-fold lower than WT, respectively (Leistikow et al. 2010). The Δ*dosRS* mutant also exhibits a growth defect in several animal models, including rabbits, guinea pigs, C3HeB/FeJ mice, and non-human primates (Mehra et al. 2015; Converse et al. 2009; Gautam et al. 2015). For instance, rabbits infected with the Δ*dosRS* mutant display significantly lower lung bacterial burdens at 8-week infection than those infected with WT. WT Mtb also stimulates formation of numerous intense and organized lesions in the lungs at week 5, whereas the mutant exhibits fewer lesions (Converse et al. 2009). In the guinea pig model of TB infection, Δ*dosRS* shows a 3-log reduction lung CFUs as compared to the WT at week 6. The mutant also causes less virulence, such as lack of formation of mature granulomas, while WT induces massive inflammation and lesions with central necrosis (Converse et al. 2009). Furthermore, in the C3HeB/FeJ mouse model of TB infection, infection with Δ*dosS* leads to 0.5- and 1.5-log lower lung CFUs than infection with WT at week 8 and 12, respectively (Gautam et al. 2015). Δ*dosS* also results in 1–1.5 log less liver CFUs at week 12 and 15, respectively, as compared to WT. In the rhesus macaques model of TB infection, all mutants, including Δ*dosR*, Δ*dosS,* and Δ*dosST*, exhibit lower bacterial burden than WT (Mehra et al. 2015). Specifically, the mutant strains have at least a 100-fold lower lung bacterial burden compared to WT. Little or no TB-related pathology and granuloma formation are observed in the animals infected with the mutant, while WT or complemented strains initiate formation of numerous granulomas with necrosis in the central area (Mehra et al. 2015). It is possible that the reduced granuloma formation is due to a lower number of bacteria in the lungs. Alternatively, changes in the immune response to the *dosR* mutants, which have altered metabolism that impacts the synthesis of immunostimulatory cell envelope lipids (Galagan et al. 2013), may function to limit granuloma formation. All these animal models form well-organized hypoxia-associated granulomas when infected with Mtb, which mimics the pathology observed in humans.

The DosR-regulated genes also play a role in modulating metabolism and drug tolerance. For example, *tgs1* is a DosR-regulated gene that is highly induced during hypoxic conditions (Rustad et al. 2008; Park et al. 2003; Zheng et al. 2017). It encodes a triacylglycerol (TAG) synthase, which is involved in the last step of TAG biosynthesis. An Mtb *tgs1* mutant strain exhibits reduced tolerance to several antibiotics, such as INH and ciprofloxacin, in vitro and in vivo (Deb et al. 2009; Baek et al. 2011). Interestingly, the *tgs*1 mutant also exhibits enhanced growth compared to the wild type during hypoxia. It was shown that the carbon that is normally used to generate TAG, is instead supplied to the TCA cycle to promote enhanced growth in the mutant. Therefore, DosR may function to slow Mtb growth by diverting carbon to TAG anabolism. Given that Mtb has limited respiration, TAG anabolism may also present a mechanism to oxidize cofactors, such as NADPH, which may accumulate when respiration is limited (Farhana et al. 2010). Following reaeration, TAG is rapidly depleted (Galagan et al. 2013), supporting that TAG accumulation is specifically associated with the NRP state.

3. Acidic pH

Mtb has long been known to tolerate and grow in rich medium at acidic pH (Chapman and Bernard 1962; Portaels and Pattyn 1982). In 7H9 OADC with 0.05% Tween-80 medium buffered at various pH, Mtb will exhibit optimal growth above pH 6.5, slowed growth between pH 6.0 and 5.5 and then no growth at pH 5.0 (Abramovitch et al. 2011). At pH 4.5, Mtb is killed, but this cell death is dependent on the presence of Tween detergent in the medium (Vandal et al. 2008). In a defined medium, however, Mtb is much more sensitive to acidification of the medium. Piddington et al. showed that in a defined sauton's medium (where glycerol is the primary carbon source) at pH 6.0, Mtb cannot grow in medium with low levels of magnesium (10 μM), but grows well under the same conditions at pH 7.0 (Piddington et al. 2000). Later, Baker et al. showed that in defined medium, growth at acidic pH is dependent on the provided carbon source (Baker et al. 2014). For example, when incubated in medium with single carbon sources that fuel glycolysis, such as glycerol or glucose, Mtb cannot grow at pH 5.7 but grows well at pH 7.0. In contrast, providing Mtb with carbon sources that fuel the PEP-pyruvate-oxaloacetate anaplerotic node (Sauer and Eikmanns 2005), such as pyruvate, acetate, or choles-terol, Mtb can grow almost equally well at pH 5.7 or pH 7.0. Indeed, key enzymes associated with anaplerosis, such as phosphoenolpyruvate carboxykinase (*pckA*), isocitrate lyase (*icl1/2*), malic enzyme, (*mez*), and pyruvate phosphate dikinase (*ppdK*) are differentially regulated by acidic pH and both *pckA* and *icl1/2* are required for optimal growth at acidic pH (Baker and Abramovitch 2018). These findings support the existence of a pH-dependent checkpoint on Mtb metabolism.

Mtb fully arrests its growth when cultured in the minimal medium at pH 5.7 with glycerol as a sole carbon source. However, the bacterium remains fully viable for at least 40 days (Baker and Abramovitch 2018), and growth can be restored by the addition of a permissive carbon source such as pyruvate (Baker et al. 2014). These observations support that Mtb establishes NRP in response to acidic environments and specific carbon sources. This model of NRP has been named "acid growth arrest." Bacteria under acid growth arrest are metabolically active as they can uptake radiolabeled glycerol and metabolize it into cell envelope and storage lipids (Baker and Abramovitch 2018). These NRP bacteria also exhibit tolerance to antibiotics such as INH and RIF, and resistance to detergent treatment (Baker and Abramovitch 2018). Transcriptional profiles of Mtb at acidic pH in rich medium and acid growth arrest (Baker et al. 2014; Fisher et al. 2002; Rohde et al. 2007b; Johnson et al. 2015), show similarities, including the induction of the PhoPR regulon (Walters et al. 2006) and the downregulation of genes associated with growth. However, the profiles are distinct from the profiles obtained from hypoxia and NO treatment (which are associated with DosRST signaling) or nutrient starvation, supporting that acid growth arrest is a distinct model of NRP.

Mtb slowed growth at acidic pH is also oxygen dependent, where bacteria have reduced growth at pH 5.5 under hypoxia and growth is improved by the addition of nitrate (Tan et al. 2010). Additionally, acidic pH modulates genes associated with the electron transport chain with downregulation of the proton-translocating NADH dehydrogenase and upregulation of the non-proton-translocating NADH dehydrogenase (Baker et al. 2014). This finding suggests that acidic pH limits growth, in part, by modulating respiration, a finding further supported by the lack of drug tolerance during acid growth arrest to the PA-824 (Baker and Abramovitch 2018), a drug that inhibits respiration by generating intracellular NO (Singh et al. 2008). During acid growth arrest, however, sufficient oxygen and glycerol are available to support growth, indicating that changes in respiration are not due to availability of a terminal electron acceptor or carbon source. Indeed, in a genetic screen, mutants were isolated that do not arrest their growth at acidic pH (Baker and Abramovitch 2018). The enhanced acid growth mutants had point mutations in the PPE51 gene, and it is hypothesized that these mutations enable Mtb improved access to glycerol or another nutrient that is required for growth at acidic pH (such as magnesium). Together, these observations support that acid growth arrest is an adaptive process by which the bacterium limits metabolism at acidic pH to establish NRP.

10.4   In Vivo Models to Study NRP in Mtb

Studying NRP and replication of Mtb in infected animals is complicated by the heterogeneous environment of the infection and ability of animal models to appropriately mimic human pathology. For example, in common mouse models, such as

BALB/C or C57Bl/6 mice, Mtb infection does not cause the formation of hypoxic, caseonecrotic granulomas that are believed to be a major reservoir of NRP, drug-tolerant bacteria in humans. Mouse models have been developed where Mtb does elicit the formation of caseonecrotic granulomas including the C3HeB/FeJ "Kramnik" mouse model (Kramnik et al. 1998, 2000), and the IL-10 knockout mouse (Cyktor et al. 2013). In the C3HeB/FeJ infection model, the granuloma becomes hypoxic, the DosR pathway is strongly induced and the bacterium becomes tolerant to antibiotics (Driver et al. 2012; Harper et al. 2012). However, the model may not adequately replicate NRP in humans, as the C3HeB/FeJ granuloma has a neutral pH (Lanoix et al. 2016), as compared to the rabbit and human granulomas which are acidic (Kempker et al. 2017; Dannenberg 2006). Other animal models that generate hypoxic, caseonecrotic granulomas appropriate for studying NRP physiologies, including the rabbit, guinea pig, and non-human primates (NHP) such as cynomolgus macaque and marmoset. Transcriptional profiling of Mtb isolated from microdissected granulomas of macaques with the active or latent disease showed enhanced induction of genes associated with hypoxia and persistence (Hudock et al. 2017).

One of the key questions of interest during chronic Mtb infection, where the bacteria cease to increase in numbers, is whether the bacteria have slowed or ceased replication, or are growing with a balanced rate of cell death. One method to address this question in vivo is to compare CFUs and the abundance of bacterial chromosomes from infected tissues using quantitative real-time PCR (Munoz-Elias et al. 2005). Using this approach, during the chronic stage of infection in C57Bl/6 mice, Mtb was shown to slow its growth with an estimated doubling time of 70 days (Munoz-Elias et al. 2005). An alternative approach to studying replication in vivo is the use of an unstable replication "clock" plasmid (Gill et al. 2009). The plasmid is lost during replication with a defined frequency; therefore, bacteria populations that are replicating faster will have reduced frequency of carrying the plasmid. Isolating bacteria from infected mouse lungs and enumerating CFUs with or without the plasmid present enables a calculation of replication rate in vivo. This model found that Mtb has a doubling time during chronic infection in C57/Bl6 mice of between 54 and 134 h (Gill et al. 2009), supporting a model where the bacteria are growing during infection and that the growth is balanced by bacterial cell death. The difference between the two methods of examining in vivo replication maybe due to the stability of genomic DNA in infected tissues. Therefore, chronic infection C57Bl/6 mice may not represent an appropriate model to study NRP. It will be important to define replication rates in animal models that form hypoxic, necrotic granulomas, to better define Mtb replication dynamics and NRP in vivo.

10.5   Therapeutic Strategies to Control Bacterial Persistence

Bacterial persisters are thought to present an important reservoir of drug-tolerant bacteria during Mtb infection. Thus, compounds that disrupt survival during persistence have the potential to shorten therapy, a sought-after property for new drugs to improve outcomes of TB therapy. There exist numerous different targets and small molecules that can be employed to kill NRP Mtb, impacting physiologies as diverse as modulating metabolism, redox homeostasis, antibiotic uptake/efflux, respiration, bacterial proteases, ATP homeostasis, cell envelope and membrane integrity, and signaling pathways. This chapter will select a few specific examples of strategies to target persisters in Mtb and the reader is directed to other recent reviews for additional information on mechanisms of controlling bacterial persistence (Nathan 2012; Gold and Nathan 2017b).

10.5.1   Reactive Oxygen Species Sensitize Persister Cells to Antibiotic Treatment

Persister cells that are present within a bacterial population have enhanced survival under a variety of stress conditions (Lewis 2007). However, several reports have shown that persisters are sensitive to specific intracellular stress signals, such as reactive oxygen species (ROS). Grant et al. showed that increasing ROS in *Mycobacterium smegmatis*, by incubating the culture under aerobic conditions with dissolved oxygen saturation of 95%, potentiates killing of spontaneously occurring persisters by antibiotics (Grant et al. 2012). The oxygen-dependent phenotype is rescued by adding the OH· scavenger thiourea, suggesting that persisters are sensitive to ROS. Supporting this model, treating *M. smegmatis* cultures with the OH· producing antibiotic clofazimine eradicates persisters. A related phenomenon is also observed in Mtb (Fig. 10.1). Treating Mtb with high concentrations of vitamin C completely sterilizes the culture (Vilcheze et al. 2013). The killing is driven by increasing ROS production through Haber-Weiss and Fenton reactions. A high concentration of vitamin C also increases the level of ferrous ion through reduction of ferric ion. Ferrous ion reacts with oxygen to produce ROS, and causes DNA damage, lipid alterations, and redox stress. INH cannot sterilize a culture due to the presence of persisters, however, when INH is used in combination with vitamin C, at sublethal doses, INH can sterilize the culture. Furthermore, a recent report by Vilcheze et al. demonstrates that treating Mtb with cysteine and INH sterilizes the bacterial culture (Vilcheze et al. 2017). Cysteine functions as a reductant that can quickly reduce ferric ion to ferrous ion, which leads to increased accumulation of ROS in the presence of oxygen. Addition of cation scavengers, such as the iron chelator deferoxamine, diminishes sterilization, and the combination of cysteine and rifampin causes no additional killing to Mtb cultures grown in anaerobic conditions.

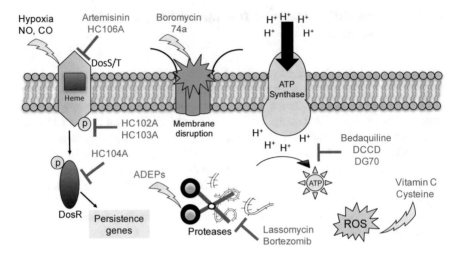

Fig. 10.1 Summary of selected pathways that can be targeted to kill persisters. Pathways that can be modulated include (1) induction of intracellular ROS overproduction; (2) activation of non-specific protease activity or inhibition of protease activity; (3) inhibition of ATP production; (4) disruption of membrane integrity; and (5) inhibition of the DosRST persistence pathway

These findings indicate that potentiation of killing by addition of cysteine is dependent on cations and oxygen. Lastly, treating cultures with cysteine and INH increases oxygen consumption of non-respiring cells, as well as shifting the balance of menaquinol/menaquinone toward menaquinol, which has been shown to control the Mtb respiration rate, thus, providing evidence that cysteine and INH can increase cellular respiration. Therefore, it is possible that cysteine can revert persister cells to metabolically active cells by stimulating their respiration. Together, these data support the hypothesis that modulating ROS production and respiration is a strategy to control persisters in mycobacterial species.

10.5.2 Modulating Respiration and Intracellular ATP Levels to Kill Persisters

Another effective strategy to eliminate persisters is to inhibit bacterial respiration and ATP synthesis (Fig. 10.1) (Bald et al. 2017). It is hypothesized that during NRP, bacteria still require some energy for survival, and further depletion of ATP synthesis will be lethal to persister cells. For instance, Rao et al. reported the intracellular ATP levels of Mtb rapidly decreases when entering NRP and then is maintained constant over 25 days of incubation in the Wayne model of hypoxia-driven NRP (Rao et al. 2008). Treating NRP Mtb bacilli with the F_0F_1 ATP synthase inhibitor bedaquiline or DCCD (N,N-dicyclohexylcarbodiimide, Fig. 10.2) dramatically decreases the ATP content, and lowers cell viability. Bedaquiline, which was FDA

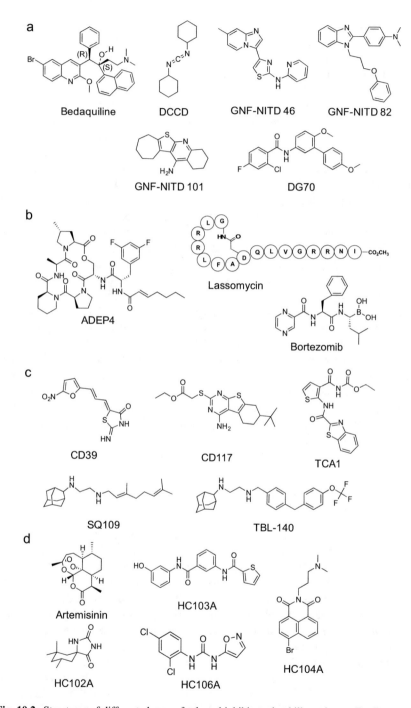

Fig. 10.2 Structures of different classes of selected inhibitors that kill persister cells. Compounds that function to (**a**) inhibit ATP synthesis (**b**) target bacterial proteases; (**c**) inhibit bacterial cell wall synthesis; and (**d**) inhibit DosRST signaling

approved for TB treatment in 2012 (Cox and Laessig 2014), is also effective in killing Mtb in a mouse model of TB infection, and sterilizes bacteria in 2 months when included with isoniazid and pyrazinamide treatment (Andries et al. 2005). The F_0F_1 ATP synthase is driven by protonmotive force (PMF). Disrupting PMF by inhibiting the membrane potential with valinomycin or disrupting the transmembrane proton concentration gradient with nigericin, also kills non-replicating Mtb (Pethe et al. 2013). This indicates that energy production is required for survival, and decreasing the ATP concentration is lethal to persisters. Similarly, Q203, which targets the cytochrome bc_1 complex of the Mtb electron transport chain, triggers rapid ATP depletion and also kills non-replicating Mtb (Pethe et al. 2013; Kalia et al. 2017). Q203 is currently in development in Phase 2 clinical trial. Additional experimental compounds targeting ATP homeostasis are in preclinical development. For instance, several inhibitors of ATP homeostasis in non-replicating Mtb were identified from high-throughput screening, including imidazopyridines (GNF-NITD 46), benzimidazole (GNF-NITD 82), and thieno [2,3-b]pyridin-4-amine (GNF-NITD 101) (Fig. 10.2) (Mak et al. 2012). All three classes of inhibitors show decreased ATP levels and bacterial survival of non-replicating Mtb. In another study, the biphenyl amide compound DG70 (Fig. 10.2) was identified from a screen that targeted non-replicating Mtb under nutrient-deprived conditions (Sukheja et al. 2017). DG70 kills both replicating and non-replicating Mtb and synergizes with other anti-mycobacterial drugs, including INH, bedaquiline, and PA824. The compound was found to inhibit oxygen consumption and ATP biosynthesis. The resistant mutants show that this compound targets the MenG protein, which is involved in the last step of menaquinone biosynthesis. This finding is confirmed by biochemical studies showing that DG70 inhibited menaquinone biosynthesis. Overall, these findings suggest that DG70 inhibits replicating and non-replicating bacteria by inhibiting Mtb respiration.

10.5.3   Targeting Bacterial Proteases to Kill Persisters

Bacterial proteases, such as Clp system caseinolytic proteases (Brotz-Oesterhelt and Sass 2014), have generated interest as new targets for antibiotic development. The protease complex generally consists of a proteolytic core, ClpP, corresponding ATP-dependent AAA+ chaperone proteins and associated adaptor proteins (Fig. 10.1). The protease targets partially synthesized and misfolded proteins, as well as cleaving specific proteins with regulatory functions. Adaptor proteins assist with binding to protease substrates, which are unfolded by the chaperone proteins and then cleaved by ClpP.

Several inhibitors of Clp have been reported to kill persisters and are in preclinical development. For instance, a newly discovered series of ClpP activators, named acyldepsipeptides (ADEPs), are potent against a broad spectrum of bacteria (Brotz-Oesterhelt et al. 2005). ADEPs activate ClpP by keeping its catalytic chamber open, allowing peptides and proteins to enter, and promoting uncontrolled protein degradation in bacterial cells. Furthermore, recent research shows that ADEP4 (Fig. 10.2) also has an effect on non-replicating persister cells (Conlon et al. 2013). Instead of triggering specific proteolytic activity, ADEP4-bound ClpP is a nonspecific protease that causes excess breakdown of proteins. *S. aureus* persisters that survive ciprofloxacin treatment are eradicated by the addition of ADEP4 (Conlon et al. 2013). ADEP4 is also effective in sterilizing stationary cultures treated with rifampicin, linezolid, or ciprofloxacin, suggesting the compound enhances the killing of persister cells (Conlon et al. 2013). Triggering nonspecific proteolytic activity is lethal to bacteria and is effective at eliminating both replicating and persister cells, indicating the idea that some essential processes can be targeted to kill persister cells.

Protease inhibitors also have been reported to function against Mtb to kill persisters. ADEPs show potential in killing Mtb, where ADEP2 was most active and shown to inhibit both Mtb enzymes ClpP1 and ClpP2, by interfering with interactions with regulatory ATPases (Ollinger et al. 2012; Famulla et al. 2016). Lassomycin (Fig. 10.2) is reported to kill both growing and non-replicating Mtb by targeting the caseinolytic protease ClpC1P1P2 (Gavrish et al. 2014). Lassomycin binds to the ATPase domain of ClpC1 and increases its ATP hydrolysis activity, but also inhibits substrate translocation from ClpC1 to the proteolytic subunits ClpP1P2 of the complex. It decreases the degradation of target cell proteins and is toxic to Mtb during stressful conditions. Additionally, the well-known human proteasome inhibitor, bortezomib (Fig. 10.2), has been shown to inhibit ClpP1P2 by covalently attaching via its boron atom to the hydroxyl group of serine at the catalytic triad (Moreira et al. 2015). Bortezomib potentiates Mtb to aminoglycoside treatment, suggesting that induction of protein mistranslation by aminoglycosides is toxic to Mtb if the proteasome is inhibited to remove incomplete translation products. To increase the selectivity of bortezomib to anti-mycobacterial activity over inhibition of the human proteasome, the boronic acid was changed to chloromethyl ketone (Moreira et al. 2017a). The newly synthesized analogs only display activity against mycobacterial ClpP1P2, but lack activity to the human proteasome. Moreover, a series of dipeptidyl boronate derivatives of bortezomib have also been synthesized (Moreira et al. 2017b). Structure relationship studies reveal several compounds with improved anti-Mtb activity and selectivity for the mycobacterial ClpP1P2 protein. Overall, these inhibitors show that ClpP protease is an attractive target that can be modulated via different mechanisms to kill bacterial persister cells.

10.5.4 Disrupting Membrane Integrity to Kill Persisters

Maintaining membrane integrity is essential for cell survival. Several studies have focused on discovering microbial membrane "disruptors" for controlling non-replicating microbes (Fig. 10.1). For instance, a screen conducted by Yang et al. identified amphiphilic indole derivatives that target *Mycobacterium bovis* BCG membrane integrity (Yang et al. 2017). These novel compounds cause BCG cell membrane depolarization and permeabilization in a time-dependent manner. The loss of membrane integrity by compound 74a is bactericidal and leads to rapid killing of replicating cells, as well as effectively killing NRP bacilli in the Wayne model of hypoxia-driven NRP. Boromycin is another example of how the cell membrane is a good target to kill persisters. This compound is a polyether macrolide antibiotic that kills Gram-positive bacteria by functioning as a potassium ionophore. Studies demonstrate that boromycin has bactericidal activity against both replicating and non-replicating Mtb under the Wayne model of hypoxia-driven NRP (Moreira et al. 2016). Like in Gram-positive bacteria, boromycin also causes a reduction of membrane potential in Mtb, as well as decreasing intracellular ATP level, suggesting it also acts as an ionophore in Mtb to collapse the potassium gradient across the membrane. A major potential drawback of membrane disruptors is the potential for host cytotoxicity, as membrane targeting agents may also interact with host membranes. Indeed, boromycin is toxic to mammals and has not been used clinically (Pache 1975; Hutter et al. 1967). Nevertheless, several compounds are in development that modulates membrane integrity, such as the approved antibiotic daptomycin (Muller et al. 2016; Hurdle et al. 2011), supporting that compounds may be identified that selectively modulate bacterial membranes.

10.5.5 Inhibition of Cell Envelope Biosynthesis Potentiates Killing of Persisters by Antibiotics

The Mtb cell envelope is composed of complex glycolipids that create a permeability barrier to the environment. The first-line antibiotic INH inhibits the enoyl-ACP reductase InhA after being activated by the catalase-peroxidase KatG to form an adduct with NAD. InhA is an essential protein involved in the synthesis of mycolic acids in Mtb. Inhibition of InhA activity causes mycobacterial cell death. Efforts to discover novel InhA inhibitors that do not require an activator identified two compounds CD39 ((Z)-2-imino-5-((E)-3-(5-nitrofuran-2-yl)allylidene)thiazolidin-4-one) and CD117 (tetrahydrobenzothienopyrimidine) (Fig. 10.2) (Vilcheze et al. 2011). They are not only bactericidal against the growing Mtb, but also active against non-replicating bacilli grown under anaerobic conditions. This finding suggests these inhibitors have different mechanisms of action from INH, because isoniazid only kills replicating bacilli (Rao et al. 2008). Both compounds enhance anti-mycobacterial activity with INH and rifampin, and inhibit mycolic acids and fatty acid biosynthesis.

TCA1 is reported to inhibit DprE1 (Fig. 10.2), a decaprenylphosphoryl-β-D-ribofuranose oxidoreductase that is involved in cell wall biosynthesis, as well as MoeW, an enzyme involved in molybdenum cofactor synthesis (Wang et al. 2013). DprE1 and DprE2 (decaprenylphosphoryl-D-2-keto erythro pentose reductase) together catalyze the epimerization of decaprenylphosphoryl ribose to decaprenylphosphoryl arabinose (Mikusova et al. 2005). Decaprenylphosphoryl arabinose is the only precursor of arabinogalactan and lipoarabinomannan poly-saccharides of the mycobacterial cell envelope. Chemical inhibition of DprE1 abolishes biosynthesis of decaprenylphosphoryl arabinose and causes cell lysis and bacterial death. There are numerous DprE1 inhibitors identified, including benzothiazinones, dinitrobenzamides, azaindoles (Shirude et al. 2013), pyrazolopyridones (Panda et al. 2014), 2-carboxyquinoxalines (Neres et al. 2015), and pyrido-benzimidazole (Warrier et al. 2016). However, TCA1 is the only inhib-itor reported to effectively kill both replicating and non-replicating Mtb in a nutrient starvation model. TCA1 also targets the MoeW protein that is involved in molyb-denum cofactor synthesis. Therefore, the activity against non-replicating Mtb may be driven by this additional activity. TCA1 sterilizes Mtb cultures treated with INH or rifampin in about 3 weeks, and shows efficacy in acute and chronic TB mouse models. Interestingly, transcriptional profiling also showed that TCA1 downregulates the persistence genes regulated by DosRST, including *rv3130c-rv3134c, fdxA*, and *hspX*, suggesting TCA1 may potentiate Mtb killing by antibiotics by inhibiting Mtb dormancy regulation or supporting a link between molybdenum cofactors and the regulation of dormancy.

The anti-mycobacterial compounds SQ109 (1,2-ethylenediamine) and TBL-140 (diphenylether-modified adamantyl 1,2-diamine, Fig. 10.2) have been shown to be bactericidal to replicating and non-replicating Mtb by modulating MmpL3 (Li et al. 2014; Foss et al. 2016). MmpL3 is a membrane-bound protein that acts as a flippase to translocate the mycolic acid precursor trehalose monomycolate (TMM) to the pseudoperiplasmic space, where TMM is further transported to the mycomembranes and modified into trehalose dimycolate (TDM) by Ag85 protein (Tahlan et al. 2012; Grzegorzewicz et al. 2012). Treating Mtb cells with SQ109 and TBL-140 inhibits the transport activity of MmpL3, and results in accumulation of TMM in the cytoplasm and thus defective TDM biosynthesis. SQ109 also inhibits membrane potential and generation of the transmembrane proton gradient, while TBL-140 inhibits membrane potential (Li et al. 2014; Foss et al. 2016). SQ109 also potentiates the killing of Mtb by first-line anti-tubercular drugs, including INH and rifampin (Chen et al. 2006). SQ109 has completed evaluation in a Phase 2b clinical trial, where it was shown to be effective and shorten the time to culture conversion (Borisov et al. 2018). Notably, several other MmpL3 inhibitors do not inhibit membrane potential, such as HC2091 (Zheng et al. 2018a), which does not kill NRP Mtb, suggesting that the membrane potential modulating activity plays a role in killing persisters.

10.5.6 Targeting Two-Component Regulatory Systems to Inhibit Bacterial Persistence

Transcriptional regulators in bacterial pathogens often play essential roles to estab-lish infection and evade host immunity. Anti-virulence therapies target virulence proteins that are not required for growth in vitro but are necessary during infection. Targeting bacterial virulence is different from conventional antibiotics that directly kill bacteria, and may reduce selection for antibiotic-resistant strains (Johnson and Abramovitch 2017).

In vitro and in vivo data support that DosRST is required for full virulence during Mtb infection and for survival during extended periods of hypoxia. Therefore, inhibiting DosRST may help reduce Mtb persistence and drug tolerance and shorten TB treatment (Fig. 10.1). Based on the homology modeling of DosR, a DosR regulon inhibitor, a phenylcoumarin derivative, was found to inhibit DosR binding to DNA (Gupta et al. 2009). Screening a phage display library allowed the discovery of short DosR mimetic peptides that inhibit the autophosphorylation activity of DosS (Kaur et al. 2014). A high throughput screen using a hypoxia and NO-inducible reporter Mtb strain has identified an additional six inhibitors, named, HC101A-HC106A that function to inhibit DosRST signaling (Fig. 10.2) (Zheng et al. 2017). HC101A is the antimalarial natural product artemisinin, which carries an endoperoxide bridge that reacts with ferrous iron in heme to form alkyl radicals that are thought to kill the malaria parasite by alkylation of parasite proteins or generation of ROS (Wang et al. 2015; Meunier and Robert 2010; Krishna et al. 2008). Chemical inhibition of the DosRST pathway by HC101A, HC102A, HC103A, and HC106A reduces Mtb persistence-associated physiologies, including TAG biosynthesis and survival (Zheng et al. 2017, 2018b); HC101A, HC102A, and HC103A also partially inhibit tolerance to INH during NRP (Zheng et al. 2017). Mechanistic studies show a specific component of the DosRST pathway is targeted by each inhibitor through distinct mechanisms. Both HC101A and HC106 target the sensor domain of DosS/T via different mechanisms, where HC101A modulates the redox status of DosS/T and alkylates the heme (Zheng et al. 2017), and HC106A likely binds directly to the heme (Zheng et al. 2018b). HC102A and HC103A are proposed to target the kinase function of DosS/T by inhibiting their autophosphorylation activities (Zheng et al. 2017). Biochemical assays indicate that HC104A functions by inhibiting DosR binding to promoter DNA (Zheng et al. 2018b). All inhibitors of the DosRST pathway are in preclinical development, although artemisinin is widely used to treat malaria and maybe potentially be repurposed for TB. These studies show that targeting the multiple domains of the DosRST signaling pathway can function to reduce Mtb signaling in response to persistence-driving cues and reduce survival of bacterial persisters.

10.6 Concluding Remarks

During the infection process, Mtb colonizes environments and stimulates immune responses that restrict Mtb growth. Mtb senses and adapts to these cues as part of pathogenesis, and a key adaptation of the bacterium is the ability to establish populations of persistent bacteria. Understanding how Mtb establishes, maintains, and exits NRP will provide us key insights into what makes Mtb such a successful pathogen. Progress has been made in understanding Mtb persistence by studying in vitro models and using reductionist approaches to define pathways associated with NRP in response to specific conditions. While it has been much more difficult to translate these findings to in vivo models, key NRP physiologies are conserved between in vitro and in vivo models. For example, in humans, strong upregulation of the DosR regulon is observed during infection (Hudock et al. 2017; Garton et al. 2008) and drugs that function against persisters in vitro are important components of a multidrug sterilizing cure in humans. A major limitation of studying persistence in vivo is the heterogeneity of the infection and the presence of both replicating and non-replicating bacteria in infected tissues. Newly developed fluorescent or luminescent reporter strains may enable in vivo studies at the single-cell level to define microenvironments that drive Mtb NRP signaling and determine the efficacy of specific antibiotics and antibiotic combinations in these NRP populations of bacteria (Abramovitch 2018; MacGilvary and Tan 2018). The combination of these reporters with animal models that develop caseonecrotic granulomas will provide an opportunity to further define host–pathogen interactions that influence Mtb persistence and drug tolerance.

References

Abramovitch, R. B. (2018). *Mycobacterium tuberculosis* reporter strains as tools for drug discovery and development. *IUBMB Life, 70*(9), 818–825. https://doi.org/10.1002/iub.1862.

Abramovitch, R. B., Rohde, K. H., Hsu, F. F., & Russell, D. G. (2011). *aprABC*: A *Mycobacterium tuberculosis* complex-specific locus that modulates pH-driven adaptation to the macrophage phagosome. *Molecular Microbiology, 80*(3), 678–694.

Adams, K. N., Takaki, K., Connolly, L. E., Wiedenhoft, H., Winglee, K., Humbert, O., Edelstein, P. H., Cosma, C. L., & Ramakrishnan, L. (2011). Drug tolerance in replicating mycobacteria mediated by a macrophage-induced efflux mechanism. *Cell, 145*(1), 39–53. https://doi.org/10.1016/j.cell.2011.02.022.

Andries, K., Verhasselt, P., Guillemont, J., Gohlmann, H. W., Neefs, J. M., Winkler, H., Van Gestel, J., Timmerman, P., Zhu, M., Lee, E., Williams, P., de Chaffoy, D., Huitric, E., Hoffner, S., Cambau, E., Truffot-Pernot, C., Lounis, N., & Jarlier, V. (2005). A diarylquinoline drug active on the ATP synthase of *Mycobacterium tuberculosis*. *Science (New York), 307*(5707), 223–227. https://doi.org/10.1126/science.1106753.

Baek, S. H., Li, A. H., & Sassetti, C. M. (2011). Metabolic regulation of mycobacterial growth and antibiotic sensitivity. *PLoS Biology, 9*(5), e1001065.

Baker, J. J., & Abramovitch, R. B. (2018). Genetic and metabolic regulation of *Mycobacterium tuberculosis* acid growth arrest. *Scientific Reports, 8*(1), 4168. https://doi.org/10.1038/s41598-018-22343-4.

Baker, J. J., Johnson, B. K., & Abramovitch, R. B. (2014). Slow growth of *Mycobacterium tuberculosis* at acidic pH is regulated by phoPR and host-associated carbon sources. *Molecular Microbiology, 94*(1), 56–69. https://doi.org/10.1111/mmi.12688.

Balaban, N. Q., Merrin, J., Chait, R., Kowalik, L., & Leibler, S. (2004). Bacterial persistence as a phenotypic switch. *Science (New York), 305*(5690), 1622–1625. https://doi.org/10.1126/science.1099390.

Bald, D., Villellas, C., Lu, P., & Koul, A. (2017). Targeting energy metabolism in *Mycobacterium tuberculosis*, a new paradigm in antimycobacterial drug discovery. *mBio, 8*(2). https://doi.org/ 10.1128/mBio.00272-17

Barry, C. E., 3rd, Boshoff, H. I., Dartois, V., Dick, T., Ehrt, S., Flynn, J., Schnappinger, D., Wilkinson, R. J., & Young, D. (2009). The spectrum of latent tuberculosis: rethinking the biology and intervention strategies. *Nature Reviews. Microbiology, 7*(12), 845–855. https://doi. org/10.1038/nrmicro2236.

Betts, J. C., Lukey, P. T., Robb, L. C., McAdam, R. A., & Duncan, K. (2002). Evaluation of a nutrient starvation model of *Mycobacterium tuberculosis* persistence by gene and protein expression profiling. *Molecular Microbiology, 43*(3), 717–731.

Bigger, J. (1944). Treatment of Staphylococcal infections with penicillin by intermittent sterilisation. *The Lancet, 244*(6320), 497–500. https://doi.org/10.1016/S0140-6736(00)74210-3.

Boon, C., & Dick, T. (2002). Mycobacterium bovis BCG response regulator essential for hypoxic dormancy. *Journal of Bacteriology, 184*(24), 6760–6767.

Borisov, S. E., Bogorodskaya, E. M., Volchenkov, G. V., Kulchavenya, E. V., Maryandyshev, A. O., Skornyakov, S. N., Talibov, O. B., Tikhonov, A. M., & Vasilyeva, I. A. (2018). Efficiency and safety of chemotherapy regimen with SQ109 in those suffering from multiple drug resistant tuberculosis. *Tuberculosis and Lung Diseases, 96*(3), 6–18.

Boshoff, H. I., & Barry, C. E., 3rd. (2005). Tuberculosis – metabolism and respiration in the absence of growth. *Nature Reviews. Microbiology, 3*(1), 70–80. https://doi.org/10.1038/ nrmicro1065.

Brotz-Oesterhelt, H., & Sass, P. (2014). Bacterial caseinolytic proteases as novel targets for antibacterial treatment. *International Journal of Medical Microbiology, 304*(1), 23–30. https:// doi.org/10.1016/j.ijmm.2013.09.001.

Brotz-Oesterhelt, H., Beyer, D., Kroll, H. P., Endermann, R., Ladel, C., Schroeder, W., Hinzen, B., Raddatz, S., Paulsen, H., Henninger, K., Bandow, J. E., Sahl, H. G., & Labischinski, H. (2005). Dysregulation of bacterial proteolytic machinery by a new class of antibiotics. *Nature Medicine, 11*(10), 1082–1087. https://doi.org/10.1038/nm1306.

Chao, M. C., & Rubin, E. J. (2010). Letting sleeping dos lie: Does dormancy play a role in tuberculosis? *Annual Review of Microbiology, 64*, 293–311. https://doi.org/10.1146/annurev. micro.112408.134043.

Chapman, J. S., & Bernard, J. S. (1962). The tolerances of unclassified mycobacteria. I. Limits of pH tolerance. *The American Review of Respiratory Disease, 86*, 582–583. https://doi.org/10. 1164/arrd.1962.86.4.582.

Chen, P., Gearhart, J., Protopopova, M., Einck, L., & Nacy, C. A. (2006). Synergistic interactions of SQ109, a new ethylene diamine, with front-line antitubercular drugs *in vitro*. *The Journal of Antimicrobial Chemotherapy, 58*(2), 332–337. https://doi.org/10.1093/jac/dkl227.

Cho, H. Y., Cho, H. J., Kim, Y. M., Oh, J. I., & Kang, B. S. (2009). Structural insight into the heme-based redox sensing by DosS from *Mycobacterium tuberculosis*. *The Journal of Biological Chemistry, 284*(19), 13057–13067. https://doi.org/10.1074/jbc.M808905200.

Cho, H. Y., Cho, H. J., Kim, M. H., & Kang, B. S. (2011). Blockage of the channel to heme by the E87 side chain in the GAF domain of *Mycobacterium tuberculosis* DosS confers the unique sensitivity of DosS to oxygen. *FEBS Letters, 585*(12), 1873–1878. https://doi.org/10.1016/j. febslet.2011.04.050.

Conlon, B. P., Nakayasu, E. S., Fleck, L. E., LaFleur, M. D., Isabella, V. M., Coleman, K., Leonard, S. N., Smith, R. D., Adkins, J. N., & Lewis, K. (2013). Activated ClpP kills persisters and eradicates a chronic biofilm infection. *Nature, 503*(7476), 365–370. https://doi.org/10.1038/ nature12790.

Converse, P. J., Karakousis, P. C., Klinkenberg, L. G., Kesavan, A. K., Ly, L. H., Allen, S. S., Grosset, J. H., Jain, S. K., Lamichhane, G., Manabe, Y. C., McMurray, D. N., Nuermberger, E. L., & Bishai, W. R. (2009). Role of the dosR-dosS two-component regulatory system in *Mycobacterium tuberculosis* virulence in three animal models. *Infection and Immunity, 77*(3), 1230–1237. https://doi.org/10.1128/IAI.01117-08.

Cox, E., & Laessig, K. (2014). FDA approval of bedaquiline – The benefit-risk balance for drug-resistant tuberculosis. *The New England Journal of Medicine, 371*(8), 689–691. https://doi.org/10.1056/NEJMp1314385.

Cyktor, J. C., Carruthers, B., Kominsky, R. A., Beamer, G. L., Stromberg, P., & Turner, J. (2013). IL-10 inhibits mature fibrotic granuloma formation during *Mycobacterium tuberculosis* infection. *Journal of Immunology.* https://doi.org/10.4049/jimmunol.1202722

Daniel, J., Maamar, H., Deb, C., Sirakova, T. D., & Kolattukudy, P. E. (2011). *Mycobacterium tuberculosis* uses host triacylglycerol to accumulate lipid droplets and acquires a dormancy-like phenotype in lipid-loaded macrophages. *PLoS Pathogens, 7*(6), e1002093.

Dannenberg, A. M. (2006). *Pathogenesis of human pulmonary tuberculosis: Insights from the rabbit model* (pp. 1–453). Washington, DC: ASM Press.

Deb, C., Lee, C. M., Dubey, V. S., Daniel, J., Abomoelak, B., Sirakova, T. D., Pawar, S., Rogers, L., & Kolattukudy, P. E. (2009). A novel in vitro multiple-stress dormancy model for *Mycobacterium tuberculosis* generates a lipid-loaded, drug-tolerant, dormant pathogen. *PLoS One, 4*(6), e6077. https://doi.org/10.1371/journal.pone.0006077.

Driver, E. R., Ryan, G. J., Hoff, D. R., Irwin, S. M., Basaraba, R. J., Kramnik, I., & Lenaerts, A. J. (2012). Evaluation of a mouse model of necrotic granuloma formation using C3HeB/FeJ mice for testing of drugs against *Mycobacterium tuberculosis*. *Antimicrobial Agents and Chemotherapy, 56*(6), 3181–3195. https://doi.org/10.1128/AAC.00217-12.

Famulla, K., Sass, P., Malik, I., Akopian, T., Kandror, O., Alber, M., Hinzen, B., Ruebsamen-Schaeff, H., Kalscheuer, R., Goldberg, A. L., & Brotz-Oesterhelt, H. (2016). Acyldepsipeptide antibiotics kill mycobacteria by preventing the physiological functions of the ClpP1P2 protease. *Molecular Microbiology, 101*(2), 194–209. https://doi.org/10.1111/mmi.13362.

Farhana, A., Guidry, L., Srivastava, A., Singh, A., Hondalus, M. K., & Steyn, A. J. (2010). Reductive stress in microbes: Implications for understanding *Mycobacterium tuberculosis* disease and persistence. *Advances in Microbial Physiology, 57*, 43–117. https://doi.org/10.1016/B978-0-12-381045-8.00002-3.

Fisher, M. A., Plikaytis, B. B., & Shinnick, T. M. (2002). Microarray analysis of the *Mycobacterium tuberculosis* transcriptional response to the acidic conditions found in phagosomes. *Journal of Bacteriology, 184*(14), 4025–4032.

Foss, M. H., Pou, S., Davidson, P. M., Dunaj, J. L., Winter, R. W., Pou, S., Licon, M. H., Doh, J. K., Li, Y., Kelly, J. X., Dodean, R. A., Koop, D. R., Riscoe, M. K., & Purdy, G. E. (2016). Diphenylether-modified 1,2-diamines with improved drug properties for development against *Mycobacterium tuberculosis*. *ACS Infectious Diseases, 2*(7), 500–508. https://doi.org/10.1021/acsinfecdis.6b00052.

Galagan, J. E., Minch, K., Peterson, M., Lyubetskaya, A., Azizi, E., Sweet, L., Gomes, A., Rustad, T., Dolganov, G., Glotova, I., Abeel, T., Mahwinney, C., Kennedy, A. D., Allard, R., Brabant, W., Krueger, A., Jaini, S., Honda, B., Yu, W. H., Hickey, M. J., Zucker, J., Garay, C., Weiner, B., Sisk, P., Stolte, C., Winkler, J. K., Van de Peer, Y., Iazzetti, P., Camacho, D., Dreyfuss, J., Liu, Y., Dorhoi, A., Mollenkopf, H. J., Drogaris, P., Lamontagne, J., Zhou, Y., Piquenot, J., Park, S. T., Raman, S., Kaufmann, S. H., Mohney, R. P., Chelsky, D., Moody, D. B., Sherman, D. R., & Schoolnik, G. K. (2013). The *Mycobacterium tuberculosis* regulatory network and hypoxia. *Nature, 499*(7457), 178–183. https://doi.org/10.1038/nature12337.

Garton, N. J., Waddell, S. J., Sherratt, A. L., Lee, S. M., Smith, R. J., Senner, C., Hinds, J., Rajakumar, K., Adegbola, R. A., Besra, G. S., Butcher, P. D., & Barer, M. R. (2008). Cytological and transcript analyses reveal fat and lazy persister-like bacilli in tuberculous sputum. *PLoS Medicine, 5*(4), 634–645.

Gautam, U. S., McGillivray, A., Mehra, S., Didier, P. J., Midkiff, C. C., Kissee, R. S., Golden, N. A., Alvarez, X., Niu, T., Rengarajan, J., Sherman, D. R., & Kaushal, D. (2015). DosS is required for the complete virulence of *Mycobacterium tuberculosis* in mice with classical granulomatous lesions. *American Journal of Respiratory Cell and Molecular Biology, 52*(6), 708–716. https://doi.org/10.1165/rcmb.2014-0230OC.

Gavrish, E., Sit, C. S., Cao, S., Kandror, O., Spoering, A., Peoples, A., Ling, L., Fetterman, A., Hughes, D., Bissell, A., Torrey, H., Akopian, T., Mueller, A., Epstein, S., Goldberg, A., Clardy, J., & Lewis, K. (2014). Lassomycin, a ribosomally synthesized cyclic peptide, kills *Mycobacterium tuberculosis* by targeting the ATP-dependent protease ClpC1P1P2. *Chemistry & Biology, 21*(4), 509–518. https://doi.org/10.1016/j.chembiol.2014.01.014.

Gengenbacher, M., & Kaufmann, S. H. (2012). *Mycobacterium tuberculosis*: Success through dormancy. *FEMS Microbiology Reviews, 36*(3), 514–532. https://doi.org/10.1111/j.1574-6976.2012.00331.x.

Gengenbacher, M., Rao, S. P., Pethe, K., & Dick, T. (2010). Nutrient-starved, non-replicating *Mycobacterium tuberculosis* requires respiration, ATP synthase and isocitrate lyase for maintenance of ATP homeostasis and viability. *Microbiology, 156*(Pt 1), 81–87. https://doi.org/10.1099/mic.0.033084-0.

Gibson, S. E. R., Harrison, J., & Cox, J. A. G. (2018) Modelling a silent epidemic: A review of the in vitro models of latent tuberculosis. *Pathogens, 7*(4). https://doi.org/10.3390/pathogens7040088

Gill, W. P., Harik, N. S., Whiddon, M. R., Liao, R. P., Mittler, J. E., & Sherman, D. R. (2009). A replication clock for *Mycobacterium tuberculosis*. *Nature Medicine, 15*(2), 211–214. https://doi.org/10.1038/nm.1915.

Gold, B., & Nathan, C. (2017a). Targeting phenotypically tolerant *Mycobacterium tuberculosis*. *Microbiology Spectrum, 5*(1). https://doi.org/10.1128/microbiolspec.TBTB2-0031-2016

Gold, B., & Nathan, C. (2017b). Targeting phenotypically tolerant *Mycobacterium tuberculosis*. *Microbiology Spectrum, 5*(1), TBTB2-0031- 2016. https://doi.org/10.1128/microbiolspec.TBTB2-0031-2016.

Gold, B., Warrier, T., & Nathan, C. (2015). A multi-stress model for high throughput screening against non-replicating *Mycobacterium tuberculosis*. *Methods in Molecular Biology, 1285*, 293–315. https://doi.org/10.1007/978-1-4939-2450-9_18.

Grant, S. S., Kaufmann, B. B., Chand, N. S., Haseley, N., & Hung, D. T. (2012). Eradication of bacterial persisters with antibiotic-generated hydroxyl radicals. *Proceedings of the National Academy of Sciences of the United States of America, 109*(30), 12147–12152. https://doi.org/10.1073/pnas.1203735109.

Grzegorzewicz, A. E., Pham, H., Gundi, V. A., Scherman, M. S., North, E. J., Hess, T., Jones, V., Gruppo, V., Born, S. E., Kordulakova, J., Chavadi, S. S., Morisseau, C., Lenaerts, A. J., Lee, R. E., McNeil, M. R., & Jackson, M. (2012). Inhibition of mycolic acid transport across the *Mycobacterium tuberculosis* plasma membrane. *Nature Chemical Biology, 8*(4), 334–341. https://doi.org/10.1038/nchembio.794.

Guerrini, V., Prideaux, B., Blanc, L., Bruiners, N., Arrigucci, R., Singh, S., Ho-Liang, H. P., Salamon, H., Chen, P. Y., Lakehal, K., Subbian, S., O'Brien, P., Via, L. E., Barry, C. E., 3rd, Dartois, V., & Gennaro, M. L. (2018). Storage lipid studies in tuberculosis reveal that foam cell biogenesis is disease-specific. *PLoS Pathogens, 14*(8), e1007223. https://doi.org/10.1371/journal.ppat.1007223.

Gupta, R. K., Thakur, T. S., Desiraju, G. R., & Tyagi, J. S. (2009). Structure-based design of DevR inhibitor active against nonreplicating *Mycobacterium tuberculosis*. *Journal of Medicinal Chemistry, 52*(20), 6324–6334. https://doi.org/10.1021/jm900358q.

Harper, J., Skerry, C., Davis, S. L., Tasneen, R., Weir, M., Kramnik, I., Bishai, W. R., Pomper, M. G., Nuermberger, E. L., & Jain, S. K. (2012). Mouse model of necrotic tuberculosis granulomas develops hypoxic lesions. *The Journal of Infectious Diseases, 205*(4), 595–602. https://doi.org/10.1093/infdis/jir786.

Hobby, G. L., Meyer, K., & Chaffee, E. (1942). Observations on the mechanism of action of penicillin. *Proceedings of the Society for Experimental Biology and Medicine, 50*(2), 281–285. https://doi.org/10.3181/00379727-50-13773.

Hudock, T. A., Foreman, T. W., Bandyopadhyay, N., Gautam, U. S., Veatch, A. V., LoBato, D. N., Gentry, K. M., Golden, N. A., Cavigli, A., Mueller, M., Hwang, S. A., Hunter, R. L., Alvarez, X., Lackner, A. A., Bader, J. S., Mehra, S., & Kaushal, D. (2017). Hypoxia sensing and persistence genes are expressed during the intragranulomatous survival of *Mycobacterium tuberculosis*. *American Journal of Respiratory Cell and Molecular Biology, 56*(5), 637–647. https://doi.org/10.1165/rcmb.2016-0239OC.

Hurdle, J. G., O'Neill, A. J., Chopra, I., & Lee, R. E. (2011). Targeting bacterial membrane function: An underexploited mechanism for treating persistent infections. *Nature Reviews. Microbiology, 9*(1), 62–75. https://doi.org/10.1038/nrmicro2474.

Hutter, R., Keller-Schierlein, W., Knusel, F., Prelog, V., Rodgers, G. C., Jr., Suter, P., Vogel, G., Voser, W., & Zahner, H. (1967). The metabolic products of microorganisms. Boromycin. *Helvetica Chimica Acta, 50*(6), 1533–1539. https://doi.org/10.1002/hlca.19670500612.

Ioanoviciu, A., Yukl, E. T., Moenne-Loccoz, P., & de Montellano, P. R. (2007). DevS, a heme-containing two-component oxygen sensor of *Mycobacterium tuberculosis*. *Biochemistry, 46*(14), 4250–4260. https://doi.org/10.1021/bi602422p.

Johnson, B. K., & Abramovitch, R. B. (2017). Small molecules that sabotage bacterial virulence. *Trends in Pharmacological Sciences, 38*(4), 339–362. https://doi.org/10.1016/j.tips.2017.01.004.

Johnson, B. K., Colvin, C. J., Needle, D. B., Mba Medie, F., Champion, P. A., & Abramovitch, R. B. (2015). The carbonic anhydrase inhibitor ethoxzolamide inhibits the *Mycobacterium tuberculosis* PhoPR regulon and Esx-1 secretion and attenuates virulence. *Antimicrobial Agents and Chemotherapy, 59*(8), 4436–4445. https://doi.org/10.1128/AAC.00719-15.

Kalia, N. P., Hasenoehrl, E. J., Ab Rahman, N. B., Koh, V. H., Ang, M. L. T., Sajorda, D. R., Hards, K., Gruber, G., Alonso, S., Cook, G. M., Berney, M., & Pethe, K. (2017). Exploiting the synthetic lethality between terminal respiratory oxidases to kill *Mycobacterium tuberculosis* and clear host infection. *Proceedings of the National Academy of Sciences of the United States of America, 114*(28), 7426–7431. https://doi.org/10.1073/pnas.1706139114.

Kaur, K., Taneja, N. K., Dhingra, S., & Tyagi, J. S. (2014). DevR (DosR) mimetic peptides impair transcriptional regulation and survival of *Mycobacterium tuberculosis* under hypoxia by inhibiting the autokinase activity of DevS sensor kinase. *BMC Microbiology, 14*(195), 1–9. https://doi.org/10.1186/1471-2180-14-195.

Kempker, R. R., Heinrichs, M. T., Nikolaishvili, K., Sabulua, I., Bablishvili, N., Gogishvili, S., Avaliani, Z., Tukvadze, N., Little, B., Bernheim, A., Read, T. D., Guarner, J., Derendorf, H., Peloquin, C. A., Blumberg, H. M., & Vashakidze, S. (2017). Lung tissue concentrations of pyrazinamide among patients with drug-resistant pulmonary tuberculosis. *Antimicrobial Agents and Chemotherapy, 61*(6). https://doi.org/10.1128/AAC.00226-17

Kint, C. I., Verstraeten, N., Fauvart, M., & Michiels, J. (2012). New-found fundamentals of bacterial persistence. *Trends in Microbiology, 20*(12), 577–585. https://doi.org/10.1016/j.tim.2012.08.009.

Kramnik, I., Demant, P., & Bloom, B. B. (1998). Susceptibility to tuberculosis as a complex genetic trait: Analysis using recombinant congenic strains of mice. *Novartis Foundation Symposium, 217*, 120–131; discussion 132-127.

Kramnik, I., Dietrich, W. F., Demant, P., & Bloom, B. R. (2000). Genetic control of resistance to experimental infection with virulent *Mycobacterium tuberculosis*. *Proceedings of the National Academy of Sciences of the United States of America, 97*(15), 8560–8565. https://doi.org/10.1073/pnas.150227197.

Krishna, S., Bustamante, L., Haynes, R. K., & Staines, H. M. (2008). Artemisinins: Their growing importance in medicine. *Trends in Pharmacological Sciences, 29*(10), 520–527. https://doi.org/10.1016/j.tips.2008.07.004.

Kumar, A., Toledo, J. C., Patel, R. P., Lancaster, J. R., Jr., & Steyn, A. J. (2007). *Mycobacterium tuberculosis* DosS is a redox sensor and DosT is a hypoxia sensor. *Proceedings of the National Academy of Sciences of the United States of America, 104*(28), 11568–11573. https://doi.org/10.1073/pnas.0705054104.

Kurthkoti, K., Amin, H., Marakalala, M. J., Ghanny, S., Subbian, S., Sakatos, A., Livny, J., Fortune, S. M., Berney, M., & Rodriguez, G. M. (2017). The capacity of *Mycobacterium tuberculosis* to survive iron starvation might enable it to persist in iron-deprived microenvironments of human granulomas. *mBio, 8*(4). https://doi.org/10.1128/mBio.01092-17

Lanoix, J. P., Ioerger, T., Ormond, A., Kaya, F., Sacchettini, J., Dartois, V., & Nuermberger, E. (2016). Selective inactivity of pyrazinamide against tuberculosis in C3HeB/FeJ mice is best explained by neutral pH of caseum. *Antimicrobial Agents and Chemotherapy, 60*(2), 735–743. https://doi.org/10.1128/AAC.01370-15.

Leistikow, R. L., Morton, R. A., Bartek, I. L., Frimpong, I., Wagner, K., & Voskuil, M. I. (2010). The *Mycobacterium tuberculosis* DosR regulon assists in metabolic homeostasis and enables rapid recovery from nonrespiring dormancy. *Journal of Bacteriology, 192*(6), 1662–1670. https://doi.org/10.1128/JB.00926-09.

Lewis, K. (2007). Persister cells, dormancy and infectious disease. *Nature Reviews Microbiology, 5*(1), 48–56. https://doi.org/10.1038/nrmicro1557.

Li, W., Upadhyay, A., Fontes, F. L., North, E. J., Wang, Y., Crans, D. C., Grzegorzewicz, A. E., Jones, V., Franzblau, S. G., Lee, R. E., Crick, D. C., & Jackson, M. (2014). Novel insights into the mechanism of inhibition of MmpL3, a target of multiple pharmacophores in *Mycobacterium tuberculosis*. *Antimicrobial Agents and Chemotherapy, 58*(11), 6413–6423. https://doi.org/10.1128/AAC.03229-14.

Lin, P. L., Dartois, V., Johnston, P. J., Janssen, C., Via, L., Goodwin, M. B., Klein, E., Barry, C. E., 3rd, & Flynn, J. L. (2012). Metronidazole prevents reactivation of latent *Mycobacterium tuberculosis* infection in macaques. *Proceedings of the National Academy of Sciences of the United States of America, 109*(35), 14188–14193. https://doi.org/10.1073/pnas.1121497109.

Liu, Y., Tan, S., Huang, L., Abramovitch, R. B., Rohde, K. H., Zimmerman, M. D., Chen, C., Dartois, V., VanderVen, B. C., & Russell, D. G. (2016). Immune activation of the host cell induces drug tolerance in *Mycobacterium tuberculosis* both in vitro and in vivo. *The Journal of Experimental Medicine, 213*(5), 809–825. https://doi.org/10.1084/jem.20151248.

Loebel, R. O., Shorr, E., & Richardson, H. B. (1933). The influence of adverse conditions upon the respiratory metabolism and growth of human tubercle bacilli. *Journal of Bacteriology, 26*(2), 167–200.

MacGilvary, N. J., & Tan, S. (2018). Fluorescent *Mycobacterium tuberculosis* reporters: Illuminating host-pathogen interactions. *Pathogens and Disease, 76*(3). https://doi.org/10.1093/femspd/fty017.

Mak, P. A., Rao, S. P., Ping Tan, M., Lin, X., Chyba, J., Tay, J., Ng, S. H., Tan, B. H., Cherian, J., Duraiswamy, J., Bifani, P., Lim, V., Lee, B. H., Ling Ma, N., Beer, D., Thayalan, P., Kuhen, K., Chatterjee, A., Supek, F., Glynne, R., Zheng, J., Boshoff, H. I., Barry, C. E., 3rd, Dick, T., Pethe, K., & Camacho, L. R. (2012). A high-throughput screen to identify inhibitors of ATP homeostasis in non-replicating *Mycobacterium tuberculosis*. *ACS Chemical Biology, 7*(7), 1190–1197. https://doi.org/10.1021/cb2004884.

Malhotra, V., Sharma, D., Ramanathan, V. D., Shakila, H., Saini, D. K., Chakravorty, S., Das, T. K., Li, Q., Silver, R. F., Narayanan, P. R., & Tyagi, J. S. (2004). Disruption of response regulator gene, devR, leads to attenuation in virulence of *Mycobacterium tuberculosis*. *FEMS Microbiology Letters, 231*(2), 237–245. https://doi.org/10.1016/S0378-1097(04)00002-3.

Manzanillo, P. S., Shiloh, M. U., Portnoy, D. A., & Cox, J. S. (2012). *Mycobacterium tuberculosis* activates the DNA-dependent cytosolic surveillance pathway within macrophages. *Cell Host & Microbe, 11*(5), 469–480. https://doi.org/10.1016/j.chom.2012.03.007.

Marakalala, M. J., Raju, R. M., Sharma, K., Zhang, Y. J., Eugenin, E. A., Prideaux, B., Daudelin, I. B., Chen, P. Y., Booty, M. G., Kim, J. H., Eum, S. Y., Via, L. E., Behar, S. M., Barry, C. E., 3rd, Mann, M., Dartois, V., & Rubin, E. J. (2016). Inflammatory signaling in human tuberculosis granulomas is spatially organized. *Nature Medicine, 22*(5), 531–538. https://doi.org/10.1038/nm.4073.

McKinney, J. D., Honer zu Bentrup, K., Munoz-Elias, E. J., Miczak, A., Chen, B., Chan, W. T., Swenson, D., Sacchettini, J. C., Jacobs, W. R., Jr., & Russell, D. G. (2000). Persistence of *Mycobacterium tuberculosis* in macrophages and mice requires the glyoxylate shunt enzyme isocitrate lyase. *Nature, 406*(6797), 735–738.

Mehra, S., Foreman, T. W., Didier, P. J., Ahsan, M. H., Hudock, T. A., Kissee, R., Golden, N. A., Gautam, U. S., Johnson, A. M., Alvarez, X., Russell-Lodrigue, K. E., Doyle, L. A., Roy, C. J., Niu, T., Blanchard, J. L., Khader, S. A., Lackner, A. A., Sherman, D. R., & Kaushal, D. (2015). The DosR regulon modulates adaptive immunity and is essential for *Mycobacterium tuberculosis* persistence. *American Journal of Respiratory and Critical Care Medicine, 191*(10), 1185–1196. https://doi.org/10.1164/rccm.201408-1502OC.

Meunier, B., & Robert, A. (2010). Heme as trigger and target for trioxane-containing antimalarial drugs. *Accounts of Chemical Research, 43*(11), 1444–1451. https://doi.org/10.1021/ar100070k.

Mikusova, K., Huang, H., Yagi, T., Holsters, M., Vereecke, D., D'Haeze, W., Scherman, M. S., Brennan, P. J., McNeil, M. R., & Crick, D. C. (2005). Decaprenylphosphoryl arabinofuranose, the donor of the D-arabinofuranosyl residues of mycobacterial arabinan, is formed via a two-step epimerization of decaprenylphosphoryl ribose. *Journal of Bacteriology, 187*(23), 8020–8025. https://doi.org/10.1128/jb.187.23.8020-8025.2005.

Moreira, W., Ngan, G. J., Low, J. L., Poulsen, A., Chia, B. C., Ang, M. J., Yap, A., Fulwood, J., Lakshmanan, U., Lim, J., Khoo, A. Y., Flotow, H., Hill, J., Raju, R. M., Rubin, E. J., & Dick, T. (2015). Target mechanism-based whole-cell screening identifies bortezomib as an inhibitor of caseinolytic protease in mycobacteria. *mBio, 6*(3), e00253–e00215. https://doi.org/10.1128/mBio.00253-15.

Moreira, W., Aziz, D. B., & Dick, T. (2016). Boromycin kills mycobacterial persisters without detectable resistance. *Frontiers in Microbiology, 7*(199), 1–7. https://doi.org/10.3389/fmicb.2016.00199.

Moreira, W., Santhanakrishnan, S., Dymock, B. W., & Dick, T. (2017a). Bortezomib warhead-switch confers dual activity against mycobacterial caseinolytic protease and proteasome and selectivity against human proteasome. *Frontiers in Microbiology, 8*(746), 1–6. https://doi.org/10.3389/fmicb.2017.00746.

Moreira, W., Santhanakrishnan, S., Ngan, G. J. Y., Low, C. B., Sangthongpitag, K., Poulsen, A., Dymock, B. W., & Dick, T. (2017b). Towards selective mycobacterial ClpP1P2 inhibitors with reduced activity against the human proteasome. *Antimicrobial Agents and Chemotherapy, 61*(5), e02307–e02316. https://doi.org/10.1128/aac.02307-16.

Muller, A., Wenzel, M., Strahl, H., Grein, F., Saaki, T. N. V., Kohl, B., Siersma, T., Bandow, J. E., Sahl, H. G., Schneider, T., & Hamoen, L. W. (2016). Daptomycin inhibits cell envelope synthesis by interfering with fluid membrane microdomains. *Proceedings of the National Academy of Sciences of the United States of America, 113*(45), E7077–E7086. https://doi.org/10.1073/pnas.1611173113.

Munoz-Elias, E. J., Timm, J., Botha, T., Chan, W. T., Gomez, J. E., & McKinney, J. D. (2005). Replication dynamics of *Mycobacterium tuberculosis* in chronically infected mice. *Infection and Immunity, 73*(1), 546–551. https://doi.org/10.1128/IAI.73.1.546-551.2005.

Nathan, C. (2012). Fresh approaches to anti-infective therapies. *Science Translational Medicine, 4*(140), 140sr142. https://doi.org/10.1126/scitranslmed.3003081.

Neres, J., Hartkoorn, R. C., Chiarelli, L. R., Gadupudi, R., Pasca, M. R., Mori, G., Venturelli, A., Savina, S., Makarov, V., Kolly, G. S., Molteni, E., Binda, C., Dhar, N., Ferrari, S., Brodin, P., Delorme, V., Landry, V., de Jesus Lopes Ribeiro, A. L., Farina, D., Saxena, P., Pojer, F., Carta, A., Luciani, R., Porta, A., Zanoni, G., De Rossi, E., Costi, M. P., Riccardi, G., & Cole, S. T. (2015). 2-Carboxyquinoxalines kill *Mycobacterium tuberculosis* through noncovalent inhibition of DprE1. *ACS Chemical Biology, 10*(3), 705–714. https://doi.org/10.1021/cb5007163.

Ohno, H., Zhu, G., Mohan, V. P., Chu, D., Kohno, S., Jacobs, W. R., Jr., & Chan, J. (2003). The effects of reactive nitrogen intermediates on gene expression in *Mycobacterium tuberculosis. Cellular Microbiology, 5*(9), 637–648.

Ollinger, J., O'Malley, T., Kesicki, E. A., Odingo, J., & Parish, T. (2012). Validation of the essential ClpP protease in *Mycobacterium tuberculosis* as a novel drug target. *Journal of Bacteriology, 194*(3), 663–668. https://doi.org/10.1128/JB.06142-11.

Pache, W. (1975). Boromycin. In J. W. Corcoran & F. E. Hahn (Eds.), *Antibiotics. Vol. III Mechanism of action of antimicrobial and antitumor agents* (pp. 585–587). Berlin: Springer.

Panda, M., Ramachandran, S., Ramachandran, V., Shirude, P. S., Humnabadkar, V., Nagalapur, K., Sharma, S., Kaur, P., Guptha, S., Narayan, A., Mahadevaswamy, J., Ambady, A., Hegde, N., Rudrapatna, S. S., Hosagrahara, V. P., Sambandamurthy, V. K., & Raichurkar, A. (2014). Discovery of pyrazolopyridones as a novel class of noncovalent DprE1 inhibitor with potent anti-mycobacterial activity. *Journal of Medicinal Chemistry, 57*(11), 4761–4771. https://doi.org/10.1021/jm5002937.

Pandey, A. K., & Sassetti, C. M. (2008). Mycobacterial persistence requires the utilization of host cholesterol. *Proceedings of the National Academy of Sciences of the United States of America, 105*(11), 4376–4380.

Park, H. D., Guinn, K. M., Harrell, M. I., Liao, R., Voskuil, M. I., Tompa, M., Schoolnik, G. K., & Sherman, D. R. (2003). Rv3133c/dosR is a transcription factor that mediates the hypoxic response of *Mycobacterium tuberculosis. Molecular Microbiology, 48*(3), 833–843.

Peddireddy, V., Doddam, S. N., & Ahmed, N. (2017). Mycobacterial dormancy systems and host responses in tuberculosis. *Frontiers in Immunology, 8*, 84. https://doi.org/10.3389/fimmu.2017.00084.

Pethe, K., Bifani, P., Jang, J., Kang, S., Park, S., Ahn, S., Jiricek, J., Jung, J., Jeon, H. K., Cechetto, J., Christophe, T., Lee, H., Kempf, M., Jackson, M., Lenaerts, A. J., Pham, H., Jones, V., Seo, M. J., Kim, Y. M., Seo, M., Seo, J. J., Park, D., Ko, Y., Choi, I., Kim, R., Kim, S. Y., Lim, S., Yim, S. A., Nam, J., Kang, H., Kwon, H., Oh, C. T., Cho, Y., Jang, Y., Kim, J., Chua, A., Tan, B. H., Nanjundappa, M. B., Rao, S. P., Barnes, W. S., Wintjens, R., Walker, J. R., Alonso, S., Lee, S., Kim, J., Oh, S., Oh, T., Nehrbass, U., Han, S. J., No, Z., Lee, J., Brodin, P., Cho, S. N., Nam, K., & Kim, J. (2013). Discovery of Q203, a potent clinical candidate for the treatment of tuberculosis. *Nature Medicine, 19*(9), 1157–1160. https://doi.org/10.1038/nm.3262.

Piddington, D. L., Kashkouli, A., & Buchmeier, N. A. (2000). Growth of *Mycobacterium tuberculosis* in a defined medium is very restricted by acid pH and Mg2+ levels. *Infection and Immunity, 68*(8), 4518–4522.

Podust, L. M., Ioanoviciu, A., & Ortiz de Montellano, P. R. (2008). 2.3 A X-ray structure of the heme-bound GAF domain of sensory histidine kinase DosT of *Mycobacterium tuberculosis. Biochemistry, 47*(47), 12523–12531. https://doi.org/10.1021/bi8012356.

Portaels, F., & Pattyn, S. R. (1982). Growth of mycobacteria in relation to the pH of the medium. *Annals of Microbiology (Paris), 133*(2), 213–221.

Prideaux, B., Via, L. E., Zimmerman, M. D., Eum, S., Sarathy, J., O'Brien, P., Chen, C., Kaya, F., Weiner, D. M., Chen, P. Y., Song, T., Lee, M., Shim, T. S., Cho, J. S., Kim, W., Cho, S. N., Olivier, K. N., Barry, C. E., 3rd, & Dartois, V. (2015). The association between sterilizing activity and drug distribution into tuberculosis lesions. *Nature Medicine, 21*(10), 1223–1227. https://doi.org/10.1038/nm.3937.

Primm, T. P., Andersen, S. J., Mizrahi, V., Avarbock, D., Rubin, H., & Barry, C. E., 3rd. (2000). The stringent response of *Mycobacterium tuberculosis* is required for long-term survival. *Journal of Bacteriology, 182*(17), 4889–4898.

Rao, S. P., Alonso, S., Rand, L., Dick, T., & Pethe, K. (2008). The protonmotive force is required for maintaining ATP homeostasis and viability of hypoxic, nonreplicating *Mycobacterium tuberculosis. Proceedings of the National Academy of Sciences of the United States of America, 105*(33), 11945–11950. https://doi.org/10.1073/pnas.0711697105.

Roberts, D. M., Liao, R. P., Wisedchaisri, G., Hol, W. G., & Sherman, D. R. (2004). Two sensor kinases contribute to the hypoxic response of *Mycobacterium tuberculosis. The Journal of Biological Chemistry, 279*(22), 23082–23087. https://doi.org/10.1074/jbc.M401230200.

Rodrigues Felix, C., Gupta, R., Geden, S., Roberts, J., Winder, P., Pomponi, S. A., Diaz, M. C., Reed, J. K., Wright, A. E., & Rohde, K. H. (2017). Selective killing of dormant *Mycobacterium tuberculosis* by marine natural products. *Antimicrobial Agents and Chemotherapy, 61*(8). https://doi.org/10.1128/AAC.00743-17

Rohde, K., Yates, R. M., Purdy, G. E., & Russell, D. G. (2007a). *Mycobacterium tuberculosis* and the environment within the phagosome. *Immunological Reviews, 219*, 37–54.

Rohde, K. H., Abramovitch, R. B., & Russell, D. G. (2007b). *Mycobacterium tuberculosis* invasion of macrophages: Linking bacterial gene expression to environmental cues. *Cell Host & Microbe, 2*(5), 352–364.

Russell, D. G. (2007). Who puts the tubercle in tuberculosis? *Nature Reviews. Microbiology, 5*(1), 39–47.

Rustad, T. R., Harrell, M. I., Liao, R., & Sherman, D. R. (2008). The enduring hypoxic response of *Mycobacterium tuberculosis*. *PLoS One, 3*(1), e1502. https://doi.org/10.1371/journal.pone. 0001502.

Rustad, T. R., Sherrid, A. M., Minch, K. J., & Sherman, D. R. (2009). Hypoxia: A window into *Mycobacterium tuberculosis* latency. *Cellular Microbiology, 11*(8), 1151–1159. https://doi.org/ 10.1111/j.1462-5822.2009.01325.x.

Saini, D. K., Malhotra, V., & Tyagi, J. S. (2004a). Cross talk between DevS sensor kinase homologue, Rv2027c, and DevR response regulator of *Mycobacterium tuberculosis*. *FEBS Letters, 565*(1–3), 75–80. https://doi.org/10.1016/j.febslet.2004.02.092.

Saini, D. K., Malhotra, V., Dey, D., Pant, N., Das, T. K., & Tyagi, J. S. (2004b). DevR-DevS is a bona fide two-component system of *Mycobacterium tuberculosis* that is hypoxia-responsive in the absence of the DNA-binding domain of DevR. *Microbiology, 150*(Pt 4), 865–875. https:// doi.org/10.1099/mic.0.26218-0.

Sarathy, J. P., Via, L. E., Weiner, D., Blanc, L., Boshoff, H., Eugenin, E. A., Barry, C. E., 3rd, & Dartois, V. A. (2018). Extreme drug tolerance of *Mycobacterium tuberculosis* in caseum. *Antimicrobial Agents and Chemotherapy, 62*(2). https://doi.org/10.1128/AAC.02266-17.

Sardiwal, S., Kendall, S. L., Movahedzadeh, F., Rison, S. C., Stoker, N. G., & Djordjevic, S. (2005). A GAF domain in the hypoxia/NO-inducible *Mycobacterium tuberculosis* DosS protein binds haem. *Journal of Molecular Biology, 353*(5), 929–936. https://doi.org/10.1016/j. jmb.2005.09.011.

Sauer, U., & Eikmanns, B. J. (2005). The PEP-pyruvate-oxaloacetate node as the switch point for carbon flux distribution in bacteria. *FEMS Microbiology Reviews, 29*(4), 765–794. https://doi. org/10.1016/j.femsre.2004.11.002.

Shirude, P. S., Shandil, R., Sadler, C., Naik, M., Hosagrahara, V., Hameed, S., Shinde, V., Bathula, C., Humnabadkar, V., Kumar, N., Reddy, J., Panduga, V., Sharma, S., Ambady, A., Hegde, N., Whiteaker, J., McLaughlin, R. E., Gardner, H., Madhavapeddi, P., Ramachandran, V., Kaur, P., Narayan, A., Guptha, S., Awasthy, D., Narayan, C., Mahadevaswamy, J., Vishwas, K. G., Ahuja, V., Srivastava, A., Prabhakar, K. R., Bharath, S., Kale, R., Ramaiah, M., Choudhury, N. R., Sambandamurthy, V. K., Solapure, S., Iyer, P. S., Narayanan, S., & Chatterji, M. (2013). Azaindoles: Noncovalent DprE1 inhibitors from scaffold morphing efforts, kill *Mycobacterium tuberculosis* and are efficacious *in vivo*. *Journal of Medicinal Chemistry, 56*(23), 9701–9708. https://doi.org/10.1021/jm401382v.

Singh, R., Manjunatha, U., Boshoff, H. I., Ha, Y. H., Niyomrattanakit, P., Ledwidge, R., Dowd, C. S., Lee, I. Y., Kim, P., Zhang, L., Kang, S., Keller, T. H., Jiricek, J., & Barry, C. E., 3rd. (2008). PA-824 kills nonreplicating *Mycobacterium tuberculosis* by intracellular NO release. *Science, 322*(5906), 1392–1395.

Sivaramakrishnan, S., & de Montellano, P. R. (2013). The DosS-DosT/DosR mycobacterial sensor system. *Biosensors, 3*(3), 259–282. https://doi.org/10.3390/bios3030259.

Sohaskey, C. D. (2008). Nitrate enhances the survival of *Mycobacterium tuberculosis* during inhibition of respiration. *Journal of Bacteriology, 190*(8), 2981–2986. https://doi.org/10.1128/ JB.01857-07.

Sousa, E. H., Tuckerman, J. R., Gonzalez, G., & Gilles-Gonzalez, M. A. (2007). DosT and DevS are oxygen-switched kinases in *Mycobacterium tuberculosis*. *Protein Science: A Publication of the Protein Society, 16*(8), 1708–1719. https://doi.org/10.1110/ps.072897707.

Sturgill-Koszycki, S., Schaible, U. E., & Russell, D. G. (1996). *Mycobacterium*-containing phagosomes are accessible to early endosomes and reflect a transitional state in normal phagosome biogenesis. *The EMBO Journal, 15*(24), 6960–6968.

Sukheja, P., Kumar, P., Mittal, N., Li, S. G., Singleton, E., Russo, R., Perryman, A. L., Shrestha, R., Awasthi, D., Husain, S., Soteropoulos, P., Brukh, R., Connell, N., Freundlich, J. S., & Alland, D. (2017). A novel small-molecule inhibitor of the *Mycobacterium tuberculosis* demethylmenaquinone methyltransferase MenG is bactericidal to both growing and nutritionally deprived persister cells. *mBio, 8*(1), e02022-02016. https://doi.org/10.1128/mBio.02022-16.

Swallow, C. J., Rotstein, O. D., & Grinstein, S. (1989). Mechanisms of cytoplasmic pH recovery in acid-loaded macrophages. *The Journal of Surgical Research, 46*(6), 588–592.

Tahlan, K., Wilson, R., Kastrinsky, D. B., Arora, K., Nair, V., Fischer, E., Barnes, S. W., Walker, J. R., Alland, D., Barry, C. E., 3rd, & Boshoff, H. I. (2012). SQ109 targets MmpL3, a membrane transporter of trehalose monomycolate involved in mycolic acid donation to the cell wall core of *Mycobacterium tuberculosis*. *Antimicrobial Agents and Chemotherapy, 56*(4), 1797–1809. https://doi.org/10.1128/AAC.05708-11.

Tan, M. P., Sequeira, P., Lin, W. W., Phong, W. Y., Cliff, P., Ng, S. H., Lee, B. H., Camacho, L., Schnappinger, D., Ehrt, S., Dick, T., Pethe, K., & Alonso, S. (2010). Nitrate respiration protects hypoxic *Mycobacterium tuberculosis* against acid- and reactive nitrogen species stresses. *PLoS One, 5*(10), e13356.

Taneja, N. K., Dhingra, S., Mittal, A., Naresh, M., & Tyagi, J. S. (2010). *Mycobacterium tuberculosis* transcriptional adaptation, growth arrest and dormancy phenotype development is triggered by vitamin C. *PLoS One, 5*(5), e10860. https://doi.org/10.1371/journal.pone. 0010860.

van der Wel, N., Hava, D., Houben, D., Fluitsma, D., van Zon, M., Pierson, J., Brenner, M., & Peters, P. J. (2007). *M. tuberculosis* and *M. leprae* translocate from the phagolysosome to the cytosol in myeloid cells. *Cell, 129*(7), 1287–1298. https://doi.org/10.1016/j.cell.2007.05.059.

Vandal, O. H., Pierini, L. M., Schnappinger, D., Nathan, C. F., & Ehrt, S. (2008). A membrane protein preserves intrabacterial pH in intraphagosomal *Mycobacterium tuberculosis*. *Nature Medicine, 14*(8), 849–854.

VanderVen, B. C., Fahey, R. J., Lee, W., Liu, Y., Abramovitch, R. B., Memmott, C., Crowe, A. M., Eltis, L. D., Perola, E., Deininger, D. D., Wang, T., Locher, C. P., & Russell, D. G. (2015). Novel inhibitors of cholesterol degradation in *Mycobacterium tuberculosis* reveal how the bacterium's metabolism is constrained by the intracellular environment. *PLoS Pathogens, 11*(2), e1004679. https://doi.org/10.1371/journal.ppat.1004679.

Via, L. E., Lin, P. L., Ray, S. M., Carrillo, J., Allen, S. S., Eum, S. Y., Taylor, K., Klein, E., Manjunatha, U., Gonzales, J., Lee, E. G., Park, S. K., Raleigh, J. A., Cho, S. N., McMurray, D. N., Flynn, J. L., & Barry, C. E., 3rd. (2008). Tuberculous granulomas are hypoxic in guinea pigs, rabbits, and nonhuman primates. *Infection and Immunity, 76*(6), 2333–2340. https://doi.org/10.1128/IAI.01515-07.

Via, L. E., England, K., Weiner, D. M., Schimel, D., Zimmerman, M. D., Dayao, E., Chen, R. Y., Dodd, L. E., Richardson, M., Robbins, K. K., Cai, Y., Hammoud, D., Herscovitch, P., Dartois, V., Flynn, J. L., & Barry, C. E., 3rd. (2015). A sterilizing tuberculosis treatment regimen is associated with faster clearance of bacteria in cavitary lesions in marmosets. *Antimicrobial Agents and Chemotherapy, 59*(7), 4181–4189. https://doi.org/10.1128/AAC.00115-15.

Vilcheze, C., Baughn, A. D., Tufariello, J., Leung, L. W., Kuo, M., Basler, C. F., Alland, D., Sacchettini, J. C., Freundlich, J. S., & Jacobs, W. R., Jr. (2011). Novel inhibitors of InhA efficiently kill *Mycobacterium tuberculosis* under aerobic and anaerobic conditions. *Antimicrobial Agents and Chemotherapy, 55*(8), 3889–3898. https://doi.org/10.1128/aac.00266-11.

Vilcheze, C., Hartman, T., Weinrick, B., & Jacobs, W. R., Jr. (2013). *Mycobacterium tuberculosis* is extraordinarily sensitive to killing by a vitamin C-induced Fenton reaction. *Nature Communications, 4*(1881), 1–10. https://doi.org/10.1038/ncomms2898.

Vilcheze, C., Hartman, T., Weinrick, B., Jain, P., Weisbrod, T. R., Leung, L. W., Freundlich, J. S., & Jacobs, W. R., Jr. (2017). Enhanced respiration prevents drug tolerance and drug resistance in *Mycobacterium tuberculosis*. *Proceedings of the National Academy of Sciences of the United States of America, 114*(17), 4495–4500. https://doi.org/10.1073/pnas.1704376114.

Vos, M. H., Bouzhir-Sima, L., Lambry, J. C., Luo, H., Eaton-Rye, J. J., Ioanoviciu, A., Ortiz de Montellano, P. R., & Liebl, U. (2012). Ultrafast ligand dynamics in the heme-based GAF sensor domains of the histidine kinases DosS and DosT from *Mycobacterium tuberculosis*. *Biochemistry, 51*(1), 159–166. https://doi.org/10.1021/bi201467c.

Voskuil, M. I., Schnappinger, D., Visconti, K. C., Harrell, M. I., Dolganov, G. M., Sherman, D. R., & Schoolnik, G. K. (2003). Inhibition of respiration by nitric oxide induces a *Mycobacterium tuberculosis* dormancy program. *The Journal of Experimental Medicine, 198*(5), 705–713. https://doi.org/10.1084/jem.20030205.

Walters, S. B., Dubnau, E., Kolesnikova, I., Laval, F., Daffe, M., & Smith, I. (2006). The *Mycobacterium tuberculosis* PhoPR two-component system regulates genes essential for virulence and complex lipid biosynthesis. *Molecular Microbiology, 60*(2), 312–330.

Wang, F., Sambandan, D., Halder, R., Wang, J., Batt, S. M., Weinrick, B., Ahmad, I., Yang, P., Zhang, Y., Kim, J., Hassani, M., Huszar, S., Trefzer, C., Ma, Z., Kaneko, T., Mdluli, K. E., Franzblau, S., Chatterjee, A. K., Johnsson, K., Mikusova, K., Besra, G. S., Futterer, K., Robbins, S. H., Barnes, S. W., Walker, J. R., Jacobs, W. R., Jr., & Schultz, P. G. (2013). Identification of a small molecule with activity against drug-resistant and persistent tuberculosis. *Proceedings of the National Academy of Sciences of the United States of America, 110*(27), E2510–E2517. https://doi.org/10.1073/pnas.1309171110.

Wang, J., Zhang, C. J., Chia, W. N., Loh, C. C., Li, Z., Lee, Y. M., He, Y., Yuan, L. X., Lim, T. K., Liu, M., Liew, C. X., Lee, Y. Q., Zhang, J., Lu, N., Lim, C. T., Hua, Z. C., Liu, B., Shen, H. M., Tan, K. S., & Lin, Q. (2015). Haem-activated promiscuous targeting of artemisinin in *Plasmodium falciparum. Nature Communications, 6*, 10111. https://doi.org/10.1038/ncomms10111.

Warrier, T., Martinez-Hoyos, M., Marin-Amieva, M., Colmenarejo, G., Porras-De Francisco, E., Alvarez-Pedraglio, A. I., Fraile-Gabaldon, M. T., Torres-Gomez, P. A., Lopez-Quezada, L., Gold, B., Roberts, J., Ling, Y., Somersan-Karakaya, S., Little, D., Cammack, N., Nathan, C., & Mendoza-Losana, A. (2015). Identification of novel anti-mycobacterial compounds by screening a pharmaceutical small-molecule library against nonreplicating *Mycobacterium tuberculosis. ACS Infectious Diseases, 1*(12), 580–585. https://doi.org/10.1021/acsinfecdis.5b00025.

Warrier, T., Kapilashrami, K., Argyrou, A., Ioerger, T. R., Little, D., Murphy, K. C., Nandakumar, M., Park, S., Gold, B., Mi, J., Zhang, T., Meiler, E., Rees, M., Somersan-Karakaya, S., Porras-De Francisco, E., Martinez-Hoyos, M., Burns-Huang, K., Roberts, J., Ling, Y., Rhee, K. Y., Mendoza-Losana, A., Luo, M., & Nathan, C. F. (2016). N-methylation of a bactericidal compound as a resistance mechanism in *Mycobacterium tuberculosis. Proceedings of the National Academy of Sciences of the United States of America, 113*(31), E4523–E4530. https://doi.org/10.1073/pnas.1606590113.

Watanabe, S., Zimmermann, M., Goodwin, M. B., Sauer, U., Barry, C. E., 3rd, & Boshoff, H. I. (2011). Fumarate reductase activity maintains an energized membrane in anaerobic *Mycobacterium tuberculosis. PLoS Pathogens, 7*(10), e1002287. https://doi.org/10.1371/journal.ppat.1002287.

Wayne, L. G., & Hayes, L. G. (1996). An in vitro model for sequential study of shiftdown of *Mycobacterium tuberculosis* through two stages of nonreplicating persistence. *Infection and Immunity, 64*(6), 2062–2069.

Wisedchaisri, G., Wu, M., Sherman, D. R., & Hol, W. G. (2008). Crystal structures of the response regulator DosR from *Mycobacterium tuberculosis* suggest a helix rearrangement mechanism for phosphorylation activation. *Journal of Molecular Biology, 378*(1), 227–242. https://doi.org/10.1016/j.jmb.2008.02.029.

Yang, T., Moreira, W., Nyantakyi, S. A., Chen, H., Aziz, D. B., Go, M. L., & Dick, T. (2017). Amphiphilic indole derivatives as antimycobacterial agents: structure-activity relationships and membrane targeting properties. *Journal of Medicinal Chemistry, 60*(7), 2745–2763. https://doi.org/10.1021/acs.jmedchem.6b01530.

Zheng, H., Colvin, C. J., Johnson, B. K., Kirchhoff, P. D., Wilson, M., Jorgensen-Muga, K., Larsen, S. D., & Abramovitch, R. B. (2017). Inhibitors of *Mycobacterium tuberculosis* DosRST signaling and persistence. *Nature Chemical Biology, 13*(2), 218–225. https://doi.org/10.1038/nchembio.2259.

Zheng, H., Williams, J. T., Coulson, G. B., Haiderer, E. R., & Abramovitch, R. B. (2018a). HC2091 kills *Mycobacterium tuberculosis* by targeting the MmpL3 mycolic acid transporter. *Antimicrobial Agents and Chemotherapy, 62*(7). https://doi.org/10.1128/AAC.02459-17

Zheng, H., Alewei, B., Ellsworth, E., & Abramovitch, R. (2018b). Inhibition of *Mycobacterium tuberculosis* DosRST two-component regulatory system signaling by targeting response regulator DNA binding and sensor kinase heme. bioRxiv. https://doi.org/10.1101/411793

Chapter 11
Drug Susceptibility of Individual Mycobacterial Cells

Maikel Boot and E. Hesper Rego

Abstract *Mycobacterium tuberculosis* causes the world's deadliest infectious disease. Part of the pathogen's success is its ability to diversify itself phenotypically and survive antibiotic therapy even in the absence of genetic resistance. Here, we will highlight the physiological aspects of the pathogen that promote tolerance and describe the mechanisms by which some of these vary in a genetically identical population. A better, molecular, understanding of this phenomenon may provide the key to improved TB therapy.

11.1 Heterogeneity in TB Treatment

With over 1.6 million deaths annually, tuberculosis (TB) is the leading cause of death in the world by a single infectious agent (Dye 2006; WHO 2018). New anti-TB therapeutic strategies are desperately needed, but not because the pathogen is extensively resistant to the drugs we currently use. This may be surprising when you consider that all the antibiotics that currently make up the core treatment were developed more than five decades ago. In fact, over 96% of new TB cases are drug *susceptible*. Part of the reason for this is because the main mechanism of acquiring drug resistance—horizontal gene transfer—is lacking in *Mycobacterium tuberculosis*, the bacterial organism that causes TB. Why, then, are mortality rates not rapidly decreasing? The current standard therapy is long and arduous: a 6–9 month-long therapeutic plan consisting of a combination of four drugs (Horsburgh et al. 2015). When completed, this treatment is around 95% effective, but relapse rates can be as high as 30% if treatment is ceased just a few months earlier (Fox et al. 1999). This long treatment plan stands in contrast to the rapid killing of the majority of bacteria during treatment. Approximately 90% are killed within days, and, for almost all patients, there are no detectable bacteria in their sputum after 2 months of therapy (Mitchison and Davies 2012). Thus, it appears, that small, undetectable numbers of bacteria can

M. Boot · E. H. Rego (✉)
Department of Microbial Pathogenesis, Yale University School of Medicine, New Haven, CT, USA
e-mail: hesper.rego@yale.edu

© Springer Nature Switzerland AG 2019
K. Lewis (ed.), *Persister Cells and Infectious Disease*,
https://doi.org/10.1007/978-3-030-25241-0_11

247

persist in the face of antibiotic therapy, in the absence of genetic drug resistance. The truth is, we do not really know what makes these tolerant populations respond differently, nor do we know how they are created. But, clearly, there is a need for new TB therapeutics that treat the infection faster and more completely. Given the heterogeneity seen during TB treatment, and the many lines of evidence that suggest heterogeneity is an intrinsic characteristic of the pathogen itself (Russell 2007; Cadena et al. 2017; Rego et al. 2017), interventions targeting pathogen heterogeneity could be the key to this goal.

To address this need, there have now been a few studies looking at the response of single mycobacterial cells to antibiotics. Surprisingly, many of the phenotypes and mechanisms involved appear different from those described in model organisms. For example, to date, the antibiotic tolerance and persistence field has been dominated by studies in model bacteria, typically *Escherichia coli*, for which surviving cells are non- or slow-growing prior to challenge with antibiotics (Balaban et al. 2004, 2013; Gefen et al. 2008). In contrast, multiple studies in mycobacteria have now demonstrated that subpopulations of mycobacterial cells are able to grow and/or divide at concentrations of antibiotics that appear bactericidal to the entire population, a phenomenon termed "dynamic persistence" (Wakamoto et al. 2013) or "phenotypic resistance" (Kester and Fortune 2014). Considering the unusual physiology of the pathogen and some of these early findings, it seems likely that the mechanisms of drug susceptibility on a single-cell level in mycobacteria could be very different from those discovered in other organisms.

This field is a nascent one. With that in mind, we will summarize the state of knowledge about the factors that influence antibiotic tolerance and resistance from population-level studies. We will then go through the sources of single-cell variation that have been described for mycobacteria, and some that have not yet been described but are likely to exist. We view this as a combinatorial problem (Fig. 11.1). Any factor that influences drug susceptibility could vary from cell-to-cell through a variety of mechanisms. Thus, the ways in which cells could vary in functionally important ways are almost limitless. Going forward, the challenge will be to define the most important factors that both create variation, and which are variable, in a mycobacterial population that allows a small number of bacteria to survive the extended TB therapeutic regimen.

11.2 Population-Level Effectors of Drug Susceptibility

Antibiotics kill cells through a variety of mechanisms. However, in general, the efficacy of an antibiotic depends critically on two things: the drug must be able to find its target and cells must be in a permissive metabolic state. Mycobacteria represent an unusual challenge on both fronts. Here, we will summarize our current knowledge about the most important factors that affect antibiotic susceptibility. There have been excellent reviews written on all these subjects (Nikaido 2001; da Silva et al. 2011, 2016; Sarathy et al. 2012; Rittershaus et al. 2013; Hartman et al. 2017; Logsdon and Aldridge 2018), which we are not attempting to supplant here. We simply wish to

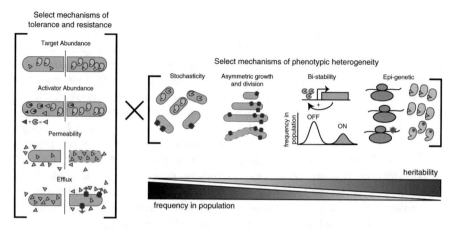

Fig. 11.1 The combinatorial problem of phenotypic heterogeneity. From population-level studies, we know that many changes in the physiology of the pathogen can affect drug susceptibility. And, there are also numerous mechanisms by which bacteria can be phenotypically different in a genetically identical population. Each mediator of susceptibility, could, in theory, vary in any—or all—of these ways, producing a highly functionally heterogeneous population. Different sources of variation produce diversity with different frequencies in the population, which is typically inversely correlated to heritability

give the reader a brief overview of the physiological features of the pathogen that have been linked to drug susceptibility on a population level. While we categorize these determinants into sections, this is not an attempt to convey that these mechanisms are mutually exclusive. Indeed, changes in one important physiological state often lead to changes in many others. This underscores the need for mechanistic studies that link changes in the physiology of the bacterium to antibiotic susceptibility at the molecular level.

11.2.1 Slow and/or No Growth

When cultured in vitro, *M. tuberculosis* divides about once a day. This stands in contrast to many other pathogens that can divide 20–50 times in that same amount of time. Early during infection, *M. tuberculosis* grows at about the same rate as it does in vitro, at least in mice. At later stages of infection, growth can be substantially slower, with doublings taking approximately 5 days (Munoz-Elias et al. 2005; Gill et al. 2009; Mcdaniel et al. 2016). This phenomenon is not exclusive to mycobacteria. Many species arrest growth in response to lack of oxygen, nutrient starvation, or even antibiotics themselves (Wayne and Hayes 1996; Ferullo and Lovett 2008; Dorr et al. 2010). *Mycobacterium tuberculosis* encounters many of these conditions during its complex life cycle within a human host. In fact, the ability of *M. tuberculosis* to downregulate its growth and metabolism might be a key part of its survival strategy: the pathogen has an unusual ability to exist in a non-replicating state for months, while remaining metabolically active (Russell 2007; Cadena et al. 2017), possibly contributing to the disease state of latency.

The connection between growth and antibiotic tolerance is well established. For *E. coli*, the rate of killing by cell-wall acting inhibitors is directly proportional to the growth rate (Tuomanen et al. 1986; Evans et al. 1991). Slow growth is the result of a decrease in metabolic activity, which makes bacteria less susceptible to antibiotics that target growth-enabling processes, such as cell-envelope biosynthesis or DNA replication. In these cases, tolerance might be explained by the fact that some antibiotics are dependent on metabolic activity for their ability to generate toxic products (de Steenwinkel et al. 2010). For example, nutrient-deprived *M. tuberculosis* is tolerant to ciprofloxacin, possibly through downregulation of gyrases (Keren et al. 2011). However, it is not always clear why cells in a lower energy state respond differently to antibiotics. For example, slow-growing cells are less metabolically active and have less ATP (Rao et al. 2008), which should reduce ATP-dependent efflux of antibiotics.

In the next sections, we will describe other mediators of antibiotic susceptibility, like efflux, permeability, and target abundance. Importantly, growth arrest differs from these as it refers to a distinct physiological state of the pathogen. Tolerance due to slow growth likely represents the complex remodeling of the pathogen's physiology, resulting in changes to the factors that mediate antibiotic susceptibility. For example, growth-arrested bacilli can have dramatic changes in permeability and metabolism that can affect the ability of the drug to reach its target or for the target to be present at all (Sarathy et al. 2013). In general, while there has been much work done on characterizing antibiotic tolerance of mycobacteria in growth-arrested states, we are lacking a comprehensive understanding of the downstream effectors that mediate tolerance and the upstream factors that lead to changes in growth rate. Nevertheless, slow growth or complete growth arrest undoubtedly contributes to the long time needed to kill a population of mycobacterial cells.

M. tuberculosis can reside for long periods of time inside macrophages, immune cells designed to kill invading pathogens by exposing them to a myriad of stressful conditions. At least some of these stresses can induce drug tolerance. *M. tuberculosis* residing within activated macrophages are less drug susceptible than those associated with resting macrophages (Liu et al. 2016). While any number of changes in pathogen physiology could explain changes in antibiotic susceptibility in vivo, including upregulation of efflux pumps (Adams et al. 2011), slow growth may be a dominating factor. Indeed, modeling many host-related stresses in vitro produces slow-growing populations that are more drug tolerant (Wayne and Hayes 1996; Xie et al. 2005; Paramasivan et al. 2005; Gengenbacher et al. 2010; de Steenwinkel et al. 2010; Thayil et al. 2011).

Are all pathways that lead to slow growth the same? Work done using in vitro models has given us robust transcriptional markers that indicate growth-arrested states (Sherman et al. 2001; Betts et al. 2002; Voskuil 2004; Balazsi et al. 2008). Surprisingly, there is little overlap in the response of the pathogen between different conditions. For example, only five genes were found to overlap when comparing the transcriptional responses that result from hypoxia, stationary phase, or nutrient starvation (Keren et al. 2011). Thus, while the pathogen grows slowly in each of these conditions, the upstream mechanisms that induce slow growth and the downstream effectors that mediate tolerance appear to be condition specific.

A particularly useful in vitro model for mimicking a condition thought to exist inside the granuloma is hypoxia (Wayne and Hayes 1996; Voskuil 2004). While *M. tuberculosis* is an obligate aerobe, it has many strategies to ensure its survival under hypoxic conditions, including respiratory networks that utilize both oxygen and nitrate as terminal electron acceptors (Sherman et al. 2001; Voskuil 2004; Boshoff and Barry 2005). The connection between hypoxia and altered antibiotic susceptibility was established soon after Lawrence Wayne introduced his model of hypoxia by restriction of headspace (Wayne and Lin 1982; Wayne and Hayes 1996). Subsequently, Wayne and others have shown that mycobacteria in a hypoxia-induced non-replicative state are far less susceptible to drugs with diverse mechanisms of action, including ciprofloxacin, isoniazid, and rifampicin (Wayne and Hayes 1996; Koul et al. 2008).

Another in vitro model that has provided useful insights, especially considering its simple implementation, is the stationary phase. During stationary phase, cells likely experience a complex environment devoid of many essential nutrients. Importantly, mycobacteria in stationary phase become more tolerant to antibiotics that target DNA replication and cell envelope biosynthesis when compared with cells that grow exponentially (Herbert et al. 1996; Paramasivan et al. 2005). There is some evidence that specific proteins expressed during stationary phase are important for the observed antibiotic tolerance. For example, DNA-binding protein 1 (MDP1) is expressed in stationary phase and confers tolerance to isoniazid in *M. smegmatis* (Niki et al. 2012). Chaperones also seem to play an important role in drug tolerance during stationary phase. Cells that lack ClpB, a chaperone that can refold aggregated structures, are defective in recovery from stationary phase and less likely to survive antibiotic treatment (Vaubourgeix et al. 2015).

Nutrient starvation, in general, increases the tolerance of *M. tuberculosis* to a wide range of anti-TB drugs (Xie et al. 2005; Gengenbacher et al. 2010). Many bacterial species, when faced with starvation, activate a global transcriptional program called the stringent response. This response is characterized by the accumulation of the signaling molecules (p)ppGpp. *Mycobacterium tuberculosis* also encodes a functional stringent response that is required for long-term survival in nutrient-limited conditions in vitro, and during infection in mice. Historically, the stringent response and elevated levels of (p)ppGpp have been associated with antibiotic tolerance in *E. coli* and other bacteria (Nguyen et al. 2011; Germain et al. 2013; Liu et al. 2017). An exception is *S. aureus* that does not rely on (p)ppGpp for the formation of drug-tolerant cells (Conlon et al. 2016). Likewise, a very recent study found that in *M. smegmatis* there is no connection between the stringent response and antibiotic tolerance (Bhaskar et al. 2018). Thus, the mechanisms that sense environmental cues and regulate growth in mycobacteria could be different as compared to other common model organisms. Indeed, even highly conserved pathways like peptidoglycan synthesis respond to starvation differently in mycobacteria. Subverting these mechanisms may help to target non-growing populations (Boutte et al. 2016).

We will cover this in more detail below, but it is worth noting here that there is little evidence supporting the notion that persistence in mycobacteria is due to pre-existing subpopulations of very slow- or non-growing cells, as has been shown to be the case for *E. coli* (Balaban et al. 2004). Part of the reason for this is technical, but biological factors could also be responsible. Indeed, established assays for generating persister cells, like a passage through stationary phase, do not result in the formation of persister-like mycobacteria (Bhaskar et al. 2018). Thus, while slow growth is likely a major contributing factor to the long time it takes to kill mycobacteria, it does not explain *per se* the multi-phasic kill curve that is observed during TB treatment.

11.2.2 *Efflux Pumps*

Many pathogenic bacteria express drug efflux pumps to actively protect against antibiotics or other foreign compounds. Canonical examples of efflux pumps include AcrB and TolC in *E. coli* or MexB in *Pseudomonas aeruginosa* (Ma et al. 1993; Li et al. 1995; Buchanan 2001). As their evolution precedes the advent of antibiotics, the primary function of these pumps is in cellular physiology, disposing of toxic products (Ho and Kim 2005), secreting signaling molecules (de Rossi et al. 2006), and exporting molecules to the cell surface (Buchanan 2001). Transportation or active efflux of antibiotics is generally considered a secondary function (Ma et al. 1993; Li et al. 1995).

The *M. tuberculosis* genome encodes an enormous array of putative transporters and efflux pumps to traffic molecules over its complex cell envelope. Of the 267 transporters present in the H37Rv genome, 45 have been predicted to be involved in drug efflux (da Silva et al. 2011). And of these putative efflux pumps, 26 have been experimentally shown to be associated with drug resistance (da Silva et al. 2011; Viveiros et al. 2012; Nasiri et al. 2017).

Given the difficulty in treating TB, this vast number of putative efflux pumps, and the role of efflux in driving resistance in other pathogens, there have been significant efforts in understanding the role of efflux in the intrinsic antibiotic resistance of the pathogen. However, although several putative efflux systems have been connected to antibiotic tolerance or resistance, the function of most of these systems remains controversial or not yet fully elucidated. For example, the *iniBAC* operon member *iniA* had been predicted to be an efflux pump that conferred resistence to isoniazid, but recent work has shown that overexpression or deletion of *iniBAC* in *Mycobacterium bovis* BCG and *Mycobacterium marinum* does not alter resistance to isoniazid (Colangeli et al. 2005; Boot et al. 2016, 2017). Likewise, MmpL3, a protein in the "mycobacterial membrane protein, large" family, was originally categorized as an efflux pump, but was recently shown to flip important cell envelope constituents, trehalose monomycolates (TMMs), over the inner membrane into the periplasm (Xu et al. 2017b). The structure of MmpL3 supports the notion that MmpL3 strictly transports TMMs, as the binding of several antibiotic compounds occurs far from the pore region (Zhang et al. 2019). Thus, while some efflux pumps could transport antibiotics directly, it is also likely that other efflux proteins that have been associated with drug resistance are only indirectly involved in the observed resistance phenotypes. Given this caveat, it is still worth noting that overexpression of many transporters confers low-level resistance in mycobacteria (Gupta et al. 2010; Balganesh et al. 2012; Dinesh et al. 2013; Kardan Yamchi et al. 2015; Caleffi-Ferracioli et al. 2016). Taking another approach, Dinesh et al. demonstrated, by a step-wise deletion of different classes of efflux pumps that loss of these pumps results in a two- to fourfold increase in sensitivity of *M. tuberculosis* to cell wall-inhibiting drugs, such as penicillin, ampicillin, meropenem, and vancomycin (Dinesh et al. 2013).

While some efflux pumps are constitutively expressed and may provide intrinsic resistance, others are specifically upregulated in response to a specific class of antibiotics, usually the one they pump over the cell membrane. In other organisms, gene regulatory circuits that control the expression of efflux pumps can lead to heterogeneity in efflux pump expression and, by consequence, variability in drug susceptibility (Schultz et al. 2017). There may be similar mechanisms at play in mycobacteria, but outside of a few cases (Morris et al. 2005; Buroni et al. 2006), the genetic circuits that control efflux pump expression have not been fully worked out. Fortunately, the advent of RNA sequencing has started to allow for an understanding of efflux pump expression in response to antibiotics on a genome-wide scale. Studies using RNA sequencing have confirmed many of the existing data on the response of *M. tuberculosis* efflux pumps to antibiotics, but have also revealed new connections between efflux pump expression and certain antibiotics (Boshoff et al. 2004; Murima et al. 2013; Boot et al. 2018). For example, it was found that many efflux pumps are not just induced by singular antibiotics, but as a general response to many antibiotics (Boot et al. 2018). A prominent example is P55 (encoded by *rv1410c*), an efflux pump involved in lipid transport (Martinot et al. 2016), which is upregulated in response to ciprofloxacin, ethambutol, isoniazid, streptomycin, and rifampicin treatment in *M. tuberculosis* (Boot et al. 2018).

Importantly, to date, there have not been any examples of drug-resistant TB disease being a result of pathogen mutations that affect the expression of efflux pumps. While some clinically resistant strains have differences in efflux pump expression, the causal link to decreased drug accumulation and acquired drug resistance is lacking. In fact, there is little evidence supporting the notion that direct inhibition of drug efflux, by efflux pump inhibitors, can increase the sensitivity of *M. tuberculosis* to antibiotic treatment (te Brake et al. 2018).

Thus, in summary, while efflux is a major, direct driver of high-level antibiotic resistance in other bacteria, it is not yet clear this is the case for mycobacteria. However, it is possible that low-level phenotypic resistance provided by the transient induction of several efflux systems, could serve as a stepping stone to higher-level genetic resistance (Brauner et al. 2016; Hicks et al. 2018). Moreover, given that the genetic circuitry controlling the induction of pumps is likely complicated and interconnected, variability in the single-cell expression of pumps might lead to increased tolerance or phenotypic resistance of subpopulations of cells during infection. Indeed, several pumps are upregulated during macrophage infection. One of them, Tap, may be upregulated in subpopulations of cells that can be eliminated when treatment is supplemented with an efflux pump inhibitor (Adams et al. 2011, 2014).

11.2.3   Cell Envelope Permeability

Mycobacteria possess a complex, thick, and lipid-rich cell envelope, which has been implicated in their natural tolerance to many drugs (Brennan and Nikaido 1995; Jankute et al. 2015). While not structurally similar to the Gram-negative cell envelope, there are distinct layers, and, likely, a periplasmic space. Like almost all bacteria, the plasma membrane of mycobacteria is surrounded by peptidoglycan, a cross-linked mesh made up of sugars and peptides. Mycobacterial peptidoglycan is covalently attached to arabinogalactan, a highly branched polysaccharide which, in turn, is covalently attached to mycolic acids—long-chained fatty acids that can be up to 90 carbon acids long. Multiple studies have revealed another layer on top of this, composed of an enormous array of free mycolates and other lipids (Graham et al. 1991; Brennan and Nikaido 1995). The importance of the cell envelope to mycobacterial physiology is illustrated by the fact that cell envelope lipids make up nearly 40% of the dry mass of the cell (Jackson 2014), and more than a quarter of the *M. tuberculosis* genome is devoted to cell envelope synthesis or regulation there of (Doerks et al. 2012). This unusual structure provides an effective barrier for both hydrophobic and hydrophilic compounds. In fact, a recent genome-wide screen using saturated transposon mutagenesis suggests that the intrinsic tolerance of *Mycobacterium tuberculosis* to several drugs is mostly determined by cell envelope permeability (Xu et al. 2017a).

How, then, are molecules transported across? Unfortunately, there is not a clear answer to this question. Whereas many Gram-negative bacteria have clear membrane-spanning porins and pumps, it is largely unclear how drug molecules traverse the *M. tuberculosis* outer membrane. Even though the *M. tuberculosis* genome encodes >100 putative OM proteins (OMPs), verification and characterization of OMP candidates has been challenging (Song et al. 2008). A major reason for this is the lack of techniques that cleanly separate the inner membrane from the outer membrane. Despite these challenges, studying the transport of molecules across this unusual structure has been an active area of research for decades and has provided us a few clues. The hydrophobic nature of the mycobacterial outer membrane suggests that hydrophobic agents can enter and pass the lipid bilayer more effectively. Work from multiple groups has shown that this is indeed the case, as hydrophobicity was found to correlate with antibiotic efficacy for several hydrophobic drugs (Wallace et al. 1979; Heifets et al. 1990; Brown et al. 1992). In fact, making the amphipathic ciprofloxacin more hydrophobic by the addition of alkyl groups makes the drug more active against *M. tuberculosis* and *M. avium* (Haemers et al. 1990). Other, more hydrophilic molecules, may be transported via porins or pore-like structures embedded in the mycobacterial membrane. Many fast-growing mycobacterial species encode the porin, MspA. Deletion of MspA results in reduced uptake of, and increased minimum inhibitory concentrations (MICs) for, several hydrophilic and hydrophobic compounds including ampicillin, chloramphenicol, norfloxacin, vancomycin, and cephaloridine (Stahl et al. 2001; Stephan et al. 2004; Danilchanka et al. 2008). Conversely, heterologous expression of MspA in *M. tuberculosis* or *M. bovis* BCG renders both species more susceptible to hydrophilic compounds, including β-lactams, isoniazid, ethambutol, and streptomycin (Mailaender et al. 2004). Although, *M. tuberculosis* does not have Msp orthologues, bioinformatics screens have revealed the presence of Omp-like proteins Rv1698 and Rv1973 (Song et al. 2008) that are specific to mycobacteria and related bacteria. Intriguingly, heterologous expression of Rv1698 can restore the sensitivity of an *M. smegmatis* mutant that lacks MspA to ampicillin and chloramphenicol.

While it is often assumed that the cell envelope composition is the same from cell-to-cell, as we will discuss below, many features of mycobacterial physiology negate the validity of this assumption. One surprising feature of the mycobacterial membrane is its low fluidity. Even when compared to bacteria with similar cell wall architecture, Fluorescence Recovery After Photobleaching (FRAP) has revealed the dramatic immobility of the outer mycobacterial cell envelope (Rodriguez-Rivera et al. 2017). This, coupled to asymmetric cell growth and division, may lead to heterogeneity even in the composition of non-covalently attached lipids across a population.

11.2.4 Drug Targets, Activators, and Modifiers

Bacteria can resist antibiotics by changing the abundance of the drug target, or modifying the drug itself. Mycobacteria encode several conserved mechanisms of drug resistance that fit into these categories, like modification of β-lactams by β-lactamases (Kasik 1965; Finch 1986). They also employ relatively specialized mechanisms, like methylation of drug targets or ribosylation of drugs, both of which effectively negate the drug–target interaction (Buriankova et al. 2004; Baysarowich et al. 2008). In addition, some anti-TB drugs are actually prodrugs that require activation by bacterial enzymes.

Naturally, any change in abundance of a drug target or activator can alter the effective intracellular concentration of the drug. For example, inactivating mutations in the gene encoding KatG, the activator of isoniazid, confer high-level resistance (Heym et al. 1993; Heym et al. 1995). However, it is not always obvious how changes in drug-target or drug-activator abundance will affect drug susceptibility. For example, overexpression of a target may lead to resistance, as more unbound drug targets are available to perform their cellular function and support survival. On the other hand, downregulation of drug targets may also lead to tolerance, as is likely the case for growth-arrested bacilli. As we discuss in the next section, variation from cell to cell in the amount of drug target or activator is one possible mechanism of diversifying drug susceptibility in a clonal population. But, how much does a drug target, activator, or modifier need to change in abundance (or across the population) in order to confer a difference in susceptibility? The answer is likely complicated and highly drug target-specific. For example, cellular depletion of dihydrofolate reductase (DHFR), the target of trimethoprim, to greater than 97% has no effect on bacterial growth. In contrast, more limited depletion of InhA and RpoB, the targets of isoniazid and rifampin, respectively, leads to rapid cell death or growth arrest (Wei et al. 2011). Thus, when considering how fluctuations in drug targets, activators, or modifiers may lead to heterogeneity in drug susceptibility, it is worth keeping in mind that not all heterogeneity is created equal. Two-fold changes across the population may be enough to make a significant difference in the susceptibility for some drugs, while other drugs may need their targets to vary by 100-fold or more to result in any appreciable difference.

11.3   Mechanisms of Phenotypic Variation in Mycobacteria

Given the vast number of factors that affect antibiotic susceptibility, perhaps it comes as no surprise that tuberculosis is difficult to treat. However, the MICs for many drugs against *M. tuberculosis* are similar to or lower than those against other pathogens. Thus, the difficulty in treating TB cannot be entirely blamed on the average tolerance of the entire bacterial population. Instead, as the pathogen is heterogeneous in terms of morphology (cell size and growth rate) and cellular processes (mistranslation) (Aldridge et al. 2012; Wakamoto et al. 2013; Rego et al. 2017; Javid et al. 2014), it is tempting to speculate that heterogeneity is an evolved mycobacterial trait. What are the most important factors that either create variation, or that vary, in a population? While we do not yet know the answer, here, we will attempt to link the mechanisms of variation that have been described in a population level to established mediators of antibiotic susceptibility (Table 11.1). We postulate that any or all of the above antibiotic susceptibility mediators could vary in a genetically identical population by a variety of mechanisms. Different sources of variation produce fluctuations at different frequencies within a population, and this is often inversely correlated with heritability (Fig. 11.1). For example, genetic changes are rare, but highly heritable, while stochastic fluctuations can be highly dynamic and not heritable over many generations. Thus, different sources of variation could aid the pathogen at different stages of the infection lifecycle. For example, high-frequency variations may be most important when bacterial numbers are small, as they are at the initial stages of infection. In contrast, rarer variants could be most important when bacterial numbers are large, as they are later in the infection lifecycle. It is also possible that, all these mechanisms are active all the time in a mycobacterial population, and the few surviving cells at the end of treatment represent the tail end of a continuum of a highly heterogeneous population (Aldridge et al. 2014; Richardson et al. 2016; Rego et al. 2017).

For the purposes of brevity, we will neglect environmental factors, including finding bacteria inside different cellular and subcellular compartments that are differentially accessible to drugs. We consider the simplest case: genetically identical cells experiencing the exact same environment, behaving differently.

Table 11.1 Established or suggested connections between a source of variation and a mediator of antibiotic susceptibility

Mediator of antibiotic susceptibility	Mechanism of single-cell variation	References
Drug activator (KatG) abundance	Stochastic pulsing	Wakamoto et al. (2013)
Drug target (RpoB) abundance	Mistranslation	Su et al. (2016)
β-Lactam target abundance	Asymmetric growth and division	Baranowski et al. (2018)
Growth arrest	Possible bistability in stringent response (?)	Sureka et al. (2008), Tiwari et al. (2010)
Cell wall permeability	Asymmetric cell growth and division (?)	Rego et al. (2017)
Efflux	Asymmetric cell growth and division (?), and unknown	Adams et al. (2011), Rego et al. (2017)
Unknown INH mediators	Changes in gene expression mediated through HupB posttranslational modifications	Sakatos et al. (2018)

11.3.1 Stochasticity

Proteins and mRNA are expressed in discrete quantities, leading to variable numbers of molecules from cell to cell. There have been a number of studies that mathematically describe this variation in model bacterial species (Tiwari et al. 2010; Eldar and Elowitz 2010), and experimentally measure its consequences for bacterial behavior especially with respect to antibiotic survival (Sureka et al. 2008; Manina et al. 2015; el Meouche et al. 2016). Gene expression in mycobacteria is governed by the same general mechanisms, yet only a few studies have linked stochastic fluctuations of important molecules to antibiotic survival. In one of the few examples, Wakamoto et al. followed individual *M. smegmatis* cells before, during, and after treatment with the prodrug isoniazid. They discovered that the slow "persistence phase" of a biphasic time–kill curve represented the dynamic balance of cell division and cell death. Cell survival was negatively correlated to the stochastic pulsing of the isoniazid activator KatG (Wakamoto et al. 2013). This provided the first evidence that stochastic fluctuations in drug targets or drug activators could be, in part, responsible for mycobacterial survival to antibiotics.

In addition to this example of "dynamic persistence" or "phenotypic resistance," multiple lines of evidence suggest that subpopulations of non-growing mycobacteria contribute to the lengthy time required for treating TB. For example, single-cell expression in ribosomal RNA, a strong correlate to growth rate (Manina et al. 2015), becomes more heterogeneous during infection, and other stressful conditions (Manina et al. 2015). Subpopulations of non-growing cells that remain metabolically active become more prominent in mice treated with isoniazid, suggesting that these rare variants could contribute to treatment failure in mice. Likewise, many bacteria respond to stress by activating a complex transcriptional program called the stringent response. At the center of this response is the (p)ppGpp synthase Rel. Surprisingly, Rel expression is bimodal in *M. smegmatis*, with stochastic fluctuations of upstream factors, contributing to the switch between high and low Rel states (Sureka et al. 2008). As Rel expression leads to drug tolerance and reduced growth rate, it is intriguing to speculate that bifurcation of the population via Rel expression could give rise to subpopulations with distinctly different fates and functions. For example, cells with high amounts of Rel could be antibiotic survivors, while those with low amounts of Rel may be biased toward growth and further host colonization (Sureka et al. 2008). However, this interpretation has recently come into question, as deletion of key stringent response proteins shows no effect on antibiotic susceptibility (Bhaskar et al. 2018).

Stochastic fluctuations allow individual cells to rapidly sample many different phenotypes with little commitment. However, there are potential mechanisms by which stochasticity can be amplified and even inherited from one generation to the next. One such mechanism is bistability. Bistability is the product of gene regulation, which typically has both positive feedback and hypersensitivity. Stochastic fluctuations in regulators can determine if a cell switches from the "off" state to the "on" state. To our knowledge, a bistable system has not been experimentally demonstrated in mycobacteria, through computational methods predict that the stress response network upstream of Rel could produce bistability (Tiwari et al. 2010). Partitioning errors that occur during cell division may be another way that stochasticity could be amplified, especially for proteins or mRNA that exist in low copy numbers (Huh and Paulsson 2011). For mycobacteria this could be an important mechanism as they both divide off-center and with less precision than other organisms, two features that could make partitioning errors more pronounced.

11.3.2 Asymmetric Cell division

In addition to stochastic mechanisms, mycobacteria take an additional, *deterministic*, route to variability through asymmetric cell division. To elongate, mycobacteria insert new cell envelope material at the cell poles. This process is asymmetric: the new pole, which was formed from the septation site from the previous round of division, grows less over the course of a cell cycle than the old pole, which was established a generation or more before (Aldridge et al. 2012). Mycobacteria also divide off-center, nearer to the new pole. Together, asymmetric growth and division establishes a heterogeneous bacterial population with respect to size, growth rate, and antibiotic susceptibility (Logsdon and Aldridge 2018). Importantly, deletion of a protein, LamA, which promotes polar growth asymmetry, leads to a faster and more uniform killing of *M. smegmatis* and *M. tuberculosis* with certain antibiotics (Rego et al. 2017), supporting the idea that growth and division asymmetry leads to diversity in drug killing (Aldridge et al. 2012).

The mechanisms by which asymmetric growth-mediated heterogeneity confers an advantage during the antibiotic challenge are poorly understood, but multiple lines of evidence suggest that important mediators of antibiotic susceptibility might be asymmetrically distributed at the time of cell division. For example, a fluorescent dye, calcein AM, whose accumulation partly predicts rifampin susceptibility, unevenly segregates or accumulates in daughter cells at the time of division (Rego et al. 2017). Mutants in proteins that influence both the import and export of molecules, like porins and efflux pumps, affect both the accumulation of calcein AM and rifampin sensitivity, suggesting that these factors may be asymmetrically distributed at the time of cell division (Rego et al. 2017).

How are proteins be positioned asymmetrically across a cell? One possibility is that they are being patterned by internal structural components like cytoskeletal elements. However, mycobacteria have no obvious homologs of cytoskeleton proteins, like MreB, which are well-conserved in laterally growing rod-shaped bacteria. Indeed, besides the septal factor FtsZ, we do not yet know of any other cytoskeletal protein(s) in mycobacteria. Another possibility is that asymmetric localization could occur through the process of polar growth itself. In contrast to growth by insertion of material along the bacterial side walls, polar growth segregates cell wall material by age: new cell wall material is inserted at the poles, and as the cell grows, older material moves toward the middle of the cell. A recent study suggests that peptidoglycan is cross-linked differently depending on cell wall age—with canonical PBP-mediated 4-3 crosslinks being abundant at the polar sites of growth, and LD-transpeptidase-mediated 3-3 crosslinks being more abundant at sites of older cell wall (Baranowski et al. 2018). The enzymes that synthesize these different crosslinks are targets for different classes of β-lactams, and, like their substrates, also localize to sites of different cell wall age. This observation underscores the idea that key differences in cell envelope constituents may arise through polar asymmetric growth and division. Fluorescent probes that are enzymatically incorporated into the outer mycobacterial membrane also show asymmetric staining patterns (Rodriguez-Rivera et al. 2017). Thus, segregation of substrate through polar growth may be a generalizable mechanism for asymmetrically partitioning cell envelope components in mycobacteria (Fig. 11.2).

In addition to asymmetric growth, mycobacteria also divide asymmetrically. Again, we do not yet know the exact mechanism by which this happens, as mycobacteria are missing conserved mechanisms for septum placement (Joyce et al. 2012). However, asymmetric polar growth seems to be a major factor, as mutants that grow more symmetrically also divide more symmetrically (Rego et al. 2017). Likewise, small physical features on the cell surface that are formed at the poles and inherited by daughter cells through polar growth are correlated to division site placement in downstream generations (Eskandarian et al. 2017). Thus, it seems likely that asymmetry in polar growth establishes asymmetry in cell division, and that local changes in the cell envelope could provide cues for septum placement.

One intriguing consequence of polar growth that has been relatively unexplored but has been postulated to exist is senescence (Kysela et al. 2013). That is, damaged components could be segregated at the time of division, rejuvenating the other daughter cells—a situation analogous to budding yeast. Supporting this idea, during

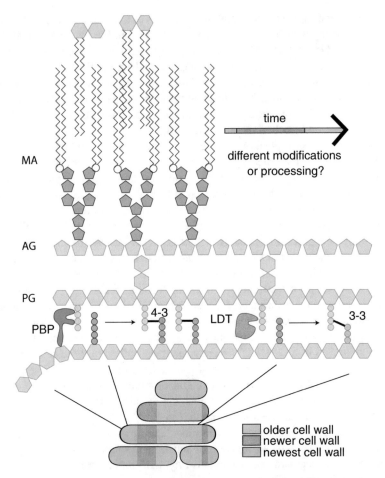

Fig. 11.2 The complex, multilayered, mycobacterial cell envelope (*PG* peptidoglycan; *AG* arabinogalactan; *MA* mycolic acids). Polar growth segregates cell envelope by age. For example, the substrates for Penicillin-Binding Proteins (PBPs), and the enzymes themselves are more abundant at the sites of new cell wall synthesis, the poles. PBPs make "canonical" 4-3 PG cross-links by attaching the fourth amino acid of one peptide side-chain to the third of another. As PG ages, and migrates toward mid-cell, it continues to be processed, eventually being cross-linked by the LD-trans peptidases (LDT), which link the third amino acid of one peptide side chain to the third amino acid of another side chain (3-3). Some lines of evidence suggest similar substrate segregation is occurring in the other layers (Rodriguez-Rivera et al. 2017). This could occur through age-related modifications, like PG, or by selectively attaching molecules to differentially cross-linked PG. At the time of division, daughter cells inherit different amounts of aged cell wall

stress, irreversibly oxidized components are segregated to one side of the mycobacterial cell and inherited by a single daughter cell (Vaubourgeix et al. 2015).

Asymmetric cell division provides the pathogen with an enormous ability for variation at a rather high frequency—cell phenotypes can change every division. This may be advantageous at times during infection when cell numbers are small.

But even when bacterial numbers are high, cell division-mediated heterogeneity could be important. In fact, reduction of asymmetric cell division seems to affect the "fast" killing phase of an *M. tuberculosis* kill curve, suggesting that even the kinetics of this phase are determined by the balance of multiple subpopulations of bacteria, some of which are able to grow at concentrations of drug typically considered bactericidal.

11.3.3 Epigenetics

"Epigenetic" is broadly defined as any non-genetic modification that influences gene expression. While many of the mechanisms we have discussed so far are, by definition, epigenetic, the term is most often applied to phenotypes which are heritable over many generations, producing states that are much more stable than the ones we have so far described. In this section, we will use "epigenetic" to describe any mechanism that produces a phenotype, which is heritable on the order of producing a colony.

Mycobacteria have many examples of semi-heritable phenotypes. In fact, some species produce multiple colony morphologies on agar plates. For example, *M. abscessus*, produces both rough and smooth colonies on standard laboratory media. These two variants have different propensities for biofilm formation, host colonization, and antibiotic tolerance (Howard et al. 2006). Switching between variants has been linked to small insertions in genes encoding for lipids abundant in the outer mycobacterial layer (Pawlik et al. 2013). Given that the frequency of switching is higher than one would expect from the basal mutation rate of the pathogen, it seems likely that these errors are caused by replication slippage of the DNA polymerase, a common mechanism for phase variation in other bacterial organisms (Bayliss 2009).

In eukaryotes, one of the most common epigenetic mechanisms is the modification of histone proteins that lead to differences in gene regulation. Mycobacteria encode the histone-like protein HupB, which, like its eukaryotic counterpart, is highly modified post-translationally (Sakatos et al. 2018). HupB is required for the formation of subpopulations of cells that can grow and form colonies on agar plates containing near-MIC concentrations of isoniazid. Interestingly, mutating a single lysine in HupB to an amino acid that cannot be modified leads to differences in gene expression and abolishes the formation of one of the phenotypically resistant subpopulations. The genes responsible for growth in the presence of INH that are differently expressed via HubB modifications are not yet known; in contrast to eukaryotes, the HupB-mediated transcriptional changes appear to be global rather than specific, thus, making the search for the responsible players challenging (Sakatos et al. 2018). Nevertheless, it appears that at least some bacteria, including *M. smegmatis*, have the potential to vary their cell state via a mechanism once thought confined to the eukaryotic kingdom.

Nobody is perfect. This is certainly true for any biological system and any enzyme. Even systems with multiple layers of proofreading can produce rare errors, and these errors can have profound downstream consequences. This is well known for DNA polymerases. Errors, either during normal cell replication, or times of stress, lead to DNA mutation, and in some instances, heritable drug resistance (Kunkel and Bebenek 2000). However, other polymerases and biosynthetic complexes in the central dogma also make errors, and these errors can lead to changes, which, while not as heritable, can be just as consequential. For example, on average, translation is 10,000 times more error-prone than DNA replication (Mohler and Ibba 2017). In fact, the error rate for certain types of translation can be as high as almost 1%. Unlike DNA, however, proteins are only semi-heritable. Yet, at least for some drug targets, a subpopulation of mutated copies may be sufficient for phenotypic drug resistance. This has been demonstrated for RpoB in mycobacteria: errors in RpoB caused by mistranslation lead to a semi-stable state of phenotypic resistance and continued growth in the presence of rifampin (Javid et al. 2014; Su et al. 2016).

RNA polymerase also makes errors. While transcription is ten times more faithful than translation, the errors that RNA polymerase causes can be highly amplified into protein: the average mRNA in an *E. coli* cell makes around 1000 copies of protein (Taniguchi et al. 2010). Thus, even though the error rate is lower than translation, mistranscription might be a large source of protein variability in a bacterial cell. To date, there have only been a few studies on this potentially important phenomenon in model organisms and none in mycobacteria (Carey 2015).

11.3.4 Where Do Classical Persisters Fit in?

The term "persistence" is broadly defined as the ability for a subpopulation of cells to survive killing by antibiotics (Brauner et al. 2016). Typically, the term has been applied to subpopulations of cells that are non-growing or slow-growing prior to challenge with antibiotics, manifesting over time as a multiphasic kill curve (Brauner et al. 2016). This framework may be sufficient to explain the killing of some, well-studied bacteria, but it is unlikely to explain all the phenomena that have been observed for mycobacteria. In fact, it is still unclear if "*E. coli*-like" mycobacterial persisters exist at all. Similar observations to those of Balaban et al. (2004), have never been made in mycobacteria. Part of the reason for this is surely technical. Until very recently, high-persistence mutants had not been identified in *M. tuberculosis* (Torrey et al. 2016), making studies using a low-dynamic range technique like microscopy very difficult. In fact, even in ideal conditions, time-lapse microscopy of *M. tuberculosis* is difficult, given its slow growth rate. This necessitates the use of a fast-growing mycobacterial model organism, like *M. smegmatis*. While *M. smegmatis* appears to be a decent model for some phenomena and mechanisms, its vastly different lifestyle as a soil-dwelling organism calls into question using this model to dissect stress-related pathways. Nevertheless, single-cell techniques require the use of a such a model system, and at least for certain mechanisms of phenotypic heterogeneity, there has been good agreement between results obtained in *M. smegmatis* and *M. tuberculosis* (Aldridge et al. 2012; Su et al. 2016; Rego et al. 2017).

In addition to these technical limitations, there are likely to be many biological differences between mycobacteria and an evolutionarily distant bacteria, like *E. coli*. Many conserved pathways, like the stringent response, are rewired differently in mycobacteria (Boutte and Crosson 2013), and there is now evidence suggesting this system is not involved in drug tolerance at all (Bhaskar et al. 2018). Passaging *M. smegmatis* through exponential phase, a sure way to eliminate "Type I" persisters in *E. coli*, does not change the abundance of persisters in mycobacteria (Bhaskar et al. 2018). Thus, we think that the jury is still out as to whether similar phenomena are at work in mycobacteria.

One topic that we have not covered here is the toxin-antitoxin (TA) systems. *M. tuberculosis* encodes approximately 70–90 TA couples, and there is virtually nothing known about these systems in relation to drug susceptibility (Ramage et al. 2009; Sala et al. 2014). While TAs have been implicated in persistence for many years, this has recently come into question (Harms et al. 2017), and we have opted not to discuss it here.

11.4   Targeting Heterogeneity

We imagine that there are two potential avenues toward targeting heterogeneity therapeutically (Fig. 11.3). The first is to use drug combinations that are active against multiple bacterial subpopulations. In fact, this might be one reason that the current TB regimen requires four drugs. With a more detailed, molecular understanding of the different subpopulations, however, we may be able to more rationally design effective drug combinations. For example, there has been substantial interest in developing interventions that target non-growing mycobacteria. In fact, the newest TB drug, bedaquiline, is highly active against *M. tuberculosis* grown under hypoxic conditions. Promisingly, some groups have successfully used non-replicating models like hypoxia or carbon starvation as a method to screen for novel compounds that target non-growing mycobacteria (Bryk et al. 2008; Grant et al. 2013; Warrier et al. 2015). Along similar lines, some, even highly related, drug targets may be non-uniformly distributed across a population. For example, enzymes that make different peptidoglycan cross-links, and which are the targets of different classes of β-lactams, are asymmetrically segregated by polar growth. Consequently, an *M. tuberculosis* population can be more rapidly killed by a drug combination (amoxicillin + meropenem + clavulanic acid) that targets both types of enzymes (Baranowski et al. 2018). In fact, the same drug combination has shown promise in a clinical trial (Diacon et al. 2016).

Another possible solution is to target the drivers of heterogeneity themselves. In this case, the burden of knowledge becomes much more apparent. While it is possible to screen for compounds that affect heterogeneity, as has been done for HIV (Dar et al. 2014), such a screen is likelier to succeed with a molecular target. For example, compounds that target LamA or the mistranslation machinery could synergize with existing therapies to more uniformly and completely kill a mycobacterial population.

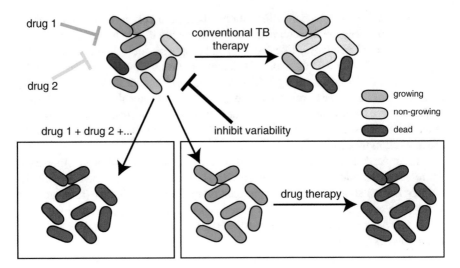

Fig. 11.3 Two ideas for improving TB therapy. Conventional therapy fails to kill all the bacteria in a population. Either by designing drug combinations that target different subpopulations, or by targeting the drivers of heterogeneity, it may be possible to more effectively kill a highly heterogeneous population of cells

Proofs of concept have recently been published supporting this idea for LamA (in vitro) and mistranslation (in vitro and in vivo) (Rego et al. 2017; Chaudhuri et al. 2018).

In this chapter, we have tried to give an overview of the aspects of mycobacterial physiology that promote survival during antibiotic treatment. While studies on large populations have taught us a lot about the physiology of the pathogen, we know much less about how the pathogen behaves on the single-cell level. There is much work to be done. We expect that future research using advanced imaging tools, fluorescent reporters, and other single-cell techniques will reveal many fascinating and important facets of mycobacterial physiology, some of which may be the key to more effective TB therapy.

References

Adams, K. N., Takaki, K., Connolly, L. E., Wiedenhoft, H., Winglee, K., Humbert, O., Edelstein, P. H., Cosma, C. L., & Ramakrishnan, L. (2011). Drug tolerance in replicating mycobacteria mediated by a macrophage-induced efflux mechanism. *Cell, 145*, 39–53.

Adams, K. N., Szumowski, J. D., & Ramakrishnan, L. (2014). Verapamil, and its metabolite norverapamil, inhibit macrophage-induced, bacterial efflux pump-mediated tolerance to multiple anti-tubercular drugs. *Journal of Infectious Diseases, 210*, 456–466.

Aldridge, B. B., Fernandez-Suarez, M., Heller, D., Ambravaneswaran, V., Irimia, D., Toner, M., & Fortune, S. M. (2012). Asymmetry and aging of mycobacterial cells lead to variable growth and antibiotic susceptibility. *Science, 335*, 100–104.

Aldridge, B. B., Keren, I., & Fortune, S. M. (2014). The spectrum of drug susceptibility in mycobacteria. *Microbiology Spectrum, 2*, 1–14.

Balaban, N. Q., Merrin, J., Chait, R., Kowalik, L., & Leibler, S. (2004). Bacterial persistence as a phenotypic switch. *Science, 305*, 1622–1625.

Balaban, N. Q., Gerdes, K., Lewis, K., & Mckinney, J. D. (2013). A problem of persistence: Still more questions than answers? *Nature Reviews Microbiology, 11*, 587–591.

Balazsi, G., Heath, A. P., Shi, L., & Gennaro, M. L. (2008). The temporal response of the *Mycobacterium tuberculosis* gene regulatory network during growth arrest. *Molecular Systems Biology, 4*, 225.

Balganesh, M., Dinesh, N., Sharma, S., Kuruppath, S., Nair, A. V., & Sharma, U. (2012). Efflux pumps of *Mycobacterium tuberculosis* play a significant role in antituberculosis activity of potential drug candidates. *Antimicrobial Agents and Chemotherapy, 56*, 2643–2651.

Baranowski, C., Sham, L.-T., Eskandarian, H. A., Welsh, M. A., Lim, H. C., Kieser, K. J., Wagner, J. C., Walker, S., Mckinney, J. D., Fantner, G. E., Ioerger, T. R., Bernhardt, T. G., Rubin, E. J., & Rego, E. H. (2018). Maturing Mycobacterium smegmatis peptidoglycan requires non-canonical crosslinks to maintain shape. eLife, 7:e37516

Bayliss, C. D. (2009). Determinants of phase variation rate and the fitness implications of differing rates for bacterial pathogens and commensals. *FEMS Microbiology Reviews, 33*, 504–520.

Baysarowich, J., Koteva, K., Hughes, D. W., Ejim, L., Griffiths, E., Zhang, K., Junop, M., & Wright, G. D. (2008). Rifamycin antibiotic resistance by ADP-ribosylation: Structure and diversity of Arr. *Proceedings of the National Academy of Sciences of the United States of America, 105*, 4886–4891.

Betts, J. C., Lukey, P. T., Robb, L. C., Mcadam, R. A., & Duncan, K. (2002). Evaluation of a nutrient starvation model of *Mycobacterium tuberculosis* persistence by gene and protein expression profiling. *Molecular Microbiology, 43*, 717–731.

Bhaskar, A., De Piano, C., Gelman, E., Mckinney, J. D., & Dhar, N. (2018). Elucidating the role of (p)ppGpp in mycobacterial persistence against antibiotics. *IUBMB Life, 70*, 836–844.

Boot, M., Sparrius, M., Jim, K. K., Commandeur, S., Speer, A., van de Weerd, R., & Bitter, W. (2016). iniBAC induction Is Vitamin B12- and MutAB-dependent in *Mycobacterium marinum*. *The Journal of Biological Chemistry, 291*, 19800–19812.

Boot, M., van Winden, V. J. C., Sparrius, M., van de Weerd, R., Speer, A., Ummels, R., Rustad, T., Sherman, D. R., & Bitter, W. (2017). Cell envelope stress in mycobacteria is regulated by the novel signal transduction ATPase IniR in response to trehalose. *PLoS Genetics, 13*, e1007131.

Boot, M., Commandeur, S., Subudhi, A. K., Bahira, M., Smith, T. C., 2nd, Abdallah, A. M., van Gemert, M., Lelievre, J., Ballell, L., Aldridge, B. B., Pain, A., Speer, A., & Bitter, W. (2018). Accelerating early antituberculosis drug discovery by creating mycobacterial indicator strains that predict mode of action. *Antimicrobial Agents and Chemotherapy, 62*.

Boshoff, H. I., & Barry, C. E., 3rd. (2005). Tuberculosis – metabolism and respiration in the absence of growth. *Nature Reviews. Microbiology, 3*, 70–80.

Boshoff, H. I., Myers, T. G., Copp, B. R., Mcneil, M. R., Wilson, M. A., Barry, C. E., & 3RD. (2004). The transcriptional responses of *Mycobacterium tuberculosis* to inhibitors of metabolism: Novel insights into drug mechanisms of action. *The Journal of Biological Chemistry, 279*, 40174–40184.

Boutte, C. C., & Crosson, S. (2013). Bacterial lifestyle shapes stringent response activation. *Trends in Microbiology, 21*, 174–180.

Boutte, C. C., Baer, C. E., Papavinasasundaram, K., Liu, W., Chase, M. R., Meniche, X., Fortune, S. M., Sassetti, C. M., Ioerger, T. R., & Rubin, E. J. (2016). A cytoplasmic peptidoglycan amidase homologue controls mycobacterial cell wall synthesis. *eLife, 5*.

Brauner, A., Fridman, O., Gefen, O., & Balaban, N. Q. (2016). Distinguishing between resistance, tolerance and persistence to antibiotic treatment. *Nature Reviews Microbiology, 14*, 320–330.

Brennan, P. J., & Nikaido, H. (1995). The envelope of mycobacteria. *Annual Review of Biochemistry, 64*, 29–63.

Brown, B. A., Wallace, R. J., Jr., Onyi, G. O., de Rosas, V., & Wallace, R. J., 3rd. (1992). Activities of four macrolides, including clarithromycin, against *Mycobacterium fortuitum, Mycobacterium chelonae*, and *M. chelonae*-like organisms. *Antimicrobial Agents and Chemotherapy, 36*, 180–184.

Bryk, R., Gold, B., Venugopal, A., Singh, J., Samy, R., Pupek, K., Cao, H., Popescu, C., Gurney, M., Hotha, S., Cherian, J., Rhee, K., Ly, L., Converse, P. J., Ehrt, S., Vandal, O., Jiang, X.,

Schneider, J., Lin, G., & Nathan, C. (2008). Selective killing of nonreplicating mycobacteria. *Cell Host & Microbe, 3*, 137–145.

Buchanan, S. K. (2001). Type I secretion and multidrug efflux: Transport through the TolC channel-tunnel. *Trends in Biochemical Sciences, 26*, 3–6.

Buriankova, K., Doucet-Populaire, F., Dorson, O., Gondran, A., Ghnassia, J. C., Weiser, J., & Pernodet, J. L. (2004). Molecular basis of intrinsic macrolide resistance in the *Mycobacterium tuberculosis* complex. *Antimicrobial Agents and Chemotherapy, 48*, 143–150.

Buroni, S., Manina, G., Guglierame, P., Pasca, M. R., Riccardi, G., & de Rossi, E. (2006). LfrR is a repressor that regulates expression of the efflux pump LfrA in Mycobacterium smegmatis. *Antimicrobial Agents and Chemotherapy, 50*, 4044–4052.

Cadena, A. M., Fortune, S. M., & Flynn, J. L. (2017). Heterogeneity in tuberculosis. *Nature Reviews Immunology, 17*, 691–702.

Caleffi-Ferracioli, K. R., Amaral, R. C., Demitto, F. O., Maltempe, F. G., Canezin, P. H., Scodro, R. B., Nakamura, C. V., Leite, C. Q., Siqueira, V. L., & Cardoso, R. F. (2016). Morphological changes and differentially expressed efflux pump genes in *Mycobacterium tuberculosis* exposed to a rifampicin and verapamil combination. *Tuberculosis (Edinburgh, Scotland), 97*, 65–72.

Carey, L. B. (2015). RNA polymerase errors cause splicing defects and can be regulated by differential expression of RNA polymerase subunits. *Elife, 4*, e09945.

Chaudhuri, S., Li, L., Zimmerman, M., Chen, Y., Chen, Y. X., Toosky, M. N., Gardner, M., Pan, M., Li, Y. Y., Kawaji, Q., Zhu, J. H., Su, H. W., Martinot, A. J., Rubin, E. J., Dartois, V. A., & Javid, B. (2018). Kasugamycin potentiates rifampicin and limits emergence of resistance in *Mycobacterium tuberculosis* by specifically decreasing mycobacterial mistranslation. *eLife, 7*, e36782.

Colangeli, R., Helb, D., Sridharan, S., Sun, J., Varma-Basil, M., Hazbon, M. H., Harbacheuski, R., Megjugorac, N. J., Jacobs, W. R., Jr., Holzenburg, A., Sacchettini, J. C., & Alland, D. (2005). The *Mycobacterium tuberculosis* iniA gene is essential for activity of an efflux pump that confers drug tolerance to both isoniazid and ethambutol. *Molecular Microbiology, 55*, 1829–1840.

Conlon, B. P., Rowe, S. E., Gandt, A. B., Nuxoll, A. S., Donegan, N. P., Zalis, E. A., Clair, G., Adkins, J. N., Cheung, A. L., & Lewis, K. (2016). Persister formation in *Staphylococcus aureus* is associated with ATP depletion. *Nature Microbiology, 1*, 16051.

da Silva, P. E., von Groll, A., Martin, A., & Palomino, J. C. (2011). Efflux as a mechanism for drug resistance in *Mycobacterium tuberculosis*. *FEMS Immunology and Medical Microbiology, 63*, 1–9.

da Silva, P. E., Machado, D., Ramos, D., Couto, I., von Groll, A., & Viveiros, M. (2016). Efflux pumps in mycobacteria: Antimicrobial resistance, physiological functions, and role in pathogenicity. In X. Z. Li (Ed.), *Efflux-mediated antimicrobial resistance in bacteria*. Cham: Springer.

Danilchanka, O., Pavlenok, M., & Niederweis, M. (2008). Role of porins for uptake of antibiotics by *Mycobacterium smegmatis*. *Antimicrobial Agents and Chemotherapy, 52*, 3127–3134.

Dar, R. D., Hosmane, N. N., Arkin, M. R., Siliciano, R. F., & Weinberger, L. S. (2014). Screening for noise in gene expression identifies drug synergies. *Science, 344*, 1392–1396.

de Rossi, E., Ainsa, J. A., & Riccardi, G. (2006). Role of mycobacterial efflux transporters in drug resistance: An unresolved question. *FEMS Microbiology Reviews, 30*, 36–52.

de Steenwinkel, J. E., de Knegt, G. J., ten Kate, M. T., van Belkum, A., Verbrugh, H. A., Kremer, K., van Soolingen, D., & Bakker-Woudenberg, I. A. (2010). Time-kill kinetics of anti-tuberculosis drugs, and emergence of resistance, in relation to metabolic activity of *Mycobacterium tuberculosis*. *The Journal of Antimicrobial Chemotherapy, 65*, 2582–2589.

Diacon, A. H., van der Merwe, L., Barnard, M., von Groote-Bidlingmaier, F., Lange, C., Garcia-Basteiro, A. L., Sevene, E., Ballell, L., & Barros-Aguirre, D. (2016). beta-lactams against tuberculosis – New trick for an old dog? *The New England Journal of Medicine, 375*, 393–394.

Dinesh, N., Sharma, S., & Balganesh, M. (2013). Involvement of efflux pumps in the resistance to peptidoglycan synthesis inhibitors in *Mycobacterium tuberculosis*. *Antimicrobial Agents and Chemotherapy, 57*, 1941–1943.

Doerks, T., van Noort, V., Minguez, P., & Bork, P. (2012). Annotation of the *M. tuberculosis* hypothetical orfeome: Adding functional information to more than half of the uncharacterized proteins. *PLoS One, 7,* e34302.

Dorr, T., Vulic, M., & Lewis, K. (2010). Ciprofloxacin causes persister formation by inducing the TisB toxin in *Escherichia coli*. *PLoS Biology, 8,* e1000317.

Dye, C. (2006). Global epidemiology of tuberculosis. *Lancet, 367,* 938–940.

el Meouche, I., Siu, Y., & Dunlop, M. J. (2016). Stochastic expression of a multiple antibiotic resistance activator confers transient resistance in single cells. *Scientific Reports, 6,* 19538.

Eldar, A., & Elowitz, M. B. (2010). Functional roles for noise in genetic circuits. *Nature, 467,* 167–173.

Eskandarian, H. A., Odermatt, P. D., Ven, J. X. Y., Hannebelle, M. T. M., Nievergelt, A. P., Dhar, N., Mckinney, J. D., & Fantner, G. E. (2017). Division site selection linked to inherited cell surface wave troughs in mycobacteria. *Nature Microbiology, 2,* 17094.

Evans, D. J., Allison, D. G., Brown, M. R., & Gilbert, P. (1991). Susceptibility of *Pseudomonas aeruginosa* and *Escherichia coli* biofilms towards ciprofloxacin: Effect of specific growth rate. *The Journal of Antimicrobial Chemotherapy, 27,* 177–184.

Ferullo, D. J., & Lovett, S. T. (2008). The stringent response and cell cycle arrest in *Escherichia coli*. *PLoS Genetics, 4,* e1000300.

Finch, R. (1986). Beta-lactam antibiotics and mycobacteria. *The Journal of Antimicrobial Chemotherapy, 18,* 6–8.

Fox, W., Ellard, G. A., & Mitchison, D. A. (1999). Studies on the treatment of tuberculosis undertaken by the British Medical Research Council tuberculosis units, 1946-1986, with relevant subsequent publications. *The International Journal of Tuberculosis and Lung Disease, 3,* S231–S279.

Gefen, O., Gabay, C., Mumcuoglu, M., Engel, G., & Balaban, N. Q. (2008). Single-cell protein induction dynamics reveals a period of vulnerability to antibiotics in persister bacteria. *Proceedings of the National Academy of Sciences of the United States of America, 105,* 6145–6149.

Gengenbacher, M., Rao, S. P., Pethe, K., & Dick, T. (2010). Nutrient-starved, non-replicating *Mycobacterium tuberculosis* requires respiration, ATP synthase and isocitrate lyase for maintenance of ATP homeostasis and viability. *Microbiology, 156,* 81–87.

Germain, E., Castro-Roa, D., Zenkin, N., & Gerdes, K. (2013). Molecular mechanism of bacterial persistence by HipA. *Molecular Cell, 52,* 248–254.

Gill, W. P., Harik, N. S., Whiddon, M. R., Liao, R. P., Mittler, J. E., & Sherman, D. R. (2009). A replication clock for *Mycobacterium tuberculosis*. *Nature Medicine, 15,* 211–214.

Graham, L. L., Beveridge, T. J., & Nanninga, N. (1991). Periplasmic space and the concept of the periplasm. *Trends in Biochemical Sciences, 16,* 328–329.

Grant, S. S., Kawate, T., Nag, P. P., Silvis, M. R., Gordon, K., Stanley, S. A., Kazyanskaya, E., Nietupski, R., Golas, A., Fitzgerald, M., Cho, S., Franzblau, S. G., & Hung, D. T. (2013). Identification of novel inhibitors of nonreplicating *Mycobacterium tuberculosis* using a carbon starvation model. *ACS Chemical Biology, 8,* 2224–2234.

Gupta, A. K., Katoch, V. M., Chauhan, D. S., Sharma, R., Singh, M., Venkatesan, K., & Sharma, V. D. (2010). Microarray analysis of efflux pump genes in multidrug-resistant *Mycobacterium tuberculosis* during stress induced by common anti-tuberculous drugs. *Microbial Drug Resistance, 16,* 21–28.

Haemers, A., Leysen, D. C., Bollaert, W., Zhang, M. Q., & Pattyn, S. R. (1990). Influence of N substitution on antimycobacterial activity of ciprofloxacin. *Antimicrobial Agents and Chemotherapy, 34,* 496–497.

Harms, A., Fino, C., Sorensen, M. A., Semsey, S., & Gerdes, K. (2017). Prophages and growth dynamics confound experimental results with antibiotic-tolerant persister cells. *MBio, 8,* e01964-17.

Hartman, T. E., Wang, Z., Jansen, R. S., Gardete, S., & Rhee, K. Y. (2017). Metabolic perspectives on persistence. *Microbiology Spectrum, 5,* TBTB2-0026-2016.

Heifets, L. B., Lindholm-Levy, P. J., & Flory, M. A. (1990). Bactericidal activity in vitro of various rifamycins against *Mycobacterium avium* and *Mycobacterium tuberculosis*. *The American Review of Respiratory Disease, 141,* 626–630.

Herbert, D., Paramasivan, C. N., Venkatesan, P., Kubendiran, G., Prabhakar, R., & Mitchison, D. A. (1996). Bactericidal action of ofloxacin, sulbactam-ampicillin, rifampin, and isoniazid on logarithmic- and stationary-phase cultures of *Mycobacterium tuberculosis*. *Antimicrobial Agents and Chemotherapy, 40*, 2296–2299.

Heym, B., Zhang, Y., Poulet, S., Young, D., & Cole, S. T. (1993). Characterization of the katG gene encoding a catalase-peroxidase required for the isoniazid susceptibility of *Mycobacterium tuberculosis*. *Journal of Bacteriology, 175*, 4255–4259.

Heym, B., Alzari, P. M., Honore, N., & Cole, S. T. (1995). Missense mutations in the catalase-peroxidase gene, katG, are associated with isoniazid resistance in *Mycobacterium tuberculosis*. *Molecular Microbiology, 15*, 235–245.

Hicks, N. D., Yang, J., Zhang, X., Zhao, B., Grad, Y. H., Liu, L., Ou, X., Chang, Z., Xia, H., Zhou, Y., Wang, S., Dong, J., Sun, L., Zhu, Y., Zhao, Y., Jin, Q., & Fortune, S. M. (2018). Clinically prevalent mutations in *Mycobacterium tuberculosis* alter propionate metabolism and mediate multidrug tolerance. *Nature Microbiology, 3*, 1032–1042.

Ho, R. H., & Kim, R. B. (2005). Transporters and drug therapy: Implications for drug disposition and disease. *Clinical Pharmacology and Therapeutics, 78*, 260–277.

Horsburgh, C. R., Jr., Barry, C. E., 3rd, & Lange, C. (2015). Treatment of tuberculosis. *The New England Journal of Medicine, 373*, 2149–2160.

Howard, S. T., Rhoades, E., Recht, J., Pang, X., Alsup, A., Kolter, R., Lyons, C. R., & Byrd, T. F. (2006). Spontaneous reversion of *Mycobacterium abscessus* from a smooth to a rough morphotype is associated with reduced expression of glycopeptidolipid and reacquisition of an invasive phenotype. *Microbiology, 152*, 1581–1590.

Huh, D., & Paulsson, J. (2011). Random partitioning of molecules at cell division. *Proceedings of the National Academy of Sciences of the United States of America, 108*, 15004–15009.

Jackson, M. (2014). The mycobacterial cell envelope-lipids. *Cold Spring Harbor Perspectives in Medicine, 4*.

Jankute, M., Cox, J. A., Harrison, J., & Besra, G. S. (2015). Assembly of the mycobacterial cell wall. *Annual Review of Microbiology, 69*, 405–423.

Javid, B., Sorrentino, F., Toosky, M., Zheng, W., Pinkham, J. T., Jain, N., Pan, M., Deighan, P., & Rubin, E. J. (2014). Mycobacterial mistranslation is necessary and sufficient for rifampicin phenotypic resistance. *Proceedings of the National Academy of Sciences of the United States of America, 111*, 1132–1137.

Joyce, G., Williams, K. J., Robb, M., Noens, E., Tizzano, B., Shahrezaei, V., & Robertson, B. D. (2012). Cell division site placement and asymmetric growth in mycobacteria. *PLoS One, 7*, e44582.

Kardan Yamchi, J., Haeili, M., Gizaw Feyisa, S., Kazemian, H., Hashemi Shahraki, A., Zahednamazi, F., Imani Fooladi, A. A., & Feizabadi, M. M. (2015). Evaluation of efflux pump gene expression among drug susceptible and drug resistant strains of *Mycobacterium tuberculosis* from Iran. *Infection, Genetics and Evolution, 36*, 23–26.

Kasik, J. E. (1965). The nature of mycobacterial penicillinase. *The American Review of Respiratory Disease, 91*, 117–119.

Keren, I., Minami, S., Rubin, E., & Lewis, K. (2011). Characterization and transcriptome analysis of *Mycobacterium tuberculosis* persisters. *MBio, 2*, e00100–e00111.

Kester, J. C., & Fortune, S. M. (2014). Persisters and beyond: Mechanisms of phenotypic drug resistance and drug tolerance in bacteria. *Critical Reviews in Biochemistry and Molecular Biology, 49*, 91–101.

Koul, A., Vranckx, L., Dendouga, N., Balemans, W., van den Wyngaert, I., Vergauwen, K., Gohlmann, H. W., Willebrords, R., Poncelet, A., Guillemont, J., Bald, D., & Andries, K. (2008). Diarylquinolines are bactericidal for dormant mycobacteria as a result of disturbed ATP homeostasis. *The Journal of Biological Chemistry, 283*, 25273–25280.

Kunkel, T. A., & Bebenek, K. (2000). DNA replication fidelity. *Annual Review of Biochemistry, 69*, 497–529.

Kysela, D. T., Brown, P. J., Huang, K. C., & Brun, Y. V. (2013). Biological consequences and advantages of asymmetric bacterial growth. *Annual Review of Microbiology, 67*, 417–435.

Li, X. Z., Nikaido, H., & Poole, K. (1995). Role of mexA-mexB-oprM in antibiotic efflux in *Pseudomonas aeruginosa*. *Antimicrobial Agents and Chemotherapy, 39*, 1948–1953.

Liu, Y., Tan, S., Huang, L., Abramovitch, R. B., Rohde, K. H., Zimmerman, M. D., Chen, C., Dartois, V., Vanderven, B. C., & Russell, D. G. (2016). Immune activation of the host cell induces drug tolerance in *Mycobacterium tuberculosis* both in vitro and in vivo. *The Journal of Experimental Medicine, 213*, 809–825.

Liu, S., Wu, N., Zhang, S., Yuan, Y., Zhang, W., & Zhang, Y. (2017). Variable persister gene interactions with (p)ppGpp for persister formation in *Escherichia coli*. *Frontiers in Microbiology, 8*, 1795.

Logsdon, M. M., & Aldridge, B. B. (2018). Stable regulation of cell cycle events in mycobacteria: Insights from inherently heterogeneous bacterial populations. *Frontiers in Microbiology, 9*, 514.

Ma, D., Cook, D. N., Alberti, M., Pon, N. G., Nikaido, H., & Hearst, J. E. (1993). Molecular cloning and characterization of acrA and acrE genes of *Escherichia coli*. *Journal of Bacteriology, 175*, 6299–6313.

Mailaender, C., Reiling, N., Engelhardt, H., Bossmann, S., Ehlers, S., & Niederweis, M. (2004). The MspA porin promotes growth and increases antibiotic susceptibility of both *Mycobacterium bovis* BCG and *Mycobacterium tuberculosis*. *Microbiology, 150*, 853–864.

Manina, G., Dhar, N., & Mckinney, J. D. (2015). Stress and host immunity amplify *Mycobacterium tuberculosis* phenotypic heterogeneity and induce nongrowing metabolically active forms. *Cell Host & Microbe, 17*, 32–46.

Martinot, A. J., Farrow, M., Bai, L., Layre, E., Cheng, T. Y., Tsai, J. H., Iqbal, J., Annand, J. W., Sullivan, Z. A., Hussain, M. M., Sacchettini, J., Moody, D. B., Seeliger, J. C., & Rubin, E. J. (2016). Mycobacterial metabolic syndrome: LprG and Rv1410 regulate triacylglyceride levels, growth rate and virulence in *Mycobacterium tuberculosis*. *PLoS Pathogens, 12*, e1005351.

Mcdaniel, M. M., Krishna, N., Handagama, W. G., Eda, S., & Ganusov, V. V. (2016). Quantifying limits on replication, death, and quiescence of *Mycobacterium tuberculosis* in mice. *Frontiers in Microbiology, 7*, 862.

Mitchison, D., & Davies, G. (2012). The chemotherapy of tuberculosis: Past, present and future. *The International Journal of Tuberculosis and Lung Disease, 16*, 724–732.

Mohler, K., & Ibba, M. (2017). Translational fidelity and mistranslation in the cellular response to stress. *Nature Microbiology, 2*, 17117.

Morris, R. P., Nguyen, L., Gatfield, J., Visconti, K., Nguyen, K., Schnappinger, D., Ehrt, S., Liu, Y., Heifets, L., Pieters, J., Schoolnik, G., & Thompson, C. J. (2005). Ancestral antibiotic resistance in *Mycobacterium tuberculosis*. *Proceedings of the National Academy of Sciences of the United States of America, 102*, 12200–12205.

Munoz-Elias, E. J., Timm, J., Botha, T., Chan, W. T., Gomez, J. E., & Mckinney, J. D. (2005). Replication dynamics of *Mycobacterium tuberculosis* in chronically infected mice. *Infection and Immunity, 73*, 546–551.

Murima, P., de Sessions, P. F., Lim, V., Naim, A. N., Bifani, P., Boshoff, H. I., Sambandamurthy, V. K., Dick, T., Hibberd, M. L., Schreiber, M., & Rao, S. P. (2013). Exploring the mode of action of bioactive compounds by microfluidic transcriptional profiling in mycobacteria. *PLoS One, 8*, e69191.

Nasiri, M. J., Haeili, M., Ghazi, M., Goudarzi, H., Pormohammad, A., Imani Fooladi, A. A., & Feizabadi, M. M. (2017). New insights in to the intrinsic and acquired drug resistance mechanisms in mycobacteria. *Frontiers in Microbiology, 8*, 681.

Nguyen, D., Joshi-Datar, A., Lepine, F., Bauerle, E., Olakanmi, O., Beer, K., Mckay, G., Siehnel, R., Schafhauser, J., Wang, Y., Britigan, B. E., & Singh, P. K. (2011). Active starvation responses mediate antibiotic tolerance in biofilms and nutrient-limited bacteria. *Science, 334*, 982–986.

Nikaido, H. (2001). Preventing drug access to targets: Cell surface permeability barriers and active efflux in bacteria. *Seminars in Cell & Developmental Biology, 12*, 215–223.

Niki, M., Niki, M., Tateishi, Y., Ozeki, Y., Kirikae, T., Lewin, A., Inoue, Y., Matsumoto, M., Dahl, J. L., Ogura, H., Kobayashi, K., & Matsumoto, S. (2012). A novel mechanism of growth phase-dependent tolerance to isoniazid in mycobacteria. *The Journal of Biological Chemistry, 287,* 27743–27752.

Paramasivan, C. N., Sulochana, S., Kubendiran, G., Venkatesan, P., & Mitchison, D. A. (2005). Bactericidal action of gatifloxacin, rifampin, and isoniazid on logarithmic- and stationary-phase cultures of *Mycobacterium tuberculosis. Antimicrobial Agents and Chemotherapy, 49,* 627–631.

Pawlik, A., Garnier, G., Orgeur, M., Tong, P., Lohan, A., le Chevalier, F., Sapriel, G., Roux, A. L., Conlon, K., Honore, N., Dillies, M. A., Ma, L., Bouchier, C., Coppee, J. Y., Gaillard, J. L., Gordon, S. V., Loftus, B., Brosch, R., & Herrmann, J. L. (2013). Identification and character-ization of the genetic changes responsible for the characteristic smooth-to-rough morphotype alterations of clinically persistent *Mycobacterium abscessus. Molecular Microbiology, 90,* 612–629.

Ramage, H. R., Connolly, L. E., & Cox, J. S. (2009). Comprehensive functional analysis of *Mycobacterium tuberculosis* toxin-antitoxin systems: Implications for pathogenesis, stress responses, and evolution. *PLoS Genetics, 5,* e1000767.

Rao, S. P., Alonso, S., Rand, L., Dick, T., & Pethe, K. (2008). The protonmotive force is required for maintaining ATP homeostasis and viability of hypoxic, nonreplicating *Mycobacterium tuberculosis. Proceedings of the National Academy of Sciences of the United States of America, 105,* 11945–11950.

Rego, E. H., Audette, R. E., & Rubin, E. J. (2017). Deletion of a mycobacterial divisome factor collapses single-cell phenotypic heterogeneity. *Nature, 546,* 153–157.

Richardson, K., Bennion, O. T., Tan, S., Hoang, A. N., Cokol, M., & Aldridge, B. B. (2016). Temporal and intrinsic factors of rifampicin tolerance in mycobacteria. *Proceedings of the National Academy of Sciences of the United States of America, 113,* 8302–8307.

Rittershaus, E. S., Baek, S. H., & Sassetti, C. M. (2013). The normalcy of dormancy: Common themes in microbial quiescence. *Cell Host & Microbe, 13,* 643–651.

Rodriguez-Rivera, F. P., Zhou, X., Theriot, J. A., & Bertozzi, C. R. (2017). Visualization of mycobacterial membrane dynamics in live cells. *Journal of the American Chemical Society, 139,* 3488–3495.

Russell, D. G. (2007). Who puts the tubercle in tuberculosis? *Nature Reviews Microbiology, 5,* 39–47.

Sakatos, A., Babunovic, G. H., Chase, M. R., Dills, A., Leszyk, J., Rosebrock, T., Bryson, B., & Fortune, S. M. (2018). Posttranslational modification of a histone-like protein regulates pheno-typic resistance to isoniazid in mycobacteria. *Science Advances, 4,* eaao1478.

Sala, A., Bordes, P., & Genevaux, P. (2014). Multiple toxin-antitoxin systems in *Mycobacterium tuberculosis. Toxins (Basel), 6,* 1002–1020.

Sarathy, J. P., Dartois, V., & Lee, E. J. (2012). The role of transport mechanisms in *Mycobacterium tuberculosis* drug resistance and tolerance. *Pharmaceuticals (Basel), 5,* 1210–1235.

Sarathy, J., Dartois, V., Dick, T., & Gengenbacher, M. (2013). Reduced drug uptake in phenotyp-ically resistant nutrient-starved nonreplicating *Mycobacterium tuberculosis. Antimicrobial Agents and Chemotherapy, 57,* 1648–1653.

Schultz, D., Palmer, A. C., & Kishony, R. (2017). Regulatory dynamics determine cell fate following abrupt antibiotic exposure. *Cell Systems, 5,* 509–517.e3.

Sherman, D. R., Voskuil, M., Schnappinger, D., Liao, R., Harrell, M. I., & Schoolnik, G. K. (2001). Regulation of the *Mycobacterium tuberculosis* hypoxic response gene encoding alpha-crystallin. *Proceedings of the National Academy of Sciences of the United States of America, 98,* 7534–7539.

Song, H., Sandie, R., Wang, Y., Andrade-Navarro, M. A., & Niederweis, M. (2008). Identification of outer membrane proteins of *Mycobacterium tuberculosis. Tuberculosis (Edinburgh, Scotland), 88,* 526–544.

Stahl, C., Kubetzko, S., Kaps, I., Seeber, S., Engelhardt, H., & Niederweis, M. (2001). MspA provides the main hydrophilic pathway through the cell wall of *Mycobacterium smegmatis. Molecular Microbiology, 40*, 451–464.

Stephan, J., Mailaender, C., Etienne, G., Daffe, M., & Niederweis, M. (2004). Multidrug resistance of a porin deletion mutant of *Mycobacterium smegmatis. Antimicrobial Agents and Chemotherapy, 48*, 4163–4170.

Su, H. W., Zhu, J. H., Li, H., Cai, R. J., Ealand, C., Wang, X., Chen, Y. X., Kayani, M. U., Zhu, T. F., Moradigaravand, D., Huang, H., Kana, B. D., & Javid, B. (2016). The essential mycobacterial amidotransferase GatCAB is a modulator of specific translational fidelity. *Nature Microbiology, 1*, 16147.

Sureka, K., Ghosh, B., Dasgupta, A., Basu, J., Kundu, M., & Bose, I. (2008). Positive feedback and noise activate the stringent response regulator rel in mycobacteria. *PLoS One, 3*, e1771.

Taniguchi, Y., Choi, P. J., Li, G. W., Chen, H., Babu, M., Hearn, J., Emili, A., & Xie, X. S. (2010). Quantifying *E. coli* proteome and transcriptome with single-molecule sensitivity in single cells. *Science, 329*, 533–538.

te Brake, L. H. M., de Knegt, G. J., de Steenwinkel, J. E., van Dam, T. J. P., Burger, D. M., Russel, F. G. M., van Crevel, R., Koenderink, J. B., & Aarnoutse, R. E. (2018). The role of efflux pumps in tuberculosis treatment and their promise as a target in drug development: Unraveling the black box. *Annual Review of Pharmacology and Toxicology, 58*, 271–291.

Thayil, S. M., Morrison, N., Schechter, N., Rubin, H., & Karakousis, P. C. (2011). The role of the novel exopolyphosphatase MT0516 in *Mycobacterium tuberculosis* drug tolerance and persistence. *PLoS One, 6*, e28076.

Tiwari, A., Balazsi, G., Gennaro, M. L., & Igoshin, O. A. (2010). The interplay of multiple feedback loops with post-translational kinetics results in bistability of mycobacterial stress response. *Physical Biology, 7*, 036005.

Torrey, H. L., Keren, I., Via, L. E., Lee, J. S., & Lewis, K. (2016). High persister mutants in *Mycobacterium tuberculosis. PLoS One, 11*, e0155127.

Tuomanen, E., Cozens, R., Tosch, W., Zak, O., & Tomasz, A. (1986). The rate of killing of *Escherichia coli* by beta-lactam antibiotics is strictly proportional to the rate of bacterial growth. *Journal of General Microbiology, 132*, 1297–1304.

Vaubourgeix, J., Lin, G., Dhar, N., Chenouard, N., Jiang, X., Botella, H., Lupoli, T., Mariani, O., Yang, G., Ouerfelli, O., Unser, M., Schnappinger, D., Mckinney, J., & Nathan, C. (2015). Stressed mycobacteria use the chaperone ClpB to sequester irreversibly oxidized proteins asymmetrically within and between cells. *Cell Host & Microbe, 17*, 178–190.

Viveiros, M., Martins, M., Rodrigues, L., Machado, D., Couto, I., Ainsa, J., & Amaral, L. (2012). Inhibitors of mycobacterial efflux pumps as potential boosters for anti-tubercular drugs. *Expert Review of Anti-Infective Therapy, 10*, 983–998.

Voskuil, M. I. (2004). *Mycobacterium tuberculosis* gene expression during environmental conditions associated with latency. *Tuberculosis (Edinburgh, Scotland), 84*, 138–143.

Wakamoto, Y., Dhar, N., Chait, R., Schneider, K., Signorino-Gelo, F., Leibler, S., & Mckinney, J. D. (2013). Dynamic persistence of antibiotic-stressed mycobacteria. *Science, 339*, 91–95.

Wallace, R. J., Jr., Dalovisio, J. R., & Pankey, G. A. (1979). Disk diffusion testing of susceptibility of *Mycobacterium fortuitum* and *Mycobacterium chelonei* to antibacterial agents. *Antimicrobial Agents and Chemotherapy, 16*, 611–614.

Warrier, T., Martinez-Hoyos, M., Marin-Amieva, M., Colmenarejo, G., Porras-de Francisco, E., Alvarez-Pedraglio, A. I., Fraile-Gabaldon, M. T., Torres-Gomez, P. A., Lopez-Quezada, L., Gold, B., Roberts, J., Ling, Y., Somersan-Karakaya, S., Little, D., Cammack, N., Nathan, C., & Mendoza-Losana, A. (2015). Identification of novel anti-mycobacterial compounds by screening a pharmaceutical small-molecule library against nonreplicating *Mycobacterium tuberculosis. ACS Infectious Diseases, 1*, 580–585.

Wayne, L. G., & Hayes, L. G. (1996). An in vitro model for sequential study of shiftdown of *Mycobacterium tuberculosis* through two stages of nonreplicating persistence. *Infection and Immunity, 64*, 2062–2069.

Wayne, L. G., & Lin, K. Y. (1982). Glyoxylate metabolism and adaptation of *Mycobacterium tuberculosis* to survival under anaerobic conditions. *Infection and Immunity, 37*, 1042–1049.

Wei, J. R., Krishnamoorthy, V., Murphy, K., Kim, J. H., Schnappinger, D., Alber, T., Sassetti, C. M., Rhee, K. Y., & Rubin, E. J. (2011). Depletion of antibiotic targets has widely varying effects on growth. *Proceedings of the National Academy of Sciences of the United States of America, 108*, 4176–4181.

WHO. (2018). *Global tuberculosis report.*

Xie, Z., Siddiqi, N., & Rubin, E. J. (2005). Differential antibiotic susceptibilities of starved *Mycobacterium tuberculosis* isolates. *Antimicrobial Agents and Chemotherapy, 49*, 4778–4780.

Xu, W., Dejesus, M. A., Rucker, N., Engelhart, C. A., Wright, M. G., Healy, C., Lin, K., Wang, R., Park, S. W., Ioerger, T. R., Schnappinger, D., & Ehrt, S. (2017a). Chemical genetic interaction profiling reveals determinants of intrinsic antibiotic resistance in *Mycobacterium tuberculosis*. *Antimicrobial Agents and Chemotherapy, 61*, e01334-17.

Xu, Z., Meshcheryakov, V. A., Poce, G., & Chng, S. S. (2017b). MmpL3 is the flippase for mycolic acids in mycobacteria. *Proceedings of the National Academy of Sciences of the United States of America, 114*, 7993–7998.

Zhang, B., Li, J., Yang, X., Wu, L., Zhang, J., Yang, Y., Zhao, Y., Zhang, L., Yang, X., Yang, X., Cheng, X., Liu, Z., Jiang, B., Jiang, H., Guddat, L. W., Yang, H., & Rao, Z. (2019). Crystal structures of membrane transporter MmpL3, an anti-TB drug target. *Cell, 176*, 636–648.e13.

Chapter 12
Antimicrobial Drug Discovery Against Persisters

Wooseong Kim, Iliana Escobar, Beth Burgwyn Fuchs, and Eleftherios Mylonakis

Abstract The efficacy of most currently prescribed antibiotics that target biosynthetic processes during cell growth or cellular uptake is energy dependent. However, because persisters are non-growing, dormant cell population with low-energy metabolic states (Conlon et al., *Nature Microbiology, 1*, 2016; Lewis, *Annual Review of Microbiology, 64*, 357, 2010; Shan et al., *MBio, 8*, 2017), conventional antibiotics fail to effectively eliminate bacterial persisters, which may lead to chronic and reoccurring infection (Lewis, *Annual Review of Microbiology, 64*, 357, 2010). The lack of antibiotics to treat infections caused by persisters entreats the urgency for developing new therapeutics effective against bacterial persisters. In response to this dire need, several strategies and anti-persister antimicrobials have been developed. Anti-persister strategies can be grouped into two approaches (1) direct killing of persisters through growth-independent targets and (2) converting persisters to antibiotic susceptible states by antibiotic adjuvants. In this chapter, we review growth-independent targets, such as bacterial proteases (Conlon, *Nature, 503*, 365–370, 2013), membrane lipid bilayers (Hurdle et al., *Nature Reviews Microbiology, 9*, 62–75, 2011), and bacterial DNA (Kwan et al., Environmental Microbiology, 2015). We also discuss a *Caenorhabditis elegans*-based screening strategy to identify membrane-active antimicrobials with relatively low cytotoxicity, which overcomes the membrane selectivity issue (Kim et al., *ACS Infectious Diseases, 4*, 1540–1545, 2018b, *Nature, 556*, 103–107, 2018c). Lastly, we review antibiotic adjuvants that resuscitate persisters to conventional antibiotic susceptible conditions (Allison et al., *Nature, 473*, 216–220, 2011). Included among these strategies, we explore the engineering of conventional antibiotics conjugated with drug carriers such as a peptide and an antibody that facilitate uptake or accessibility of antibiotics (Brezden et al., *Journal of the American Chemical Society, 138*, 10945–10949, 2016; Lehar et al., *Nature, 527*, 323–328, 2015; Schmidt et al., *ACS Nano, 8*, 8786–8793, 2014).

W. Kim · I. Escobar · B. B. Fuchs · E. Mylonakis (✉)
Division of Infectious Diseases, Rhode Island Hospital, Department of Medicine, Warren Alpert Medical School of Brown University, Providence, RI, USA
e-mail: emylonakis@lifespan.org

© Springer Nature Switzerland AG 2019
K. Lewis (ed.), *Persister Cells and Infectious Disease*,
https://doi.org/10.1007/978-3-030-25241-0_12

273

12.1 Direct Killing of Persisters by Aiming at Growth-Independent Targets

12.1.1 Bacterial Protease ClpP Activators, ADEPs

Acyldepsipeptides (ADEPs) are antimicrobial peptides that form bacterial protease complexes allowing them to degrade cellular proteins (Lee et al. 2010; Li et al. 2010). They work independently of cellular metabolism or cell division making them strong therapeutic candidates to combat infections due to persister cells (Conlon et al. 2013). ADEPs bind cytoplasmic serine protease (ClpP), a tetradecameric complex of the caseinolytic protease system composed of ClpP and its ATPase chaperones. This complex is able to regulate the rate of protein degradation in an ATP-dependent manner (Brötz-Oesterhelt et al. 2005). However, when coupled with ADEPs, the protease complex becomes ATPase independent, resulting in uncontrolled cellular protein degradation (Lee et al. 2010; Li et al. 2010). Brötz-Qesterhect et al. confirmed the binding of ADEP analogs to ClpP using affinity chromatography and chemical crosslinking (Brötz-Oesterhelt et al. 2005). This binding changed the quaternary structure of the ClpP tetradecamer, exposing its axial pore and rendering it ATPase independent (Lee et al. 2010; Li et al. 2010).

Throughout the years, the ADEP complex has gone through many synthetic improvements geared to increase its overall drug properties and biological activity (Fig. 12.1). For instance, in order to optimize its poor solubility and fast system clearance, the N-methylalanine group was replaced with pipecolate, which reduced the entropic energy barrier for binding to ClpP (Hinzen et al. 2006). To improve ADEP's biological activity, its polyunsaturated side chain was replaced with two fluorines at positions 3 and 5 of the phenyl moiety (Fig. 12.1), creating the new analog ADEP4 (Hinzen et al. 2006).

Conlon et al. reasoned that since ADEP activity was cell growth independent, the improvements found on ADEP4 would be robust enough to treat methicillin-resistant *Staphylococcus aureus* (MRSA) persisters (Conlon et al. 2013). Indeed, after treating 10^9 CFU/mL of stationary-phase MRSA persisters with 5 µg/mL ADEP4, the researchers observed a total decrease of persister viability up to 4 logs in 2 days (Conlon et al. 2013). This result was tempered by the fact that resistance to ADEP4 was seen in as little as 3 days. Nevertheless, Conlon et al. were able to demonstrate

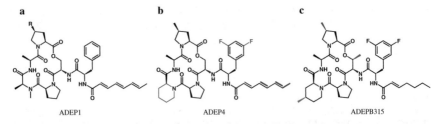

Fig. 12.1 Acyldepsipeptide analogs increase solubility and biological activity. Red highlights: modified structures. Blue highlights: loss or subtraction from the previous analog

that addition of 0.4 µg/mL of rifampicin in combination with ADEP4 was able to completely eradicate all persisters in less than 3 days. This group went on to show that ADEP4 and rifampicin combined treatment was also able to kill persisters in the context of a biofilm as well as clear infection in a deep-seated mouse thigh infection model within 3 days (Conlon et al. 2013).

More recently, ADEP4 was further optimized by Carney et al. who replaced the serine residue of the macrocycle with allo-threonine and substituted 4-methylpipecoate for the pipecolated residue to create the analog ADEP B315 (Carney et al. 2014) (Fig. 12.1). These improvements resulted in a significant increase in antimicrobial activity against *Staphylococcus aureus* from a MIC of 0.098 to 0.024 µg/mL (Carney et al. 2014). This was further supported when Arvanitis et al. demonstrated that ADEP B315 was effective against both methicillin-sensitive *S. aureus* (MSSA) and MRSA mouse infection models when compared to vancomycin treatment (Arvanitis et al. 2016). Encouragingly, the authors also reported a lack of toxicity on murine kidney or liver cells at a dose of 50 mg/kg (Arvanitis et al. 2016). These results suggest that ADEP therapy may be a promising antibiotic treatment for chronic persister infections.

12.1.2 Membrane-Active Antimicrobial Agents

The lipid bilayer of the bacterial membrane can be a promising target to kill persisters because it is not only growth-independent but also indispensable for bacterial survival (Hurdle et al. 2011). Indeed, the bacterial membrane has already been selected by evolution as a target by the host defense systems of other organisms. For instance, the innate immune system in higher eukaryotes secretes antimicrobial peptides (AMPs), such as defensins and cathelicidins that kill bacteria by disrupting lipid bilayers. AMPs and their modified analogs have bactericidal activity against not only metabolically active bacteria but also persisters, a subject which has been explored in many recent reviews (Defraine et al. 2018; Mishra et al. 2017; Mohammad et al. 2015; Patel and Akhtar 2017).

Despite their potential as anti-persister agents, AMPs have disadvantages including the high manufacturing cost, reduced activity in physiological salt conditions, and cytotoxicity (Marr et al. 2006). Knowing the value of this target that has already been selected naturally, small molecules targeting lipid bilayers have been identified and optimized to treat bacterial persisters (Defraine et al. 2018; Kim et al. 2018a; Mylonakis et al. 2016). Here, we discuss systemic approaches to identify membrane-active small molecules, their potency against persisters, their molecular mechanisms of actions and structural optimization to improve potency.

12.1.2.1 In Silico Screening Strategy

The first systemic approach to identify antimicrobial agents specifically against bacterial persisters was conducted by the Coates group (Hu et al. 2010). Based on a previous

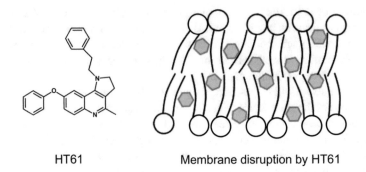

HT61   Membrane disruption by HT61

Fig. 12.2 HT61 disrupts bacterial lipid bilayers. The chemical structure of HT61 and its putative mode of action are represented. The membrane damage caused by HT61 is proportional to negative charge density

study showing fluoroquinolones were potent against persistent *Mycobacterium tuberculosis*, they searched compounds having similar structure to quinolones among 952,601 commercially available, drug-like compounds. Using a computer-based virtual screening technique, they selected 57 quinolone-like compounds and tested their potency against *S. aureus* persisters. Among them, two compounds having similar structure were effective against *S. aureus* persisters. Hu et al. synthesized over 300 analogs of these 2 compounds, tested their anti-persister activity, and subsequently identified HT61 as a promising candidate (Fig. 12.2). Briefly, Hu et al. observed that *S. aureus* cells grown in nutrient broth reached stationary phase (~10^9 CFU/mL) at 24 h of growth and showed constant cell concentrations up to 6 days, indicating that *S. aureus* is in a non-multiplying state (Hu et al. 2010). To test antibiotic tolerance of these stationary-phase non-multiplying cells, they first removed growth media by washing with phosphate-buffered saline (PBS), adjusted the cell concentration to ~10^7 CFU/mL, and then treated with several antibiotics including azithromycin, vancomycin, and linezolid (Hu et al. 2010). They observed that almost all stationary-phase MSSA and MRSA cells were persisters showing high tolerance to conventional antibiotics targeting biosynthesis (Hu et al. 2010), which is consistent with other group reports (Allison et al. 2011; Keren et al. 2004; Kim et al. 2015). Within 24 h, 12.5 µg/mL HT61 eliminated ~10^7 CFU/mL of both MSSA and MRSA persister cells showing tolerance to a panel of antibiotics, including vancomycin and mupirocin at 100 µg/mL (Hu et al. 2010). Its minimum stationary-phase bactericidal concentration 50 (MSC$_{50}$) (Coates et al. 2002) was 2.5 µg/mL and MSC$_{99}$ was 4.5 µg/mL. Further investigations with HT61 revealed that this compound had significant bactericidal activity against persisters formed by 103 clinical MRSA isolates and other Gram-positive bacteria including *Streptococcus pyogenes*, *Streptococcus agalactiae*, and *Propionibacterium acnes* (Hu et al. 2010).

Initially, Hu et al. found that the mode of action of HT61 was the depolarization and physical disruption of the bacterial cell membrane (Hu et al. 2010). Later, using artificial lipid bilayers combined with cell-based leakage assays, Hubbard et al.

showed that HT61 directly interacts with bacterial lipid bilayers and induces the alternation of lipid bilayer structure, which consequently leads to membrane disruptions (Fig. 12.2) (Hubbard et al. 2017b). From their findings, they proposed that the physical membrane damage is the primary killing mechanism against persisters, whereas membrane depolarization and ATP leakage is a consequential result of the membrane disruption (Hubbard et al. 2017b). Several studies showed that membrane depolarizing agents, such as ionophores do not affect the viability of *S. aureus* persisters (Grassi et al. 2017; Kim et al. 2018c), but rather induce persister formation by blocking ATP synthesis (Grassi et al. 2017; Narayanaswamy et al. 2018).

HT61 exhibited several advantages as a potential anti-persister agent. For example, *S. aureus* did not develop resistance to HT61 after 50 passages of exposure to HT61 (Hu et al. 2010), indicating the low probability of resistance development. Also, 1% HT61 in gel formulation exhibited efficacy against MRSA in a mouse skin infection model (Hu et al. 2010). At this level, treatment of HT61 for 14 days did not cause any adverse side effects, such as irritation, inflammation, itching, or weight loss. Currently, HT61 is in clinical trials to determine the compound efficacy as a therapeutic agent (Hubbard et al. 2017a). However, its clinical use is limited to topical applications due to its hydrophobicity and toxicity.

12.1.2.2 Whole Animal Infection-Based Screening Strategy

The challenge to screen membrane-active antimicrobial agents is that most hits are toxic to host cells due to lack of selectivity between bacterial and mammalian membranes (Hurdle et al. 2011). To overcome toxicity issues, our group focused on hit compounds from a whole animal *C. elegans*-based screen for identifying anti-infectives that rescue *C. elegans* from MRSA infection (Kim et al. 2018c; Rajamuthiah et al. 2014). The advantage of a *C. elegans*-based drug screening strategy is that compounds toxic to worms are simultaneously excluded because hits are determined based on the survival of *C. elegans* (Kim et al. 2017, 2018a). We screened approximately 82,000 small molecules using *C. elegans*-MRSA killing assay in a 384-well plate format and identified 185 compounds that significantly prolonged the life span of MRSA infected *C. elegans* (Kim et al. 2018a). Among them, we identified four membrane-active antimicrobials, such as NH125, two synthetic retinoids (CD437, CD1530), and nTZDpa that are effective against MRSA persisters (Kim et al. 2015, 2016, 2018b, c). Through a series of studies, we established methodologies to elucidate the mechanisms of action, and, through structure–activity relationship (SAR), we were able to optimize the lead compounds. Here, we share information on some of the lead compounds.

NH125 (1-Hexadecyl-2-methyl-3-(phenylmethyl)-1H-imidazolium iodide (Fig. 12.3) is an antimicrobial agent known to inhibit bacterial histidine kinase, WalK. It is highly conserved in Gram-positive bacteria and essential for survival (Yamamoto et al. 2000, 2001). We found that NH125 causes rapid membrane permeabilization, which correlates with its bactericidal activity against MRSA persisters (Kim et al. 2015). To examine the interaction between NH125 and lipid bilayer, we employed giant unilamellar vesicles (GUVs), a widely used biomembrane-mimicking lipid bilayer system (Walde et al.

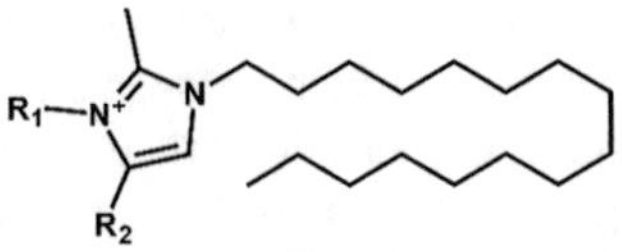

Compound	R_1	R_2	MIC (μM)	MBEC (μM)	HC_{50} (μM)
NH125	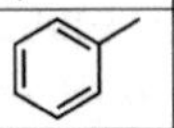		2.35	46.9	12.3
Analog 1			1.56	23.5	7.8
Analog 2	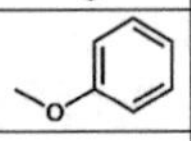		3.13	11.7	13.4
Analog 8			0.39	31.3	13.0
Analog 11	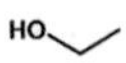		0.39	46.9	6.8
Analog 30			3.13	23.5	12.6

Fig. 12.3 Antimicrobial activity and membrane selectivity of NH125 and its analogs. Structures, antimicrobial activity, and hemolytic activity of NH125 and its analogs are displayed. *MIC* minimum inhibitory concentration, *MBEC* minimum biofilm eradication concentration, HC_{50} media hemolytic concentration

2010). Using this method, we were able to show that NH125 directly interacts with and disrupts membrane lipid bilayers (Kim et al. 2016). Notably, its bacterial histidine kinase inhibitory activity did not affect the viability of MRSA persisters (Kim et al. 2016), indicating that membrane disruption is a key mechanism in killing MRSA persisters. NH125 was able to eradicate 5×10^7 CFU/mL stationary-phase persisters formed by a range of *S. aureus* clinical isolates within 4 h at 5 μg/mL (Kim et al. 2015, 2016). NH125 killed over 99% of MRSA biofilm persisters at 10 μg/mL and completely eliminated mature MRSA biofilms at 80 μg/mL (Kim et al. 2015).

Due to its excellent anti-persister activity, the Huigens group conducted structure–activity relationship studies to improve its potency (Abouelhassan et al. 2017; Basak et al. 2017). Since the length of NH125 side chain was already optimized (Yamamoto et al. 2000, 2001), they modified its head group and consequently obtained analogs with enhanced potency (Fig. 12.3) (Abouelhassan et al. 2017; Basak et al. 2017). For instance, Analogs 1 and 2 (Fig. 12.3) that are *N*-arylated NH125 analogs had improved potency against biofilm MRSA persisters with minimum biofilm eradication concentrations (MBECs) of 23.5 μM and 11.7 μM, respectively (Abouelhassan et al. 2017; Basak et al. 2017).

Despite its strong anti-persister activity, NH125 showed relatively low selectivity between bacterial and mammalian membranes. Its median hemolytic concentrations (HC_{50}) was 38 μg/mL (Kim et al. 2016). The generated analogs also exhibited no significant improvement to membrane selectivity (Fig. 12.3) (Abouelhassan et al. 2017; Basak et al. 2017). Encouragingly, NH125 exhibited greater selectivity than

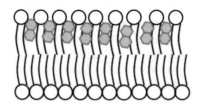

	CD437	CD1530	Analog 2	nTZDpa	Compound 14
MIC (μg/ml)	1	1	2	4	1
PKC (μg/ml)	8	8	8	64	16
HC_{50} (μg/ml)	>32	>32	>32	47	>64

Membrane disruption by retinoids or nTZDpa

Fig. 12.4 Structures and biological properties of retinoids, nTZDpa and its improved analog. Both retinoids and nTZDpa are embedded into the outer leaflet of membrane lipid bilayers. *MIC* minimum inhibitory concentration, *PKC* persister killing concentration to completely eradicate 5×10^7 CFU/mL MRSA persisters with 4 h, HC_{50} media hemolytic concentration

benzalkonium chloride, a widely used topical antiseptic and an eye drop preservative (Kim et al. 2016). Therefore, NH125 may still hold potential as a topical antimicrobial to treat chronic skin infections.

In spite of its shortcomings, the successful identification of NH125 among the hits from the *C. elegans*-MRSA screen motivated us to find other membrane-active antimicrobials having high membrane selectivity. We next focused on two synthetic retinoids, CD437 and CD1530 owing to their structural similarity (Fig. 12.4). Retinoids are a class of compounds that include vitamin A and its synthetic analogs. They are able to regulate several important cellular processes including embryonic development, cell proliferation, cell differentiation, immune function, and neuronal function (Álvarez et al. 2014). Because retinoids exhibit multiple types of bioactivities, many retinoid analogs have been synthesized to improve potency and lower toxicity profiles and are used as therapeutics to treat skin diseases and cancers in the clinic (Álvarez et al. 2014). CD437 is also known to induce apoptosis of cancer cells by binding DNA polymerase alpha subunit (Han et al. 2016). However, the antimicrobial activity of retinoids has not been reported. Like NH125, CD437 and CD1530 induced rapid membrane permeabilization, which correlated with their anti-persister activity (Kim et al. 2018c). CD437 and CD1530 completely eradicated ~10^7 CFU/ mL persister cells isolated from various stationary-phase *S. aureus* strains, including

MRSA, vancomycin-resistant *S. aureus* (VRSA), and 11 *S. aureus* clinical isolates within 4 h at 10 μg/mL. In this series of experiments, overnight cultures of *S. aureus* grew to stationary phase with essentially 100% of cells showing tolerance to 100X MIC vancomycin, gentamicin, and ciprofloxacin. For consistency, we in this assay diluted 10^9 CFU/mL persister cells to 10^7 CFU/mL for the SYTOX Green membrane permeability assay. Furthermore, the two retinoids completely eradicated MRSA persisters formed in biofilms at 32 μg/mL. Importantly, they did not induce significant human red blood cell lysis up to 64 μg/mL, indicating high membrane selectivity (Kim et al. 2018c). Encouragingly, MRSA MW2 did not develop CD437 resistance after 100-day serial passage in media containing sub-MIC levels of the compound, while cells did develop 256-fold greater resistance to ciprofloxacin during the same time period (Kim et al. 2018c).

Using multiple experimental methods including cell-based permeability assays, GUVs, and molecular dynamics (MD) simulations, we demonstrated that CD437 and CD1530 kill MRSA persisters by disrupting membrane lipid bilayers. This was achieved when two polar branch groups, such as carboxylic acid and phenolic hydroxyl moieties bound hydrophilic heads of lipid bilayers and then retinoids penetrated into the outer leaflet of the lipid bilayers via hydrophobic interactions between their aromatic backbone and lipid tails. This interaction caused permanent damage to membrane lipid bilayers (Fig. 12.4) (Kim et al. 2018c).

Since CD437 was originally synthesized as an antineoplastic agent, we modified its chemical structure to reduce its anti-cancer activity while retaining its anti-persister activity. Among 16 CD437 analogs, we found that Analog 2 having a less polar primary alcohol at the carboxylic acid moiety (Fig. 12.4) exhibits significantly reduced anti-cancer activity with median lethal concentration (LC_{50}) of >32 μg/mL against human hepatoma HepG2 (vs. CD437's LC_{50} of 3 μg/mL). Moreover, Analog 2 showed improved cytotoxicity profiles in primary hepatic and renal cell lines compared to CD437 while retaining its anti-persister activity. Notably, Analog 2 alone or in combination with gentamicin showed ~4- and ~23-fold decrease in bacterial burden in a mouse deep-seated MRSA infection model, respectively (Kim et al. 2018c). Considering that retinoid chemistry has been well established and ~4000 retinoids have been synthesized, these results combined with the established retinoid synthetic methods support further optimization of retinoids.

From these retinoid studies (Kim et al. 2018c), we have learned that the potency and cytotoxicity of membrane-active compounds can be optimized based on the understandings of mode of action and structure–activity relationships. To this end, we chose another membrane-active antimicrobial, nTZDpa (Fig. 12.4) that exhibited less potency and membrane-selectivity, and attempted to improve the antimicrobial activity and membrane selectivity (Kim et al. 2018b). nTZDpa was originally developed as a non-thiazolidinedione peroxisome proliferator-activated receptor gamma (PPARγ) partial agonist and showed in vivo efficacy in a mouse model of obesity and insulin-resistant diabetes (Berger et al. 2003). Its antibiotic activity was not previously explored.

nTZDpa rescued more than 90% of *C. elegans* infected with MRSA when testing a range from 1 to 16 μg/mL (Kim et al. 2018b). However, worm survival decreased up to

~70% at 32 µg/mL of nTZDpa, indicating nTZDpa was toxic at higher concentrations (Kim et al. 2018b). nTZDpa showed antimicrobial activity with a MIC of 4 µg/mL against various *S. aureus* and *Enterococcus faecium* strains, including MRSA, VRSA, and vancomycin-resistant *E. faecium* (VRE). nTZDpa at 64 µg/mL was able to eradicate ~10^8 CFU/mL MRSA persister within 2 h. However, it also caused ~30% and ~67% human red blood cell hemolysis at 32 µg/mL and 64 µg/mL, respectively, indicating a lack of membrane selectivity at high concentrations (Kim et al. 2018b). Therefore, we aimed to improve its anti-persister activity and membrane selectivity based on the combination of synthetic chemistry with MD simulations.

Molecular Dynamics (MD) simulations revealed that nTZDpa binds strongly to hydrophilic lipid heads via the carboxylic acid and two chlorine moieties (Kim et al. 2018b). The binding affinities of these three polar groups conferred attachment of the chlorinated benzene and chlorinated indole groups to the membrane surface, while the remaining unchlorinated benzene group dangled from the membrane due to entropic repulsion. These sustained contacts enabled nTZDpa to overcome the energy barrier for penetration into the outer leaflet of the membrane via hydrophobic interactions between its aromatic rings and the hydrophobic tails of the membrane lipids. At equilibrium, because of its multiple polar sites, nTZDpa molecules are embedded in the outer leaflet of the membrane with an inclined orientation with respect to the acyl chains of lipids. As a result, the neighboring lipids deform to accommodate the invading nTZDpa molecules, inducing significant membrane perturbation.

Gram-positive bacterial membranes including *S. aureus* possess substantial (~25%) anionic lipids, such as cardiolipin and phosphatidylglycerol while mammalian membranes consist of zwitterionic neutral lipids with a large amount of cholesterol (Brender et al. 2012; Strahl and Errington 2017; Zasloff 2002). The electrostatic interaction between cationic peptides and the negatively charged bacterial membrane, and the presence of cholesterol in mammalian membranes that protects the cell from those cationic peptides, are known to be key factors for cell selectivity of antimicrobial agents (Brender et al. 2012; Matsuzaki 2009). Considering these key aspects of membrane selectivity and the MD simulation results, 39 nTZDpa analogs were synthesized by modifying three polar branch groups or the unchlorinated arylthioether moiety (Kim et al. 2018b). This SAR study demonstrated that the addition of a larger halogen group at the arylthioether moiety increased antimicrobial potency through more severe membrane perturbation. In addition, the substitution of oxygen for sulfur at the arylthioether moiety resulted in improved membrane selectivity. Although the exact mechanism is unknown, we think a smaller oxygen atom may have minimum interaction with mammalian membranes compared to a larger sulfur atom.

Finally, the optimized nTZDpa analog compound **14**, with oxygen substituted for sulfur and additional iodine at the arylthioether moiety (Fig. 12.4), exhibited a MIC of 1 µg/mL against MRSA and eliminated 5×10^7 CFU/mL MRSA persisters within 4 h at 16 µg/mL. Additionally, it did not induce human red blood cell hemolysis up to 64 µg/mL. Compound **14** also presented a LC_{50} of >32 µg/mL against human hepatic cell line HepG2 and human renal proximal tubular cell line HKC-8 (Kim et al. 2018b). Considering its antimicrobial activity, high membrane selectivity and its unique structure, compound **14** has the potential for further development as a human antibacterial therapeutic. Furthermore, mechanism studies combining SAR and molecular dynamics simulations provide insights for the future design of non-toxic, membrane-active antibiotics.

12.1.3   DNA Cross-Linking Agents

DNA cross-linking agents cause permanent damage to microbial DNA resulting in cell death. The Wood group reasoned that since mitomycin C (MMC) is able to spontaneously cross-link DNA in a cell growth-independent fashion, this FDA-approved anticancer drug would also be effective against persisters (Kwan et al. 2015). The authors supported this hypothesis by first testing the efficacy of MMC against in vitro planktonic *E. coli* K-12 persister cells. When *E. coli* K-12 persister cells were treated with 10 µg/mL of MMC for 3 h persister cell count was reduced from 8×10^8 to 2×10^3 CFU/mL (Kwan et al. 2015). Further validation of these results, Kwan et al. also showed that persisters formed by other pathogens were susceptible to MMC. In these experiments mid to late-stationary phase *E. coli* 0157 (EHEC), *P. aeruginosa*, and *S. aureus* cells were either fully eradicated (EHEC, *S. aureus*) or reduced from 1×10^9 to 5×10^3 CFU/mL (*P. aeruginosa*) when treated with 10 µg/mL of MMC for 24 h (Kwan et al. 2015).

With evidence that MMC could effectively kill persister cells found in a planktonic setting, the researchers then queried whether MMC could be effective against a biofilm (Lewis 2010). When MMC was tested against *E. coli* K-12 persister biofilms, almost full eradication (<99.999%) was observed in 24 h. Furthermore, the efficacy of MMC was tested using Lubbock chronic wound pathogenic biofilm model, which mimics polymicrobial biofilm infections (Sun et al. 2008). MMC treatment for 5 h showed significant reduction against pathogenic *E. coli* EHEC at 10 µg/mL, *P. aeruginosa* PAO1 at 15 µg/mL, and *S. aureus* at 15 µg/mL (Kwan et al. 2015). In addition, MMC at 15 µg/mL had a similar effect on *S. aureus* and *P. aeruginosa* co-cultured biofilms as well (Kwan et al. 2015).

Lastly, to test MMC efficacy in vivo, Kwan et al. used a *C. elegans* whole animal infection model to test the ability of MMC to inhibit bacterial infection. This model showed that worms infected with EHEC for 48 h lived longer if transferred to a plate containing 10 µg/mL of MMC than worms transferred to a plate containing 5 µg/mL of ciprofloxacin (Kwan et al. 2015). While the *C. elegans* infection model is not solely confined to persister cells, the authors weakly argued that persisters, potentially found within the bacterial population were unable to overcome the antimicrobial effect of MMC.

The concept of DNA damage as a way to eliminate persisters was further expanded by Chowdhury et al. who tested seven additional DNA cross-linking drugs (Chowdhury et al. 2016). Within the seven candidates, they discovered the anticancer drug cisplatin was effective against *E. coli* and *S. aureus* persisters (Chowdhury et al. 2016). Similar to MMC, cisplatin works by binding adjacent guanines to purines thereby cross-linking DNA to itself (Eastman 1987). In the study by Chowdhury et al., *E. coli* stationary-phase cells were fully eradicated when treated with 500 μg/mL of cisplatin for a minimum of 12 h (Chowdhury et al. 2016). Similar results were seen in other pathogenic strains such as *E. coli* EHEC (500 μg/mL of cisplatin), *P. aeruginosa* strain PA14 (250 μg/mL of cisplatin), and *S. aureus* clinical isolates (500 μg/mL of cisplatin) (Chowdhury et al. 2016). Unfortunately, given cisplatins high MIC and ability to cause nephrotoxicity at high doses (Miller et al. 2010), its development as an antimicrobial drug will most likely be limited to topical applications if any.

It may seem encouraging to find that these FDA approved, DNA cross-linker drugs, are not species specific, as researchers have shown them to be effective against a multitude of bacteria: *E. coli*, *P. aeruginosa*, *S. aureus*, *Borrelia burgdorferi*, and *Acinetobacter baumannii* persister cells (Chowdhury et al. 2016; Cruz-Muñiz et al. 2017; Kwan et al. 2015; Sharma et al. 2015). Nevertheless, most of the DNA cross-linking drugs are chemotherapeutic. Their mechanism of action is intrinsically toxic to both bacterial and mammal cells. By lowering their toxicity, their efficacy to fight infection would lower as well. This constraint hinders further optimization for clinical use to treat systemic bacterial infections and would limit their use to topical applications.

12.2 Resuscitation of Persisters to Be Antibiotic Susceptible by Adjuvants

Finding an efficient way to potentiate an already known antibiotic can be a safer and a quicker route to persister cell infection treatment. In the following section, we will discuss adjuvant-antibiotic pairs (Table 12.1) in the scope of three overarching mechanistic themes: (1) proton motor force (PMF)-driven potentiation, (2) antibiotic adjuvants, and (3) quorum sensing.

12.2.1 Proton Motive Force-Driven Potentiation

Aminoglycosides are a class of antibiotics that are known to inhibit protein translation by binding to active ribosomes in the cytoplasm (Weisblum and Davies 1968). Although the exact mechanism through which these antibiotics are physically transported through the cell membrane is unknown, it is well established that such transportation is proton motive force (PMF) dependent (Taber et al. 1987). Persister cells are in a low-energy state (Conlon et al. 2016; Shan et al. 2017) and have low PMF activity (Lewis 2010). Therefore, aminoglycosides have been ineffective at combating persister cell infections. Allison et al. hypothesized that adding carbon source metabolites to a population of persister cells would activate their PMF which, in turn, would potentiate the uptake of aminoglycosides and subsequently augment their antimicrobial effect (Allison et al. 2011).

Table 12.1 Antibiotic and metabolite adjuvant combinations effective against persister cell bacteria

Adjuvant	Concentration	Antibiotic	Concentration	Bacteria	References
Mannitol	40 mM	Tobramycin	80 µg/mL	P. aeruginosa	Barraud et al. (2013)
Mannitol	10 µM	Gentamicin	10 µg/mL	E. coli	Allison et al. (2011)
Glucose	10 µM	Gentamicin	10 µg/mL	E. coli	Allison et al. (2011)
Pyruvate	20 µM	Gentamicin	10 µg/mL	E. coli	Allison et al. (2011)
Fructose	10 µM	Gentamicin	10 µg/mL	E. coli	Allison et al. (2011)
Fructose	10 µM	Gentamicin	10 µg/mL	S. aureus	Allison et al. (2011)
Triclosan	100 µM	Tobramycin	50 µM	P. aeruginosa	Maiden et al. (2018)
Triclosan	100 µM	Gentamicin	100 µM	P. aeruginosa	Maiden et al. (2018)
Triclosan	100 µM	Streptomycin	100 µM	P. aeruginosa	Maiden et al. (2018)
BF8	5 µg/mL	Ciprofloxacin	25 µg/mL	P. aeruginosa	Pan et al. (2012)
BF8	5 µg/mL	Tobramycin	25 µg/mL	P. aeruginosa	Pan et al. (2012)
BF8	5 µg/mL	Ofloxacin	5 µg/mL	E. coli	Pan et al. (2013)
BF8	5 µg/mL	Tetracycline	25 µg/mL	E. coli	Pan et al. (2013)
BF8	5 µg/mL	Tobramycin	25 µg/mL	E. coli	Pan et al. (2013)
BF8	5 µg/mL	Gentamicin	25 µg/mL	E. coli	Pan et al. (2013)
Silver	30 µM	Gentamicin	5 µg/mL	E. coli	Morones-Ramirez et al. (2013)
Silver	30 µM	Ofloxacin	3 µg/mL	E. coli	Morones-Ramirez et al. (2013)
Silver	30 µM	Ampicillin	10 µg/mL	E. coli	Morones-Ramirez et al. (2013)
Glycerol	60 mM	Kanamycin	25 µg/mL	E. coli	Orman and Brynildsen (2013)
Pyruvate	60 mM	Kanamycin	25 µg/mL	E. coli	Orman and Brynildsen (2013)
Mannitol	60 mM	Kanamycin	25 µg/mL	E. coli	Orman and Brynildsen (2013)
Glucose	60 mM	Kanamycin	25 µg/mL	E. coli	Orman and Brynildsen (2013)
Glucose	60 mM	Kanamycin	25 µg/mL	E. coli	Orman and Brynildsen (2013)

The authors tested this hypothesis using ten carbon sources in combination with 10 µg/mL of gentamicin. This experiment revealed that the addition of 10 mM of mannitol, glucose, fructose, or 20 mM pyruvate was sufficient to decrease the survival of *E. coli* persisters by 99.9% after 2 h of gentamicin treatment (Allison et al. 2011). To illustrate that those adjuvants in pair with gentamicin were not only effective against *E. coli* bacteria, additional bacteria including *S. aureus* were tested. In this experiment, *S. aureus* exhibited similar susceptibly to gentamicin (10 µg/mL) after treatment with fructose (10 µM). Interestingly, gentamicin potentiation was not seen when *S. aureus* persister cells were treated with other carbon source metabolites such as glucose, mannitol, or pyruvate (Allison et al. 2011). The authors reasoned this lack of potentiation was due to low expression of metabolic transporters in *S. aureus* persisters, which they corroborated via microarray analysis.

To confirm that this phenotype was facilitated by aminoglycoside uptake, Texas Red conjugated gentamicin was measured via fluorescence-activated cell sorting (FACS) (Allison et al. 2011) through which the researchers observed fluorescence increases upon gentamicin treatment. Additionally, these results demonstrated cell uptake was specific to aminoglycosides, given that when cells were treated with another class of antibiotics such as ampicillin and ofloxacin they did not yield similar results (Allison et al. 2011). Conversely, Allison and colleagues reasoned that by dissipating PMF via a proton ionophore such as carbonyl cyanide m-chlorophenyl hydrazone (CCCP), metabolite treatment would no longer have an effect on the survival of persister cells. Indeed, after treatment with CCCP, metabolites, and gentamicin, *E. coli* persister cells were no longer susceptible to antibiotic treatment (Allison et al. 2011).

Orman et al. supported these findings in their study that examined persister cell metabolism (Orman and Brynildsen 2013). They found that treating stationary-phase *E. coli* persister cells with 60 mM glycerol, pyruvate, mannitol, glucose, or fructose had an adjuvant antimicrobial effect ($\geq$99.9% clearance) with kanamycin (25 µg/mL), but not ampicillin (100 µg/mL).

To test these findings in vivo, researchers employed a chronic urinary tract infection mouse model to demonstrated that metabolite treatment with mannitol (1.5 g/kg), in conjunction with gentamicin (1 mg/kg), was able to reduce infection burden by approximately 95% after 3 days of treatment (Allison et al. 2011). These findings were able to demonstrate that metabolically inactive persister cells can be sensitized to aminoglycoside antibiotics through reinvigorated uptake when given an appropriate carbon source.

12.2.2 Antimicrobial Agents Facilitating Aminoglycoside Uptake into Persisters

In addition to agents inducing PMF activation, recent studies have shown that known antimicrobial agents, such as triclosan and silver can also facilitate the uptake of aminoglycosides into persister cells. Triclosan is an antimicrobial itself, which functions as a fatty acid synthesis inhibitor (Heath et al. 1999; McMurry et al. 1998). It binds directly to enoyl-acyl carrier protein reductase FabI to prevent fatty acid synthesis, which plays an important role in many cellular metabolic functions (Heath et al. 1999). Triclosan's adjuvant effect was discovered by the Water group in 2018 when searching for potentiates of tobramycin, a common antibiotic used against cystic fibrosis (CF)-related *P. aeruginosa* infections (Maiden et al. 2018). In this study, triclosan was identified via a high-throughput screen looking for bactericidal activity against *P. aeruginosa* biofilms in conjunction with tobramycin (Maiden et al. 2018). Although their work focused mainly on persisters found within a biofilm environment, they were able to demonstrate a 1000-fold reduction from 10^9 to 10^6 CFU/mL in a 20-h-old stationary-phase of *P. aeruginosa* persister cells after only 8 h of treatment with 100 µM triclosan and 50 µM tobramycin, and complete eradication within 24 h (Maiden et al. 2018). Surprisingly, this phenotype was not FabI-dependent and the mechanism by which this synergy occurs is yet to be discovered. Notably, triclosan is bactericidal and toxic at higher concentrations. A potential use could be at lower concentration, such as 30 µM, in conjunction with tobramycin as an aerosol to treat chronic lung infections in cystic fibrosis patients. Further studies to elucidate the exact mechanism of action are needed.

Silver is another reagent known to have antimicrobial activity through various mechanisms of action. Exposure leads to formation of reactive oxygen species, which can deregulate iron metabolism through the direct interaction with Fe-S clusters. Silver can also directly interact with Fe-S clusters resulting in an increased release of Fe^{2+} and further iron metabolism deregulation (Morones-Ramirez et al. 2013). In addition, silver can also cause cell death by disrupting disulfide bonds found within proteins. These proteins are misfolded and mistransported to the plasma membrane decreasing its integrity while increasing its permeability (Morones-Ramirez et al. 2013). Given these membrane-targeting antimicrobial properties, Morones-Ramirez et al. hypothesized that silver may have an adjuvant effect with other antibiotics that poorly penetrate into the cell membrane of persister bacteria. To test this, *E. coli* persisters were treated with 30 µM of Ag^+ and 10 µg/mL of ampicillin, 3 µg/mL of ofloxacin, or 5 µg/mL of gentamicin. After treatment, CFU/mL counts confirmed that silver in conjunction with these antibiotics indeed lowered persister cell viability from 1×10^8 to 1×10^7 (ampicillin), 5×10^6 (ofloxacin), or 1×10^4 (gentamicin) CFU/mL (Morones-Ramirez et al. 2013).

Additionally, Morones-Ramirez et al. demonstrated that silver, alone or in combination with gentamicin, exhibits in vivo efficacy in a mouse urinary catheter biofilm infection model. In this model, biofilms were grown in catheters that were surgically implanted subcutaneously in mice. After 48 h the mice received no treatment or intraperitoneally-delivered gentamicin, Ag^+, or gentamicin plus Ag^+. Silver alone at 6 mg $AgNO_3$/kg body weight (35 µM) had a 10-fold CFU/mL reduction in total while silver plus gentamicin (2.5 mg/kg) had almost a 100-fold reduction. Although this data highlights the potential of silver as an antibiotic adjuvant capable of treating persister cells in vivo, high levels of silver are toxic and no interest has been seen in developing silver as a systemic antibiotic.

12.2.3 Quorum Sensing Inhibitory Adjuvants

During sub-optimal growth conditions, bacterial cells are able to produce environmental ques inducing them into a persister state. This allows them to survive during harsh growing conditions or maintain a hold on their environmental niche. Bacteria are able to signal these environmental ques via quorum sensing (QS). QS is a mechanism by which bacteria are able to signal density conditions in their environment such as in the biofilm state. QS molecules accumulate during stationary phase of bacterial growth. Stationary phase supernatant, or spent media, of *P. aeruginosa* PAO1 is known to increase persister cell populations during the exponential phase (Möker et al. 2010). Given these observations, Pan et al. reasoned that QS may be important in biofilm formation and subsequently persister cell function making QS inhibitors a good candidate for treating bacterial persisters.

Among these QS inhibitors (Z)-4-Bromo-5-(bromomethylene)-3-methylfuran-2 (5H)-one (BF8) is known to inhibit *E. coli* and *P. aeruginosa* biofilm formation (Han et al. 2008; Pan et al. 2012). Pan et al. tested and discovered that BF8 was able to sensitize *P. aeruginosa* PAO1 persisters to multiple antibiotics (Pan et al. 2012). Specifically, they found that BF8 at 5 µg/mL plus ciprofloxacin at 25 µg/mL or tobramycin at 25 µg/mL significantly reduced PAO1 persister viability. However, this phenomenon was not seen when treating cells with 25 µg/mL tetracycline, 25 µg/mL gentamicin, or 500 µg/mL carbenicillin (Pan et al. 2012). Additionally, Pan et al. showed that BF8 had a similar effect on *E. coli* persisters (Pan et al. 2013). They further demonstrated that treatment of *E. coli* persisters with BF8 at 5 µg/mL significantly reduced persister cell viability after treatment with ofloxacin (5 µg/mL), gentamicin (25 µg/mL), tobramycin (25 µg/mL), or tetracycline (25 µg/mL), but not ampicillin (100 µg/mL) (Pan et al. 2013).

To date, the Pan group was unable to delineate a clear mechanism of action for BF8. Instead, in light of DNA microarray data comparing BF8 treated and not treated cells, they hypothesized that BF8 may be working via protein transport and membrane potential. Such cellular activities require energy, which may possibly lead to a partial cellular metabolic awakening, therefore making persisters susceptible to only some antibiotics but not all.

12.3 Engineering Antibiotics

As discussed above, enhancing the uptake of aminoglycosides is an effective strategy to kill bacterial persisters (Allison et al. 2011). Instead of using adjuvants, the Wong group engineered aminoglycosides by conjugating tobramycin with a drug carrier, which would facilitate aminoglycoside uptake into bacterial persisters (Schmidt et al. 2014). Previously, the Wong group discovered that antimicrobial peptides and cell-penetrating peptides capable of permeating or translocating across bacterial membranes commonly generate saddle-splay (also known as negative

Gaussian) curvature in the membranes, which causes bacterial membrane destabilization (Mishra et al. 2011; Schmidt et al. 2011, 2012; Schmidt and Wong 2013). They found that these peptides contain a conserved domain consisting of less than 20 amino acids containing arginine, lysine, and hydrophobic contents, which is responsible for interacting with bacterial membranes and generating the saddle-splay curvature (Mishra et al. 2011; Schmidt et al. 2011; Schmidt and Wong 2013).

The authors conjugated penetratin-originated 12 amino acid peptide (RQIKIWFQNRRW) to tobramycin, which was named pentobra (Fig. 12.5) (Schmidt et al. 2014). While tobramycin alone was not effective against persister cells, pentobra was able to penetrate into bacterial cells and kill both *S. aureus* and *E. coli* persisters (Schmidt et al. 2014). The treatment of *S. aureus* persisters with 25.7 μM pentobra resulted in 5-log reduction in viability from $\sim10^8$ to $\sim10^3$ CFU/mL; the treatment of *E. coli* with 51.3 μM pentobra led to 4-log reduction from $\sim10^6$ to $\sim10^2$ CFU/mL (Schmidt et al. 2014). Moreover, pentobra did not cause damage to eukaryotic cell membrane or cytotoxicity up to 100 μM.

In addition to extracellular persisters, some pathogens such as *S. aureus*, can survive inside host cells by converting to dormant states. Since conventional antibiotics show a low penetration rate into host cells or poor anti-persister activity, it is hard to treat intracellular bacterial persisters (Mariathasan and Tan 2017). For instance, *S. aureus* persisters formed in murine macrophages are tolerant to high concentrations of vancomycin, linezolid, and daptomycin, which are usually used as antibiotics of last resort (Lehar et al. 2015). Lehar et al. applied the antibody–drug conjugate concept for killing intracellular bacterial persisters (Lehar et al. 2015). The antibody–drug conjugate is composed of the antibody, linker, and drug. Since the antibody functions to selectively deliver the drug to a target and the linker modulates drug activity, the antibody–drug conjugate has therapeutic advantages, such as improved efficacy and reduced cytotoxicity (Chari et al. 2014). To efficiently deliver an antibiotic to bacterial persisters, they employed the antibody targeting *S. aureus* wall-teichoic acids, which showed highest binding affinity among over 40 tested *S. aureus* antibodies. They chose a rifamycin derivative called rifalogue as an antibiotic because it is suitable for connecting to the linker through its tertiary amine and shows high potency against MRSA persisters and stability in an intracellular environment (Lehar et al. 2015). The antibody and rifalogue were connected by a cathepsin-cleavable linker (Fig. 12.5), which is cleaved by an intracellular protease. In the extracellular environment, this antibody–antibiotic conjugate (AAC) binds to *S. aureus*, however, it does not show antimicrobial activity due to its large size. Once AAC-opsonized *S. aureus* cells are phagocytosed by host cells, rifalogue is released from the AAC and subsequently eradicates intracellular *S. aureus* persisters. Indeed, AAC was potent and killed MRSA persisters formed in a variety of host cells, such as human macrophages, endothelial, and epithelial cell lines. For example, when murine macrophages are infected with 4×10^6 CFU/mL MRSA USA300, the addition of 100 μg/mL AAC to the culture media led to a 4-log reduction in the number of viable intracellular bacteria (from 10^5 CFU/well to 10^1 CFU/well) (Lehar et al. 2015). Further, AACs at a daily dose of 50 mg/kg resulted in $\sim$6-log decrease (from $\sim10^8$ to 10^2 CFU/2 kidneys) in viable bacterial cells in a murine model of bacteremia (Lehar et al. 2015). It is noteworthy that the replacement of rifalogue with

Fig. 12.5 Structures of engineered antibiotics effective against bacterial persisters. (**a**) Pentobra, (**b**) antibody–antibiotic conjugate (AAC), (**c**) Kanamycin–P14LRR conjugate (P14KanS)

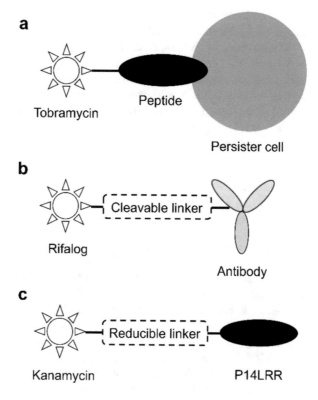

its analog rifampicin which is unable to kill MRSA persisters abolishes bactericidal potency against intracellular MRSA (Lehar et al. 2015). This result indicates that the ability for AAC to kill intracellular MRSA persisters is dependent on the persister killing potency of the antibiotic as well as its intercellular accumulation (Lehar et al. 2015).

The Seleem and Chmielewski group focused on the potential of short peptides translocating across mammalian cell membranes as drug carriers to deliver antibiotics into host cells. They designed a proline-rich short antimicrobial peptide designated P14LRR that can cross the mammalian membrane without causing damage (Kuriakose et al. 2013). This group synthesized the P14LRR–kanamycin conjugate (P14KanS in Fig. 12.5) containing a reducible disulfide linker, which is cleaved in a reducing intracellular environment (Brezden et al. 2016). Unlike the AAC (Lehar et al. 2015), P14KanS showed extracellular antimicrobial activity against various Gram-positive and Gram-negative bacteria including *Mycobacterium tuberculosis* with MICs of 0.12–2 µM, which is a significantly improved potency compared to kanamycin or P14LLR alone (Brezden et al. 2016; Mohamed et al. 2017). Importantly, P14KanS was able to kill intracellular *S. aureus* persisters. When human keratinocytes infected with MSSA or MRSA were treated with 15 µM P14KanS for 24 h, the viability of MSSA and MRSA showed ~2.5 log and ~1.24-log reduction, respectively (Mohamed et al.

2017). Further, treatment with 10 μM P14KanS for 72 h rescued all *C. elegans* infected with MRSA (Brezden et al. 2016).

The success of Pentobra, AAC, and P14KanS suggests that efficacy of conventional antibiotics can be improved by conjugation with drug carriers. In addition to antibodies and peptides, several other antibiotic delivery systems using polymers, lipids, and nanoparticles are currently being developed to improve efficacy and reduce side effects (Cal et al. 2017). Therefore, apart from discovering new anti-persister agents, engineering conventional antibiotics still holds therapeutic potential against bacterial persisters.

12.4 Conclusions

Although the identification of bacterial persisters was first reported in 1944, active research on persisters has been reinitiated in the 2000s, when evidence that persisters are responsible for recalcitrance of chronic infections began to accumulate. Since then, understanding of the molecular mechanisms of persisters formation and antibiotic tolerance has been expanded, and several strategies and anti-persister antimicrobial agents have been developed. Key findings and developments include (1) metabolite-mediated uptake of gentamicin into persister cells, (2) activation of an unconventional target, ClpP protease by ADEP4 in bacterial persisters, (3) conjugation of conventional antibiotics with a peptide or an antibody to enhance the uptake or accessibility of drugs to persisters, and (4) identification of membrane-active synthetic retinoid antibiotics. Although these antimicrobial agents or adjuvants still have deficiencies, such as cytotoxicity at high concentrations and probability of resistance development, these drawbacks can be resolved by a combination of other antibiotics and further chemical modifications. The proportion of chronic and recurrent infections caused by bacterial persisters will continue to increase due to the growing number of immunocompromised patients and the use of indwelling medical devices. Therefore, development of new therapeutics effective against bacterial persisters is urgently needed. The knowledge from pioneering work, thus far will provide important insights into developing the next generation of anti-persister therapeutics.

References

Abouelhassan, Y., Basak, A., Yousaf, H., & Huigens, R. W. (2017). Identification of n-arylated NH125 analogues as rapid eradicating agents against MRSA persister cells and potent biofilm killers of gram-positive pathogens. *Chembiochem, 18,* 352–357. https://doi.org/10.1002/cbic.201600622.

Allison, K. R., Brynildsen, M. P., & Collins, J. J. (2011). Metabolite-enabled eradication of bacterial persisters by aminoglycosides. *Nature, 473,* 216–220. https://doi.org/10.1038/nature10069.

Álvarez, R., Vaz, B., Gronemeyer, H., & de Lera, A. R. (2014). Functions, therapeutic applications, and synthesis of retinoids and carotenoids. *Chemical Reviews, 114*, 1–125. https://doi.org/10.1021/cr400126u.

Arvanitis, M., Li, G., Li, D.-D., Cotnoir, D., Ganley-Leal, L., Carney, D. W., Sello, J. K., & Mylonakis, E. (2016). A conformationally constrained cyclic acyldepsipeptide is highly effective in mice infected with methicillin-susceptible and -resistant *Staphylococcus aureus*. *PLoS One, 11*, e0153912. https://doi.org/10.1371/journal.pone.0153912.

Barraud, N., Buson, A., Jarolimek, W., & Rice, S. A. (2013). Mannitol enhances antibiotic sensitivity of persister bacteria in *Pseudomonas aeruginosa biofilms*. *PLoS One, 8*, e84220.

Basak, A., Abouelhassan, Y., Zuo, R., Yousaf, H., Ding, Y., & Huigens, R. W. (2017). Antimicrobial peptide-inspired NH125 analogues: Bacterial and fungal biofilm-eradicating agents and rapid killers of MRSA persisters. *Organic & Biomolecular Chemistry, 40*, 277. https://doi.org/10.1039/c7ob01028a.

Berger, J. P., Petro, A. E., Macnaul, K. L., Kelly, L. J., Zhang, B. B., Richards, K., Elbrecht, A., Johnson, B. A., Zhou, G., Doebber, T. W., Biswas, C., Parikh, M., Sharma, N., Tanen, M. R., Thompson, G. M., Ventre, J., Adams, A. D., Mosley, R., Surwit, R. S., & Moller, D. E. (2003). Distinct properties and advantages of a novel peroxisome proliferator-activated protein [gamma] selective modulator. *Molecular Endocrinology, 17*, 662–676. https://doi.org/10.1210/me.2002-0217.

Brender, J. R., McHenry, A. J., & Ramamoorthy, A. (2012). Does cholesterol play a role in the bacterial selectivity of antimicrobial peptides? *Frontiers in Immunology, 3*. https://doi.org/10.3389/fimmu.2012.00195

Brezden, A., Mohamed, M. F., Nepal, M., Harwood, J. S., Kuriakose, J., Seleem, M. N., & Chmielewski, J. (2016). Dual targeting of intracellular pathogenic bacteria with a cleavable conjugate of kanamycin and an antibacterial cell-penetrating peptide. *Journal of the American Chemical Society, 138*, 10945–10949. https://doi.org/10.1021/jacs.6b04831.

Brötz-Oesterhelt, H., Beyer, D., Kroll, H.-P., Endermann, R., Ladel, C., Schroeder, W., Hinzen, B., Raddatz, S., Paulsen, H., Henninger, K., Bandow, J. E., Sahl, H.-G., & Labischinski, H. (2005). Dysregulation of bacterial proteolytic machinery by a new class of antibiotics. *Nature Medicine, 11*, 1082–1087. https://doi.org/10.1038/nm1306.

Cal, P. M. S. D., Matos, M. J., & Bernardes, G. J. L. (2017). Trends in therapeutic drug conjugates for bacterial diseases: A patent review. *Expert Opinion on Therapeutic Patents, 27*, 179–189. https://doi.org/10.1080/13543776.2017.1259411.

Carney, D. W., Schmitz, K. R., Truong, J. V., Sauer, R. T., & Sello, J. K. (2014). Restriction of the conformational dynamics of the cyclic acyldepsipeptide antibiotics improves their antibacterial activity. *Journal of the American Chemical Society, 136*, 1922–1929. https://doi.org/10.1021/ja410385c.

Chari, R. V. J., Miller, M. L., & Widdison, W. C. (2014). Antibody-drug conjugates: An emerging concept in cancer therapy. *Angewandte Chemie (International Ed. in English), 53*, 3796–3827. https://doi.org/10.1002/anie.201307628.

Chowdhury, N., Wood, T. L., Martínez Vázquez, M., García Contreras, R., & Wood, T. K. (2016). DNA-crosslinker cisplatin eradicates bacterial persister cells. *Biotechnology and Bioengineering, 113*, 1984–1992. https://doi.org/10.1002/bit.25963.

Coates, A., Hu, Y., Bax, R., & Page, C. (2002). The future challenges facing the development of new antimicrobial drugs. *Nature Reviews. Drug Discovery, 1*, 895–910. https://doi.org/10.1038/nrd940.

Conlon, B. P., Nakayasu, E. S., Fleck, L. E., LaFleur, M. D., Isabella, V. M., Coleman, K., Leonard, S. N., Smith, R. D., Adkins, J. N., & Lewis, K. (2013). Activated ClpP kills persisters and eradicates a chronic biofilm infection. *Nature, 503*, 365–370. https://doi.org/10.1038/nature12790.

Conlon, B. P., Rowe, S. E., Gandt, A. B., Nuxoll, A. S., Donegan, N. P., Zalis, E. A., Clair, G., Adkins, J. N., Cheung, A. L., & Lewis, K. (2016). Persister formation in *Staphylococcus aureus* is associated with ATP depletion. *Nature Microbiology, 1*, 16051. https://doi.org/10.1038/nmicrobiol.2016.51.

Cruz-Muñiz, M. Y., López-Jacome, L. E., Hernández-Durán, M., Franco-Cendejas, R., Licona-Limón, P., Ramos-Balderas, J. L., Martínez Vázquez, M., Belmont-Díaz, J. A., Wood, T. K., & García Contreras, R. (2017). Repurposing the anticancer drug mitomycin C for the treatment of persistent *Acinetobacter baumannii* infections. *International Journal of Antimicrobial Agents, 49*, 88–92. https://doi.org/10.1016/j.ijantimicag.2016.08.022.

Defraine, V., Fauvart, M., & Michiels, J. (2018). Fighting bacterial persistence: Current and emerging anti-persister strategies and therapeutics. *Drug Resistance Updates, 38*, 12–26. https://doi.org/10.1016/j.drup.2018.03.002.

Eastman, A. (1987). The formation, isolation and characterization of DNA adducts produced by anticancer platinum complexes. *Pharmacology & Therapeutics, 34*, 155–166.

Grassi, L., Di Luca, M., Maisetta, G., Rinaldi, A. C., Esin, S., Trampuz, A., & Batoni, G. (2017). Generation of persister cells of *Pseudomonas aeruginosa* and *Staphylococcus aureus* by chemical treatment and evaluation of their susceptibility to membrane-targeting agents. *Frontiers in Microbiology, 8*, 1917. https://doi.org/10.3389/fmicb.2017.01917.

Han, Y., Hou, S., Simon, K. A., Ren, D., & Luk, Y.-Y. (2008). Identifying the important structural elements of brominated furanones for inhibiting biofilm formation by *Escherichia coli*. *Bioorganic & Medicinal Chemistry Letters, 18*, 1006–1010. https://doi.org/10.1016/j.bmcl.2007.12.032.

Han, T., Goralski, M., Capota, E., Padrick, S. B., Kim, J., Xie, Y., & Nijhawan, D. (2016). The antitumor toxin CD437 is a direct inhibitor of DNA polymerase [alpha]. *Nature Chemical Biology, 12*, 511–515. https://doi.org/10.1038/nchembio.2082.

Heath, R. J., Rubin, J. R., Holland, D. R., Zhang, E., Snow, M. E., & Rock, C. O. (1999). Mechanism of triclosan inhibition of bacterial fatty acid synthesis. *The Journal of Biological Chemistry, 274*, 11110–11114.

Hinzen, B., Raddatz, S., Paulsen, H., Lampe, T., Schumacher, A., Häbich, D., Hellwig, V., Benet-Buchholz, J., Endermann, R., Labischinski, H., & Brötz-Oesterhelt, H. (2006). Medicinal chemistry optimization of acyldepsipeptides of the enopeptin class antibiotics. *ChemMedChem, 1*, 689–693. https://doi.org/10.1002/cmdc.200600055.

Hu, Y., Shamaei-Tousi, A., Liu, Y., & Coates, A. (2010). A new approach for the discovery of antibiotics by targeting non-multiplying bacteria: A novel topical antibiotic for Staphylococcal infections. *PLoS One, 5*, e11818. https://doi.org/10.1371/journal.pone.0011818.

Hubbard, A. T., Coates, A. R., & Harvey, R. D. (2017a). Comparing the action of HT61 and chlorhexidine on natural and model *Staphylococcus aureus* membranes. *The Journal of Antibiotics, 70*, 1020–1025. https://doi.org/10.1038/ja.2017.90.

Hubbard, A. T. M., Barker, R., Rehal, R., Vandera, K.-K. A., Harvey, R. D., & Coates, A. R. M. (2017b). Mechanism of action of a membrane-active quinoline-based antimicrobial on natural and model bacterial membranes. *Biochemistry, 56*, 1163–1174. https://doi.org/10.1021/acs.biochem.6b01135.

Hurdle, J. G., O'Neill, A. J., Chopra, I., & Lee, R. E. (2011). Targeting bacterial membrane function: An underexploited mechanism for treating persistent infections. *Nature Reviews Microbiology, 9*, 62–75. https://doi.org/10.1038/nrmicro2474.

Keren, I., Kaldalu, N., Spoering, A., Wang, Y., & Lewis, K. (2004). Persister cells and tolerance to antimicrobials. *FEMS Microbiology Letters, 230*, 13–18. https://doi.org/10.1016/S0378-1097(03)00856-5.

Kim, W., Conery, A. L., Rajamuthiah, R., Fuchs, B. B., Ausubel, F. M., & Mylonakis, E. (2015). Identification of an antimicrobial agent effective against methicillin-resistant *Staphylococcus aureus* persisters using a fluorescence-based screening strategy. *PLoS One, 10*, e0127640. https://doi.org/10.1371/journal.pone.0127640.

Kim, W., Fricke, N., Conery, A. L., Fuchs, B. B., Rajamuthiah, R., Jayamani, E., Vlahovska, P. M., Ausubel, F. M., & Mylonakis, E. (2016). NH125 kills methicillin-resistant *Staphylococcus aureus* persisters by lipid bilayer disruption. *Future Medicinal Chemistry, 8*, 257–269. https://doi.org/10.4155/fmc.15.189.

Kim, W., Hendricks, G. L., Lee, K., & Mylonakis, E. (2017). An update on the use of *C. elegans* for preclinical drug discovery: Screening and identifying anti-infective drugs. *Expert Opinion on Drug Discovery, 12*, 625–633. https://doi.org/10.1080/17460441.2017.1319358.

Kim, W., Hendricks, G. L., Tori, K., Fuchs, B. B., & Mylonakis, E. (2018a). Strategies against methicillin-resistant *Staphylococcus aureus* persisters. *Future Medicinal Chemistry, 10*, e0127640–e0127794. https://doi.org/10.4155/fmc-2017-0199.

Kim, W., Steele, A. D., Zhu, W., Csatary, E. E., Fricke, N., Dekarske, M. M., Jayamani, E., Pan, W., Kwon, B., Sinitsa, I. F., Rosen, J. L., Conery, A. L., Fuchs, B. B., Vlahovska, P. M., Ausubel, F. M., Gao, H., Wuest, W. M., & Mylonakis, E. (2018b). Discovery and optimization of nTZDpa as an antibiotic effective against bacterial persisters. *ACS Infectious Diseases, 4*, 1540–1545. https://doi.org/10.1021/acsinfecdis.8b00161.

Kim, W., Zhu, W., Hendricks, G. L., Van Tyne, D., Steele, A. D., Keohane, C. E., Fricke, N., Conery, A. L., Shen, S., Pan, W., Lee, K., Rajamuthiah, R., Fuchs, B. B., Vlahovska, P. M., Wuest, W. M., Gilmore, M. S., Gao, H., Ausubel, F. M., & Mylonakis, E. (2018c). A new class of synthetic retinoid antibiotics effective against bacterial persisters. *Nature, 556*, 103–107. https://doi.org/10.1038/nature26157.

Kuriakose, J., Hernandez-Gordillo, V., Nepal, M., Brezden, A., Pozzi, V., Seleem, M. N., & Chmielewski, J. (2013). Targeting intracellular pathogenic bacteria with unnatural proline-rich peptides: Coupling antibacterial activity with macrophage penetration. *Angewandte Chemie (International Ed. in English), 52*, 9664–9667. https://doi.org/10.1002/anie.201302693.

Kwan, B. W., Chowdhury, N., & Wood, T. K. (2015). Combatting bacterial infections by killing persister cells with mitomycin C. *Environmental Microbiology.* https://doi.org/10.1111/1462-2920.12873

Lee, B.-G., Park, E. Y., Lee, K.-E., Jeon, H., Sung, K. H., Paulsen, H., Rübsamen-Schaeff, H., Brötz-Oesterhelt, H., & Song, H. K. (2010). Structures of ClpP in complex with acyldepsipeptide antibiotics reveal its activation mechanism. *Nature Structural & Molecular Biology, 17*, 471–478. https://doi.org/10.1038/nsmb.1787.

Lehar, S. M., Pillow, T., Xu, M., Staben, L., Kajihara, K. K., Vandlen, R., DePalatis, L., Raab, H., Hazenbos, W. L., Morisaki, J. H., Kim, J., Park, S., Darwish, M., Lee, B.-C., Hernandez, H., Loyet, K. M., Lupardus, P., Fong, R., Yan, D., Chalouni, C., Luis, E., Khalfin, Y., Plise, E., Cheong, J., Lyssikatos, J. P., Strandh, M., Koefoed, K., Andersen, P. S., Flygare, J. A., Wah Tan, M., Brown, E. J., & Mariathasan, S. (2015). Novel antibody-antibiotic conjugate eliminates intracellular *S. aureus. Nature, 527*, 323–328. https://doi.org/10.1038/nature16057.

Lewis, K. (2010). Persister cells. *Annual Review of Microbiology, 64*, 357–372. https://doi.org/10.1146/annurev.micro.112408.134306.

Li, D. H. S., Chung, Y. S., Gloyd, M., Joseph, E., Ghirlando, R., Wright, G. D., Cheng, Y.-Q., Maurizi, M. R., Guarné, A., & Ortega, J. (2010). Acyldepsipeptide antibiotics induce the formation of a structured axial channel in ClpP: A model for the ClpX/ClpA-bound state of ClpP. *Chemistry & Biology, 17*, 959–969. https://doi.org/10.1016/j.chembiol.2010.07.008.

Maiden, M. M., Hunt, A. M. A., Zachos, M. P., Gibson, J. A., Hurwitz, M. E., Mulks, M. H., & Waters, C. M. (2018). Triclosan is an aminoglycoside adjuvant for eradication of *Pseudomonas aeruginosa* biofilms. *Antimicrobial Agents and Chemotherapy, 62*, e00146–e00118. https://doi.org/10.1128/AAC.00146-18.

Mariathasan, S., & Tan, M.-W. (2017). Antibody-antibiotic conjugates: A novel therapeutic platform against bacterial infections. *Trends in Molecular Medicine, 23*, 135–149. https://doi.org/10.1016/j.molmed.2016.12.008.

Marr, A. K., Gooderham, W. J., & Hancock, R. E. (2006). Antibacterial peptides for therapeutic use: Obstacles and realistic outlook. *Current Opinion in Pharmacology, 6*, 468–472. https://doi.org/10.1016/j.coph.2006.04.006.

Matsuzaki, K. (2009). Control of cell selectivity of antimicrobial peptides. *Biochimica et Biophysica Acta, 1788*, 1687–1692. https://doi.org/10.1016/j.bbamem.2008.09.013.

McMurry, L. M., Oethinger, M., & Levy, S. B. (1998). Triclosan targets lipid synthesis. *Nature, 394*, 531–532. https://doi.org/10.1038/28970.

Miller, R. P., Tadagavadi, R. K., Ramesh, G., & Reeves, W. B. (2010). Mechanisms of cisplatin nephrotoxicity. *Toxins (Basel), 2*, 2490–2518. https://doi.org/10.3390/toxins2112490.

Mishra, A., Lai, G. H., Schmidt, N. W., Sun, V. Z., Rodriguez, A. R., Tong, R., Tang, L., Cheng, J., Deming, T. J., Kamei, D. T., & Wong, G. C. L. (2011). Translocation of HIV TAT peptide and analogues induced by multiplexed membrane and cytoskeletal interactions. *Proceedings of the National Academy of Sciences of the United States of America, 108*, 16883–16888. https://doi.org/10.1073/pnas.1108795108.

Mishra, B., Reiling, S., Zarena, D., & Wang, G. (2017). Host defense antimicrobial peptides as antibiotics: Design and application strategies. *Current Opinion in Chemical Biology, 38*, 87–96. https://doi.org/10.1016/j.cbpa.2017.03.014.

Mohamed, M. F., Brezden, A., Mohammad, H., Chmielewski, J., & Seleem, M. N. (2017). Targeting biofilms and persisters of ESKAPE pathogens with P14KanS, a kanamycin peptide conjugate. *Biochimica et Biophysica Acta, 1861*, 848–859. https://doi.org/10.1016/j.bbagen.2017.01.029.

Mohammad, H., Thangamani, S., & Seleem, M. N. (2015). Antimicrobial peptides and peptidomimetics – Potent therapeutic allies for staphylococcal infections. *Current Pharmaceutical Design, 21*, 2073–2088.

Möker, N., Dean, C. R., & Tao, J. (2010). *Pseudomonas aeruginosa* increases formation of multidrug-tolerant persister cells in response to quorum-sensing signaling molecules. *Journal of Bacteriology, 192*, 1946–1955. https://doi.org/10.1128/JB.01231-09.

Morones-Ramirez, J. R., Winkler, J. A., Spina, C. S., & Collins, J. J. (2013). Silver enhances antibiotic activity against gram-negative bacteria. *Science Translational Medicine, 5*, 190ra81–190ra81. https://doi.org/10.1126/scitranslmed.3006276.

Mylonakis, E., Podsiadlowski, L., Muhammed, M., & Vilcinskas, A. (2016). Diversity, evolution and medical applications of insect antimicrobial peptides. *Philosophical Transactions of the Royal Society London B: Biological Sciences, 371*, 20150290. https://doi.org/10.1098/rstb.2015.0290.

Narayanaswamy, V. P., Keagy, L. L., Duris, K., Wiesmann, W., Loughran, A. J., Townsend, S. M., & Baker, S. (2018). Novel glycopolymer eradicates antibiotic- and CCCP-induced persister cells in *Pseudomonas aeruginosa*. *Frontiers in Microbiology, 9*, 1724. https://doi.org/10.3389/fmicb.2018.01724.

Orman, M. A., & Brynildsen, M. P. (2013). Establishment of a method to rapidly assay bacterial persister metabolism. *Antimicrobial Agents and Chemotherapy, 57*, 4398–4409. https://doi.org/10.1128/AAC.00372-13.

Pan, J., Bahar, A. A., Syed, H., & Ren, D. (2012). Reverting antibiotic tolerance of *Pseudomonas aeruginosa* PAO1 persister cells by (Z)-4-bromo-5-(bromomethylene)-3-methylfuran-2(5H)-one. *PLoS One, 7*, e45778. https://doi.org/10.1371/journal.pone.0045778.

Pan, J., Xie, X., Tian, W., Bahar, A. A., Lin, N., Song, F., An, J., & Ren, D. (2013). (Z)-4-bromo-5-(bromomethylene)-3-methylfuran-2(5H)-one sensitizes *Escherichia coli* persister cells to antibiotics. *Applied Microbiology and Biotechnology, 97*, 9145–9154. https://doi.org/10.1007/s00253-013-5185-2.

Patel, S., & Akhtar, N. (2017). Antimicrobial peptides (AMPs): The quintessential "offense and defense" molecules are more than antimicrobials. *Biomedicine & Pharmacotherapy, 95*, 1276–1283. https://doi.org/10.1016/j.biopha.2017.09.042.

Rajamuthiah, R., Fuchs, B. B., Jayamani, E., Kim, Y., Larkins-Ford, J., Conery, A., Ausubel, F. M., & Mylonakis, E. (2014). Whole animal automated platform for drug discovery against multidrug resistant *Staphylococcus aureus*. *PLoS One, 9*, e89189. https://doi.org/10.1371/journal.pone.0089189.

Schmidt, N. W., & Wong, G. C. L. (2013). Antimicrobial peptides and induced membrane curvature: Geometry, coordination chemistry, and molecular engineering. *Current Opinion in Solid State & Materials Science, 17*, 151–163. https://doi.org/10.1016/j.cossms.2013.09.004.

Schmidt, N. W., Mishra, A., Lai, G. H., Davis, M., Sanders, L. K., Tran, D., Garcia, A., Tai, K. P., McCray, P. B., Ouellette, A. J., Selsted, M. E., & Wong, G. C. L. (2011). Criterion for amino acid composition of defensins and antimicrobial peptides based on geometry of membrane destabilization. *Journal of the American Chemical Society, 133*, 6720–6727. https://doi.org/10.1021/ja200079a.

Schmidt, N. W., Lis, M., Zhao, K., Lai, G. H., Alexandrova, A. N., Tew, G. N., & Wong, G. C. L. (2012). Molecular basis for nanoscopic membrane curvature generation from quantum mechanical models and synthetic transporter sequences. *Journal of the American Chemical Society, 134*, 19207–19216. https://doi.org/10.1021/ja308459j.

Schmidt, N. W., Deshayes, S., Hawker, S., Blacker, A., Kasko, A. M., & Wong, G. C. L. (2014). Engineering persister-specific antibiotics with synergistic antimicrobial functions. *ACS Nano, 8*, 8786–8793. https://doi.org/10.1021/nn502201a.

Shan, Y., Brown Gandt, A., Rowe, S. E., Deisinger, J. P., Conlon, B. P., & Lewis, K. (2017). ATP-dependent persister formation in *Escherichia coli*. *MBio, 8*, e02267–16. https://doi.org/10.1128/mBio.02267-16.

Sharma, B., Brown, A. V., Matluck, N. E., Hu, L. T., & Lewis, K. (2015). *Borrelia burgdorferi*, the causative agent of lyme disease, forms drug-tolerant persister cells. *Antimicrobial Agents and Chemotherapy, 59*, 4616–4624. https://doi.org/10.1128/AAC.00864-15.

Strahl, H., & Errington, J. (2017). Bacterial membranes: Structure, domains, and function. *Annual Review of Microbiology, 71*, 519–538. https://doi.org/10.1146/annurev-micro-102215-095630.

Sun, Y., Dowd, S. E., Smith, E., Rhoads, D. D., & Wolcott, R. D. (2008). In vitro multispecies Lubbock chronic wound biofilm model. *Wound Repair and Regeneration, 16*, 805–813. https://doi.org/10.1111/j.1524-475X.2008.00434.x.

Taber, H. W., Mueller, J. P., Miller, P. F., & Arrow, A. S. (1987). Bacterial uptake of aminoglycoside antibiotics. *Microbiological Reviews, 51*, 439–457.

Walde, P., Cosentino, K., Engel, H., & Stano, P. (2010). Giant vesicles: Preparations and applications. *Chembiochem, 11*, 848–865. https://doi.org/10.1002/cbic.201000010.

Weisblum, B., & Davies, J. (1968). Antibiotic inhibitors of the bacterial ribosome. *Bacteriological Reviews, 32*, 493–528.

Yamamoto, K., Kitayama, T., Ishida, N., Watanabe, T., Tanabe, H., Takatani, M., Okamoto, T., & Utsumi, R. (2000). Identification and characterization of a potent antibacterial agent, NH125 against drug-resistant bacteria. *Bioscience, Biotechnology, and Biochemistry, 64*, 919–923. https://doi.org/10.1271/bbb.64.919.

Yamamoto, K., Kitayama, T., Minagawa, S., Watanabe, T., Sawada, S., Okamoto, T., & Utsumi, R. (2001). Antibacterial agents that inhibit histidine protein kinase YycG of *Bacillus subtilis*. *Bioscience, Biotechnology, and Biochemistry, 65*, 2306–2310.

Zasloff, M. (2002). Antimicrobial peptides of multicellular organisms. *Nature, 415*, 389–395. https://doi.org/10.1038/415389a.

Printed in the United States
By Bookmasters